The Elusive Embryo

The Elusive Embryo

How Women and Men Approach
New Reproductive Technologies

Gay Becker

UNIVERSITY OF CALIFORNIA PRESS
Berkeley · *Los Angeles* · *London*

University of California Press
Berkeley and Los Angeles, California

University of California Press, Ltd.
London, England

© 2000 by the Regents of the University of
California

Material from Gay Becker and Robert D.
Nachtigall, " 'Born to Be a Mother': The Cultural
Construction of Risk in Infertility Treatment in the
U.S.," *Social Science and Medicine* 39, no. 4
(1994), is reprinted with permission from Elsevier
Science, Ltd.

Library of Congress Cataloging-in-Publication Data

Becker, Gaylene.
    The elusive embryo : how women and men
approach new reproductive technologies /
Gay Becker.
        p.   cm.
    Includes bibliographical references and index.
    ISBN 0-520-22430-2 (cloth : alk. paper)—
    ISBN 0-520-22431-0 (pbk. : alk paper)
    1. Human reproductive technology—Case
studies.   2. Infertility—Patients—Interviews.
I. Title.

    RG133.5 .B434   2000
    616.6'9206—dc21   00-055967

Manufactured in the United States of America

09 08 07 06 05 04 03 02 01 00

10 9 8 7 6 5 4 3 2 1

The paper used in this publication meets the
minimum requirements of ANSI/NISO Z39.48-
1992 (R 1997) (*Permanence of Paper*).

For Roger

Contents

Acknowledgments

This book could not have been written without the participation of several hundred women and men who volunteered to be interviewed not once but several times. They did so with the knowledge that answering our questions would likely cause them emotional pain. They did it anyway, because they believed it might help other people confronting infertility to understand the issues and decisions, as well as the feelings, that arise for those undergoing medical treatment. Their commitment to this project reinforced my own determination to bring their stories to light. My first thanks go to them.

This study was made possible by funding from the National Institute on Aging (NIA), National Institutes of Health, Gender and the Disruption of Life Course Structure, RO1 AGO8973. An earlier pilot study was funded by the Academic Senate of the University of California, San Francisco.

I am indebted to my research partner, Robert Nachtigall, for his long-term support of my efforts. His medical expertise and his many insights into reproductive medicine and the growth of medical technology have greatly enriched this work. Responsibility for its content, however, is mine alone.

Research of this scope and length cannot be conducted without the participation of a dedicated team of researchers. Edwina Newsom, project manager for this and subsequent studies, gave this project her all, and I greatly appreciate her insights, her interviewing and organizational skills, and her commitment. I am also grateful to those who interviewed people for this study with skill and sensitivity: Gary Cook, Jeff Harmon, Seline Szkupinski Quiroga, and Diane Tober. LaSonya Chatman diligently transcribed interviews. Leilani Cuizon-Canalita and Nury Mayen printed endless drafts of this manuscript and helped me with the final assembly. Their unflagging commitment to anthropological research such as this is deeply appreciated. I also acknowledge and thank the organizations that helped to recruit participants for this study: Catholic Charities Adoption Services, Northern California Resolve, and PACT—An Adoption Alliance. The enthusiastic support of health professionals for this project is greatly appreciated, especially that of David Adamson, Mary Martin Cadieux, Simon Henderson, and Cecile Lampton.

Many thanks to the reviewers for this book, Kristine Bertelsen, Robert Nachtigall, Virginia Olesen, Frances Winddance Twine, and an anonymous reviewer, for their valuable comments and suggestions. I am indebted to Steve Sturdy, who made extremely helpful suggestions about this research that I have incorporated. I also thank Jane Grimes and Alice Miner, who read the work for me to determine its intelligibility for a general readership.

Naomi Schneider, my editor at the University of California Press, has kept me moving forward with her relentless enthusiasm for this project. I appreciate her astute advice and support. Many thanks to editors Erika Büky and Sue Heinemann for their careful production of the manuscript.

Finally, special thanks go to my husband, Roger Van Craeynest, who lived through the experience of infertility with me and who has wholeheartedly supported my subsequent work on this topic, contributing many insights along the way.

Introduction

From Personal Experience to Research

I began studying infertility after spending several years addressing my own. It was the first time I had chosen a research topic I was personally involved with.[1] Looking back more than fifteen years, my experience of infertility and its treatment seems much different today from the way it did at the time. In part this is because reproductive technology has changed and expanded so much. The medical procedures that seemed so intrusive to me at the time were low-key compared with those in use today.

Yet one important aspect has changed very little: the underlying cultural phenomena that conspire to make infertility so agonizing for many women and men. Although the intervening years have seen greater awareness of infertility among the general public and greater acceptance of practices such as adoption, the people I interviewed for this study face the same issues I confronted. Those issues revolve around questions of *normalcy* normalcy—for one's body and one's life. Parenthood equals normalcy for people in their middle years.

As Roger and I entered our thirties, friends who were having children began pressuring us to do the same. We were in no hurry, but we began a dialogue about the cultural dimensions of parenthood and how it would fit into our own lives. Most of our friends already had children; increasingly, we felt different from our peers. The peer pressure was uncomfortable, but we were resistant to having children simply to fit in. A few years later, we saw things differently and decided that children would enrich our lives. Having considered this decision long and care-fully, we nevertheless were no better prepared for infertility than anyone ever is. When we did not conceive and turned to medical treatment for help, we were swept into a maelstrom of new concerns from which we emerged rather unsteadily a few years later.

One thing I have learned from my subsequent research on infertility is that women demonstrate a very wide range of tolerance for medical treatment. Some women can endure prolonged treatment over many years, while others find that they can't tolerate much. I was one of the latter. Even so, I went past my comfortable limits. Infertility treatment completely upset my sense of inner balance, and it took me a long time to regain my equilibrium. Stopping the effort to conceive forces women to scrutinize their gender identity with respect to womanhood, moth-erhood, family, and a range of related issues. I was no exception.

My own experience of the disruption to life from infertility was only one in a long series of disruptions that had punctuated my life.[2] By the time Roger and I decided to have children, I was very tired of such disruptions. Having worked hard to maintain my equilibrium through medical treatment, it came as a shock to find that once I called it quits, this disruption wasn't over. It took another five years, a series of other difficult life experiences that were not connected but somehow seemed to be, and a lot of psychotherapy before infertility began to seem like part of the past. The anthropological analysis of biological parenthood that had been part of our decision making gradually gave way to more finely tuned discussions—this time about what constituted normalcy and gender identity and, ultimately, what it might mean for our lives if we never had children. We began rethinking the directions of our lives.

When I decided to study infertility instead of living it, I began by applying my perspective as an anthropologist in earnest. Roger and I had been reflecting on infertility from an anthropological point of view all along because it helped us to keep our experience in perspective. Once I stopped medical treatment, I saw just how useful this cultural lens was. For one thing, awareness of the cultural forces at work lessened my sense of personal responsibility and made me realize I was up against "cul-ture" writ large—that it wasn't I who was at fault. I had stumbled into a morass of broad social and cultural issues that were bigger than any individual.

For another, medical treatment had forced me to look on my body in new—and alien—ways. My work as a medical anthropologist helped me understand the dynamics at play in biomedicine. Having just completed a hospital-based study of how practitioners think about chronic illness and disability, I had learned a great deal about medical detachment, seen repeated instances of bodies being treated as objects, and witnessed the effects of depersonalization on people who lived with chronic conditions. From this vantage point there was nothing special about infertility, except for one thing: it wasn't an illness at all. I already had one chronic illness. During infertility treatment, I felt I had acquired another. It was only after medical treatment that I realized this illness wasn't real; it was manufactured.

With this insight I began to look at bodies and at illness in new ways and to ask myself how I could pass my newfound perceptions on to others. Studying infertility renewed my interest in bodily distress, in questions about how people deal with disruption, and in how people experience a sense of difference from others. I became especially intrigued by how people take power into their own hands and resist ideas that are undesirable or impossible to live out. Indeed, once I began working seriously to uncover the cultural elements of infertility and reproductive technologies, I found myself mining a rich vein of societal conflicts. This work dovetailed with my lifelong interest in how people define what is normal, how they fit themselves inside that definition— or do not—and how vast the difference can be between cultural ideals, or ideologies, and the realities of people's lives. What people do in order to live with this disparity is, of course, the most salient question of all.

As the initial study began, I tried to distance myself emotionally. I was trained to keep a strict separation between my life and the lives of people involved in my research. Of course, anthropologists today acknowledge that such detachment is not possible or even desirable. And as soon as I started interviewing other people experiencing infertility I realized the futility—even ludicrousness—of such a position. I realized that this study was helping me to work my way through the personal issues infertility had raised for me. Sometimes I was a few steps ahead of the people I interviewed, simply because I was finished with medical treatment, but sometimes they were ahead of me. I learned from the women and men I interviewed, and in the process I regained my inner sense of balance and refocused my life.

CHAPTER 1

Consuming Technologies

Laura, a thirty-five-year-old woman, and her husband, Joe, had undergone infertility treatment for several years.[1] Infertility problems had been
identified in both. In vitro fertilization (IVF) was the last resort.[2] As
Laura explained:

*We did the IVF. We went through the process. I responded quickly, so
it went quicker than they expected. We went in and we were real up.
About as up as you could be. It was what he [Joe] had to look forward to. And we were feeling real good about it. They got eighteen
eggs and nothing fertilized. So we sat here afterwards waiting for the
calls. Went back the next day and tried to inseminate them again—
still nothing. So that was it. That chance was the end of the road.*

*Amazingly enough, we made the best of it. We sat here at the table
realizing it wasn't going to work. We shed some tears. He [Joe] sat
there [pointing to chair] and there was a PC set up there, and he
started writing our letter for adoption. I couldn't help him. I couldn't
find anything that I was good at right then. I said, "You know, when
people write those letters, they talk about their hobbies. My hobby is
infertility."*

Laura's story captures the emotional highs and lows people experience
when IVF is unsuccessful. Her hopes and those of her husband, so high
initially, crashed when the cycle failed. Laura is not only struggling with
lost hope; she is also dealing with infertility's assault on her identity.

4

Being unable to think of anything good about herself for an adoption letter or to think of anything she does with her spare time besides deal with infertility conveys not just the depth of her despair but also the profound impact on her sense of self of the loss of any hope for a biological child. In the midst of addressing these difficult issues of personal identity, Laura is being forced to confront another: her position as a consumer-patient in the rapidly developing industry of advanced reproductive technology.

When I started to study infertility almost twenty years ago, there was little public recognition of its effect on people's lives. Although scientists had been researching human fertility in the lab for a number of years, little of this work had found its way into clinical practice.[3] In vitro fertilization had been introduced just a few years earlier. Reproductive endocrinology, the subspecialty of medicine that deals with fertility, was in its infancy, and treatments for infertility were minimal. Moreover, almost no media attention was paid to infertility or any related phenomenon such as adoption. It was this dearth of attention that led me to study the topic: first, because I believed people needed to be educated about infertility; second, because I sensed that major changes in social attitudes toward infertility were just around the corner; and third, because infertility is entwined with many cultural phenomena that intrigue anthropologists such as myself, and there is no better time to study those phenomena than in a period of change. I did not, however, anticipate just how profound those changes would be or how deeply new reproductive technologies would affect the ways in which people think about fertility.

Because I am an anthropologist, I look at developments in reproductive technology through the lens of culture. Culture is pervasive in human actions; it is embedded in everything human.[4] In this book I explore how reproductive technologies embody cultural phenomena and become entwined with people's lives.[5] I examine technologies designed to bring about conception from the perspective of the women and men who use them. Drawing on two studies of infertility with over three hundred women and men in the United States who were interviewed several times over one or two years, I tell their stories of the effect of reproductive technologies on their lives.

I am concerned with understanding how women and men navigate their way through a complex life passage in which they must come to grips with deeply embedded cultural expectations about biological reproduction. I examine how people seek solutions while resisting the heavy moral force of such expectations. I explore how women and men negotiate gender and gender relations, how they tease apart and analyze the various elements of the cultural ideal of biological parenthood, and how they assess the biomedical system in which they ambivalently participate. I trace how that experience becomes increasingly politicized as they confront the powerful social, cultural, and economic forces that shape this industry, and how they act to influence the process in which they are engaged.

CHANGING NOTIONS OF NATURE AND CULTURE

Advances in reproductive technologies are reshaping the ways in which women and men—but especially women—experience their bodies and their lives. As that technology expands, cultural notions of what constitutes the natural body are changing.[6] Since the late twentieth century, the process of redefining nature has accelerated along with the pace of technological development; yet the changes have revealed a lack of synchrony between technological advance and people's experiences and understanding of their bodies. The female body, in particular, has been reconceived as a site of technological advance. In consequence the body itself becomes a site of disruption,[7] as Laura learned when she adjusted first to the idea of using in vitro fertilization at all, then to the retrieval of eighteen eggs from within her body, and finally to the realization that the process had not worked.

Practicality—the need for results—is the primary force that propels women and men deeper and deeper into treatment, but this attitude is always tinged with regret that conception could not have occurred without any intervention. Indeed, one of the main themes they express is the loss of what they consider to be natural. This pervasive sense of sadness was countered by the need, as they saw it, to remedy their childlessness.[8]

No one in this study felt that the reproductive technologies they turned to were in any way natural. Women and men in this study viewed the use of reproductive technologies as a necessary but unpleasant step toward having a biological family.[9] As they remind us repeatedly, what they considered natural was to conceive in private, without the knowledge, participation, or help of any third party or any kind of technology. While they sometimes reported going through parts of the medical treatment process automatically, that was often because they felt worn down by treatment. Any excitement they expressed about the process was related to the hoped-for outcome, a child. Sometimes immersion in the technological details offered an escape from facing the bigger issues, but it did not lead them to regard any part of the process as pleasant. Yet when a pregnancy did occur because of technological intervention, the parents often made a concerted effort to treat the process *as if* it were natural.[10] This tendency is part of the larger phenomenon of modernity and an outgrowth of industrialization. Anthony Giddens notes that although in most parts of the globe people now live in created environments subject to human control,[11] in everyday life people continue to view their bodies as natural, resisting the idea that the body reflects cultural notions of bodiliness, even when that body has been modified by implants and other technological changes.[12]

This shift from nature to culture is accentuated by the presence of new reproductive technologies. While going through infertility treatment with his wife, Charlie predicted: "Twenty years from now people will automatically bank their sperm and their eggs in their early twenties, then go on with their lives until they are much older, when they are ready to have kids. The issue [infertility] you are studying now will disappear. We will think of biological reproduction differently. It will be shaped by advances in technology."

This portrait of the future dissolves the split between nature and culture in daily life. If Charlie's prediction comes true, not only is the current disruption resulting from infertility a temporary phenomenon, but technology's role in reproduction will become even more prominent than it is now. We are in the midst of change: these technologies can be seen as fundamentally transformative.[13]

By showing the complexity of the task these women and men are engaged in, I aim to break down stereotypes of women in blind pursuit of medical technology. What, precisely, is at stake for them? The list is long, but at the top are having a family, charting the direction of their lives, and preserving their gender identity. The challenges are profound: creating a family while making the right decisions—whether to pursue medical treatment rather than adoption, for example—maintaining a solid relationship with one's partner, being assertive and autonomous in dealings with the health care system, weathering family friction, and keeping careers afloat. Their situations can have diverse repercussions on their lives.

Exploring and managing changes in oneself is part of modern social activity.[14] The discovery of infertility can be one trigger of this process. In writing this book, I want to make what I learned in my study available to people undergoing or contemplating reproductive technologies. I believe knowledge is power, and the more we know about something, the better equipped we are to grapple with it. I am not simply concerned, however, with reporting people's responses to medical treatment; I want to examine the social and cultural forces that have created the current situation and that continue to nurture the growth of technology. Exploring these processes from the consumer's perspective can illuminate those cultural dynamics for the benefit of consumers, social scientists, and practitioners of all sorts.

Social scientists and practitioners are currently very interested in technological innovation and its ramifications for social life, and my goal is to speak to them as well as to consumers because reproductive technologies and their use have great potential to inform our understanding of cultural processes in modern life. To engage the widest possible audience, I pause in the text periodically to define my terms. I also make ample use of notes for further technical and analytic discussion.

THE GROWTH OF AN INDUSTRY

In the twenty-some years since Louise Brown, the first "test tube" baby, was born in England, in vitro fertilization and other assisted reproductive technologies have moved from a highly experimental status to options that are mentioned routinely to patients during the first office visit for infertility treatment. Initially developed specifically to treat women with damaged fallopian tubes, IVF and related technologies are now used to treat all types of infertility, including male infertility and that catchall diagnosis, "unexplained infertility." As the range of medical options has changed, consumers' responses to them have changed also. Louise Brown was six years old when we began studying infertility in 1984. Her birth was a media event with few apparent reverberations among people living with infertility; they saw little or no connection between that birth and their own lives.

The studies I have conducted with Robert Nachtigall have explored, specifically, how the discovery of infertility disrupts cultural expectations about the structure of life and how men and women differ in their responses to unwanted childlessness. After conducting a pilot study with 36 couples, we carried out a second, larger study with 134 couples and 9 women without their partners who were either undergoing medical treatment at the time of the first interview or had completed medical treatment during the preceding three years.[15]

Only one of the twenty-eight couples interviewed in 1984, the first year of the research, considered IVF an option. Of the few IVF programs in the United States at that time, none was in our geographic area. The "take-home baby" rate at the most successful clinic in the United States was approximately 15 percent, and the average cost of a single cycle of IVF was approximately $5,000, which was a lot of money at the time and was unlikely to be offset by insurance. Moreover, such programs screened patients carefully to protect their success rates: they targeted women who had specific tubal problems, and they seldom accepted women over the age of thirty-five. Most couples in the study viewed the cost as prohibitive, the treatment as experimental, and the success rates as insufficient to justify the cost. Moreover, they believed that IVF was an extreme version of a medical process that was already emotionally difficult. If they did not conceive through more traditional means, the majority expected to pursue adoption, which they regarded as less costly and more likely to succeed.

The one couple who did apply to an IVF program, after fourteen years of medical treatment, was turned down. They were considered by the clinic to have a low probability of success: each partner had an infertility factor, they were close to the age limit of thirty-five, and the female partner failed the clinic's psychological tests, ostensibly because she was too emotional about her infertility.

By 1987, when I interviewed an additional eight couples and seven women, several IVF programs had been initiated locally, and others had sprung up around the United States. How did this increase in IVF programs affect people's responses to infertility treatment and their attitudes about IVF? Four of these couples were receptive to IVF. Two had already undergone IVF: one had conceived after three cycles of treatment, while the other had undergone numerous cycles without success. Two other couples were pursuing IVF: one couple was turned down because of the financial constraints of their health maintenance organization (HMO), and the other planned to undergo the treatment. The remaining couples dismissed IVF treatment for the same reasons as couples did in 1984, emphasizing that they could adopt a child for the cost of a single IVF cycle and that success rates in IVF programs had not significantly improved.

When our new study began in 1991, dramatic changes were apparent. There were now seven IVF clinics in the area, the majority of which were affiliated with local hospitals or medical centers. Criteria for entry into IVF programs had been relaxed greatly. While some programs had an age limit of forty, others had none; all programs treated various types of infertility. In some programs the only criterion for participation was the ability to pay.[16] These changes have persisted; the ability to pay remains the primary arbiter of whether people consider IVF feasible.

DRIVING FORCES IN CONSUMER CULTURE

Regardless of the outcome, new reproductive technologies may take a toll on people's lives because people invest them with so much power. But it is only through human actions that such technologies are engaged. To understand their effects on the lives of people who use them and on society generally, we need to understand technologies as expedients of human actions, tools in the interplay of culture. These technologies may appear to take on power over people's lives, but that is only because society infuses them with power. Not only is technology an expression of culture; technology affords a prime example of consumer culture— how people handle the relationship between the social order and the intimate spheres of their lives.[17]

Reproductive technologies have entered the mainstream of medical treatment. Both the public and medical practitioners identify them as socially and culturally desirable, reflecting the way that society's priorities are reproduced in the institution of biomedicine and in business practices. This is consumer culture at work. According to Don Slater, understanding consumer culture entails more than studying individual choice and consciousness, wants and desires; it means examining these qualities in the context of social relations, structures, institutions, and systems. If we want to understand why new reproductive technologies have taken hold, we must look at the social conditions under which personal and social wants and the organization of social resources are negotiated.[18]

Consumption can be seen as meaningful social practice. Consumer culture reveals individuals' power of disposal over their lives and over the resources they identify as necessary.[19] For the consumer of new reproductive technologies, for example, exercising discretion over their use is an expression of power in an apparently intractable situation. Consumption is replete with cultural meanings, and people use technologies in accordance with those meanings. In doing so, people experience the social order as a compelling moral order and reproduce it in everyday life.[20] For example, health promotion in the United States can be seen as an instance of middle-class morality, in which people feel responsible for eating right, exercising, and avoiding activities that are viewed as unhealthy, such as smoking.[21]

Examining people's experiences with new reproductive technologies can tell us much about how the consumption of technology evolves as a cultural process: that is, how it emanates from social forces. This process is occurring at a time when technological advances are appearing in quick succession, when cultural meanings are in flux, when gender is in a state of continuous negotiation, and when technology itself can be seen as culture.

Consumer culture revolves around specific objects of consumption that are meaningful because they reproduce social identities.[22] For Laura, IVF held out the hope of motherhood, an identity for which she longed. Technologies derive from and are created by cultural priorities. Parenthood is one such priority. It is easy to see why new reproductive technologies have caught on so quickly: they hold the potential to allow people to reproduce themselves by having a child. Consumer culture thus connects questions about how we want to or should live with questions of entitlement, addressing the wants and needs of individuals. Consumers have played a central role in promoting and sustaining the new reproductive technologies. As we will see, consumer experiences with these technologies are the key to understanding the cultural dynamics at work.

The growth of technology is closely tied to a society's central tenets. The United States can be characterized by its cultural diversity, but it can also be characterized by cultural ideologies originating from its early roots as a colony of dissidents and free thinkers who immigrated from Great Britain. Subsequently, Enlightenment ideals such as freedom and rationality, originating in the philosophy of rational determinism,[23] were institutionalized in a distinctively American form in the U.S. Constitution and became the basis for cultural values and ideologies that persist today.[24] They include progress, productivity, individualism, control over the environment, perseverance, and an orientation toward the future.[25] Such ideals continue to dominate U.S. society despite its cultural diversity, in part because they reflect rights and responsibilities as they devolve on the individual and in part because they are embedded in social institutions.[26]

The ethos of radical individualism is essential to technological growth in the United States and can even be viewed as an ideology, one particularly prominent among the middle class.[27] Not everyone subscribes to this cultural ideology, which is sometimes distinctly at odds with the beliefs of people from other cultural backgrounds and social classes. Indeed, people may often feel at odds with the moral responsibilities that adhere to particular ideologies and may rebel against the social constraints that such ideologies impose on them. Nevertheless, such ideologies shape how people think about their lives and the problems they face, whether or not the individuals are conscious of their influence.[28] For example, when patients and physicians decide to undertake a last-ditch effort for a cure, they usually proceed for reasons related to the importance of maintaining control over the environment and overcoming obstacles through persistence.[29] These beliefs underpin the drive to create and promote ever more effective technologies. Social institutions, such as biomedicine, in turn reflect these cultural expectations.

Progress is one of the cultural ideologies of the United States. Indeed, the dominant modernist ideology of progress is spreading worldwide. Long associated with American concepts of expansion in realms such as industrialization and the "taming" of the West, notions of progress also inform the field of medicine, which can be viewed as one of the primary frontiers in contemporary American society. Biomedicine is replete with metaphors of progress. For example, television newscasters frequently state, "Researchers report that we are making progress in winning the fight against [disease]," and then recount the latest development in a specific area of medicine. This emphasis is nowhere more apparent than in new reproductive technologies. Despite recent postmodern challenges, the belief in linear progress, absolute truths, and rational planning of ideal social orders under standardized conditions of knowledge and production persisted during much of the twentieth century.[30] Such notions continue to underpin both individual ideas and institutional ideologies about how the world works, and those ideas infuse people's actions with meaning.

Media coverage of high-technology innovations facilitates public receptivity and the process of commodification: for example, the public has gradually shifted from viewing assisted reproductive technologies as esoteric and overpriced to considering them commonplace. Women and men often reported that their ideas about reproductive technologies altered after viewing television news reports, talk shows, and informational programs in which new developments were portrayed. At the same time, people remain wary of technology taking over their lives.[31] Such ambivalence was expressed in a recent statement on television sponsored by the Media Foundation which used captions stating, "The product is you," and "Cast off the chains of market-structured consciousness." This book shows such sentiments mirrored in people's repeated expressions of ambivalence about new reproductive technologies. Ashley conveys her ambivalence about doing IVF:

You sort of feel that you have gotten every bad break that you can get. They gave me a 20 percent chance in one cycle, and I am a pessimist anyway so I see it as an 80 percent chance of failure, and I would be totally blown away if it worked. But I feel like I need to go through the motions, partially because I think I would look back on it and always wonder, and feel like I hadn't tried everything. But I don't know if I can stand it—I don't know how awful the shots and all that stuff is going to be. But if it is tolerable, I can see maybe doing another cycle while we are waiting around for the adoption stuff. But the money—we are not covered by insurance, and our savings are just going. And I want to have enough money to do adoption. I don't want to totally wipe us out. I think we are going to see how bad it is.

In a medical field that is unregulated, as assisted reproduction largely has been, technology may drive treatment, especially when reinforced by strong cultural priorities. When a specific medical technology is no longer viewed by medicine as experimental, that technological innovation may be increasingly accepted by the public and may eventually be viewed as commonplace.[32] As a technology becomes accepted as routine, the cost may provoke debate about the allocation of resources.

CONTROLLING CONSUMPTION

Who uses these new technologies? Consumer culture raises questions about whether resources are allocated equitably or whether social systems (including, for example, market forces, private corporations, media and cultural institutions, modern "knowledge," science, and expertise) have the power to dictate people's needs or to reduce some people's access to resources.[33]

Practitioners have flocked to new reproductive technologies aimed at the middle and upper classes. The actual cost of new reproductive technologies to the consumer is determined by several factors: the expense of operating a program and its laboratory, the labor involved in the procedures themselves, and the availability, or lack, of insurance to underwrite the cost.[34] The median cost of a single cycle of IVF is now approximately $10,000; the incorporation of donor egg technology adds $5,000 or more to the cost of a cycle. Costs have escalated as complex technical variations have proliferated. New reproductive technologies are now estimated to be a $350-million-a year business, while infertility care overall has been estimated at $2 billion a year.[35] The greatest profit lies in performing new reproductive technologies.

In contrast to the profits to be made, consumers who contemplate these technologies feel hard-pressed to find the money. Claire and Morrie examine what it would mean to them financially if they undertook IVF:

CLAIRE: *I think it's the way to go. But if we have any problems or if it doesn't work the first time, then we have to spend more money.*

MORRIE: *We don't have the money for the first time.*

CLAIRE: *We have a credit card [laughter].*

MORRIE: *It'll take us twenty years to pay off. We don't even have savings for a retirement fund, let alone for one time.*

CLAIRE: *My doctor thinks I'm a real good candidate for it. I don't feel the same way about the money as Morrie does. We could borrow it from a credit card, and the interest rates have gone down, so it's not as bad as it was.*

MORRIE: *Three tries at $10,000 apiece—that would be our retirement.*

CLAIRE: *I think $30,000 wouldn't be feasible. There would be no way that we could afford to do that.*

MORRIE: *I'm not complaining about it, but . . .*

CLAIRE: *I know you're not, but the way that I feel about what I want in my life is that I've lived so long without having much materially. It's just been a struggle to have what we do have, and I don't ever see it changing very much, so making payments on another $15,000 doesn't faze me because I don't ever see that we're going to get out of the rut that we're in financially. So I want to live my life the way I want to live it, regardless of how much money I have. The value I place on what I want in my life is my family. I've always wanted children. That's what means the most to me because it's a lifelong investment into somebody that you have close to you for your whole life.*

Like Claire and Morrie, everyone in this book who contemplated IVF was forced to weigh the importance of children in their lives against the financial costs of attempting to conceive with reproductive technologies. But it is not simply a question of money versus children. Many other factors are involved, and the decisions couples face are complex.

The cost of such technologies, no matter how high, may appear increasingly justifiable as the success rate improves. The economic cost is culturally refigured, for example, if people want a biological child at any price. Indeed, the cost—which is almost prohibitive for most middle-class families—may become part of the allure. Being *almost* out of reach reinforces the idea that because these technologies are so esoteric, they may work where nothing else has.[36]

As specific technological advances become more widespread, they create a competitive medical marketplace. For example, when local medical practices began to offer new reproductive technologies in the early 1990s, they competed with each other for patients, advertising lower prices, nonmedical support services, and other enticements. In this new marketplace, offers of package deals, discount plans, and money-back guarantees were calculated to make treatment seem affordable. The recent development of investor-owned, expansion-oriented chains of IVF programs raises the question of whether patients are being pushed toward certain highly profitable reproductive technologies rather than to alternatives that are less risky, less complex, and less expensive.[37] Concerns have been raised by the American Society for Reproductive Medicine about the exploitation of infertility patients.[38]

Cataloguing the players who generate, maintain, and benefit from technological proliferation gives us another way to look at the relationship of consumption, control, and medical technology. Those with vested interests in new medical technologies are likely to be the same whether we are talking about new reproductive technologies, bone marrow transplants, or new treatments for HIV. The players represent, in addition to patient-consumers, the powerful institutional interests that vie for dominance. Consumers of new reproductive technologies represent only one set of interests competing among many.[39] The others include the companies who market their drugs and equipment to physicians and consumers, the entrepreneurs who offer stock in medical corporations, the sperm banks that store donor gametes, the universities and medical centers that conduct research and training (as well as the webs of affiliations that provide patient referrals), the professional medical associations that provide continuing education and self-policing of reproductive technologies, the insurance companies that mandate policies about payment, the government that promulgates social and research policies, and the legislators and advocates who develop relevant legislation.

This long list of competing interests demonstrates how much power and money are at stake.[40] The new technologies represent big business. As we can see from this list of vested interests, biomedicine, the realm people usually think of when they think of new reproductive technologies, is one realm among many. With respect to the new reproductive technologies, biomedicine is not necessarily the most powerful institution, although it continues to be the *symbolic* realm of action. Indeed, corporate interests appear to play an increasingly powerful role. New reproductive technologies are thus of special interest as an example of the amalgamation of biomedical and business interests in a rapidly growing field. As we will see, consumers are wary of this kind of amalgamation.

THE EMERGENCE OF NEW REPRODUCTIVE TECHNOLOGIES AS THE GOLD STANDARD

The introduction and development of assisted reproductive technologies has revolutionized the ways in which physicians think about the treatment of infertility. New reproductive technologies have become "the gold standard," to use a phrase often repeated by physicians in this study. Definitive diagnoses of specific infertility problems are often possible only with new reproductive technologies. But, ironically, the proliferation of assisted reproductive technologies has led to a paradigm shift in which infertility care is driven not by the diagnosis but by the treatment. The emphasis has shifted from diagnosing and correcting abnormal physiology to achieving a pregnancy in the fastest and most direct manner possible, regardless of the cost or invasiveness. This approach aggressively augments the natural reproductive cycle, or bypasses it altogether, and aims for results regardless of the underlying infertility diagnosis.

Women and men balk at this approach and are skeptical of it. After attending an informational evening program in which several infertility specialists discussed the specifics of IVF, Milt complained:

When you clear away all of the smoke and all of the rhetoric, they don't have any answers. There are no answers out there. And one of

*the things that I thought was most poignant and that I carry away in
my memory, and that I still state to myself when we talk about these
things, is that in vitro is the gold standard. That's the benchmark
against what everything else is measured against, and that's because
they can watch it through a microscope and they know exactly what's
going on every minute.*

Karen interjected:

*Some of the things that they said were very enlightening. But what it
seemed to be was that all they were talking about is tests. "We can do
this test, we can do that test." "This test tells us this, this test tells us
that." But the answer of what you do next, every time, is in vitro. The
tests just gave a little more information about performing in vitro. But
they didn't have any other suggestions as to what to do as a therapy.
And I actually asked them. I asked a question which was completely
ignored. I asked, "Is there anything else besides in vitro?" When they
heard my question, they all laughed, and nobody answered it. My
question was totally serious.*

The specialized nature of modern expertise contributes to the run-
away character of technology.[41] Although in the past infertility treatment rarely lasted longer than a few years or cost more than a few
thousand dollars, it now lasts until the couple's emotional and financial
resources are exhausted. Although it holds out the promise of shorter
treatments, the sometimes bewildering array of high-technology options
may extend the time that a couple remains in treatment.[42]

Paradoxically, too, despite this aggressive approach, some of the diagnostic techniques utilized in the early stages of treatment are incon-
clusive, and empirical therapy—all-purpose treatment regimens that do
not depend on a specific diagnosis—is the rule of thumb of most early
treatment. Patients often lose precious time—sometimes years—on empirical therapies, the effectiveness of which cannot easily be gauged for
a specific patient.[43] Because a woman's age is a significant determinant
of the effectiveness of treatment, such delays undermine the expensive
and sophisticated efforts made to achieve a pregnancy. Why?

Infertility specialists sometimes do not offer new reproductive technologies to patients immediately because of the great expense. If cost
were not an issue, physicians would undoubtedly suggest that patients
turn to the new technologies sooner, as they do in Great Britain (where
the government covers the cost), because from a medical perspective they

yield better results in a shorter time. But there are reasons besides cost
why people do not pursue new reproductive technologies sooner. First,
they are more invasive than other types of treatment, entailing multiple
medical procedures and long courses of hormones that control women's
reproductive cycles. Women experience more side effects and have more
concerns about medical risks. Second, socialization to being an infertility
patient takes time. Except for some women in their forties who begin
treatment with donor eggs right away, people are seldom ready to accept
aggressive new reproductive technologies early in treatment, preferring
to take a less invasive approach at first and hope it will be effective.

Ashley and Scott have been trying to conceive for four years. They
have gradually moved from the most basic treatments to being on the
verge of IVF. Ashley talks about what it has been like:

*For me, it has been just total frustration because we are not covered
by insurance, and it is kind of like if somebody wanted to design a
program to drive me literally insane, this is it. We did a lot of small
diagnostic tests, then I was put on drugs, then I had surgery for
fibroids, then we were supposed to do six cycles with more drugs, but
I didn't respond to it. So they gave me more drugs, and then I got
hyperstimulated and had to stop the drugs completely. So then I was
having to do these urine tests at work and rush them to the doctor's
office in rush hour traffic. You know, you have to do everything exactly, and under rush and stress, and I would do all that, and then
they would say, "Sorry, we can't try this month, but maybe next
month." And next month and next month. So the whole thing has
been so frustrating, plus expensive because they want to monitor you
real closely. They gave me ultrasound after ultrasound.*

*So the shit hit the fan about a month ago when I just felt like,
"This is ridiculous," and we had a powwow with our doctor. Now,
given my age [thirty-nine], he said, "If you are going to do IVF, you
better just schedule it." But we don't know if we want to get into the
whole rat race again. The most frustrating thing is the time wasted,
the expense, not being able to try because of the condition of my ovaries, and sort of being pushed into this really extreme solution which
we don't know that we want to do. So the whole thing has been really
frustrating, and it has totally disgusted me with the medical world.*

The physician's role in infertility treatment has changed. Whereas
twenty years ago basic infertility testing and early treatment typically

took place in the gynecologist's office, today infertility specialists have become treatment managers because of the proliferation of specialized techniques and equipment. Reproductive endocrinologists (subspecialists in infertility treatment) increasingly employ Ph.D.-trained laboratory specialists, such as andrologists and embryologists, and the techniques employed include the micromanipulation of sperm and eggs and preimplantation genetic diagnosis.[44] Expert systems such as this are designed to be responsive to, and interact with, consumption. That is, they are prepared to address in a timely manner a host of medical concerns that may arise. The cost of new reproductive technologies is therefore closely related to the constant monitoring of these systems by laboratory personnel. Although a variety of clinical strategies are employed to minimize the utilization of services on weekends, IVF centers are obligated to meet the needs of patients at specific points in the reproductive cycle. This requires staffing by physicians, nurses, and office and laboratory personnel seven days a week. Because laboratory procedures are often critically time-sensitive, staffing must allow for twenty-four hour coverage when necessary.

The process of technological development in medicine culminates with the naturalization of a technology and its acceptance by the public.[45] Today babies such as Louise Brown are seen as a normal part of life. People have adjusted to the idea that conception may take place in the lab, not in the womb. In twenty years new reproductive technologies have not only come full circle, they have come to be viewed around the world as simply another means of conception.

WHO IS LEFT OUT?

Technologies may create or perpetuate social inequalities. New medical technologies are generally expensive, and in the United States access to such treatments is often limited to patients who can pay. The small number of people in this study who had low incomes had almost no medical options, and they dropped out of medical treatment in the early stages. Couples sometimes decided, after some brief diagnostic testing, that they could not afford to proceed with medical treatment, and began exploring ways of adopting a child that would not be costly. Jackie, who could not afford any medical care whatsoever, concentrated on making her body as healthy as possible through diet, exercise, and "positive thinking":

*I was tested. I went to a clinic. But I was tested—the dye through the
tubes and all that stuff, and I was told that I had scarring and that
one of my tubes was a little crooked and that my chances of getting
pregnant were pretty slim. In fact, I remember them telling me that it
could get caught in there. The scarring was caused by an IUD, and
PID. Constant PID.*

*I am kind of letting nature take its course. I would like to seek some
treatment but because I am unemployed, if I am not working, I really
can't. I remember this woman—she was a psychic—and I remember
her telling me that when I learned to love myself, then that is when I
will have a baby. So I know that I am going to have one. A baby is
going to come out of this body. And it is in God's time, and it is going
to be a miracle child. Because, like I said, I have one tube left, and it
has some scarring in there, but I believe in miracles.*

Karen, having just learned about IVF, complained:

*It's $10,000 a cycle, and the chances of it working are pretty slim. We
would have to save a long time to get $10,000. I'd spend $10,000 on
adoption before I'd spend it on in vitro because the price tag is about
the same, and that way you get a baby. And with in vitro, who knows
what you get? Nothing, probably. There need to be some options for
people like us who don't have money sitting in the bank.*

Who uses these technologies is not simply a function of who wants
to use them but also of whom society permits to use them. Access to
medical treatment for infertility has emerged as a class-based phenomenon, and, to the extent that class is linked to ethnicity, works to reduce
access for women and men of color.[46] Historical patterns of access and
discrimination provide important clues to the power relations of a particular era. It is therefore not surprising that the United States, with its
history of limited access for low-income women seeking reproductive
health care and of medical techniques used punitively against specific
groups of people (as with the sterilization of African American women),
has taken no action to give low-income women access to new reproductive technologies.[47] This phenomenon represents another, albeit subtle, form of discrimination, making it more difficult for women and
families who are poor to have children.[48]

That these technologies are more accessible to some people in society
than to others reflects the underlying moral economy of the United
States. By this I mean that not only is the economy political, but it is

shaped by specific social views as well. Moral economy refers to popu-
larly shared moral assumptions underlying certain societal practices.[49]
These technologies engage a moral dilemma about who shall have access
to them. Implicit in the moral economy that guides the consumption of
new reproductive technologies is the idea that some people are more
deserving than others, and that entitlement is related to productivity,
and hence to wealth—in short, to the ability to find the financial resources to pay for these technologies.

THE GLOBAL CONSUMPTION OF NEW
REPRODUCTIVE TECHNOLOGIES

Although our studies were conducted in a single locale in the United
States, new reproductive technologies are very much a global phenomenon, characterized everywhere by hierarchical relations and power con-
stellations.[50] Comparing the consumption of new reproductive technologies and the policies created to regulate them in various parts of the
globe can provide a view of cultural practices and power dynamics in a
given society.

Practitioners in this field focus not only on international medical advances but also on the social implications of those advances. For example, when the technique of transferring a woman's donor gametes
(eggs) into another woman was first developed, recipients over forty
were rare. But over time the age ceiling has shifted upward. When a
woman in Italy gave birth at the age of sixty-two a few years ago, the
event triggered an international debate among fertility practitioners and
bioethicists, one that intensified with the birth of a child to a sixty-three-
year-old woman in the United States. This is but one example of the
power of consumers in subverting technologies to be used in ways that
were not intended.[51]

Consumers of new reproductive technologies may travel internationally to seek them out. For example, two couples in our study went
home—to Israel and India—for IVF treatment because it was more affordable there. A technology may be developed in one nation but more
avidly used elsewhere because it fits particularly well with the social
mores of another society. For example, sperm donation is not practiced
in Egypt for religious reasons. Consequently the technique of intracytoplasmic sperm injection (ICSI), whereby the sperm of a man with a
low sperm count may be collected and effectively used for in vitro fertilization, has led to its widespread use in Egypt.[52] Some other countries,

such as China, have created population policies that interact with the use of reproductive technologies.[53]

New reproductive technologies also interact with other industries, such as the international adoption business. For example, the support organization Resolve provides information about both reproductive technologies and adoption, and many people in this study were contemplating both at the same time. Prospective adoptive parents are often people who have used new reproductive technologies without success or are waiting to gain access to them.[54] International adoptions can be characterized most often by the transfer of children from poor people to those who are well off and from countries that are poor to countries that are resource-rich, such as the United States and the countries of Western Europe. Under these conditions children may be commodified.

In the United States, most people who use new reproductive technologies must pay for them out of pocket, in contrast with the situation in some other countries, where socialized medicine prevails. As we will see, the financial strain this causes plays a role in the politicization of these technologies. At the same time, the use of reproductive technologies remains relatively unregulated in the United States, largely because of the prevailing ideology of autonomy.[55] In other nations these technologies are regulated, with the state therefore taking an overt role in social engineering. Many countries, for example, restrict access to these technologies to heterosexual, married couples, and some prohibit the use of certain technologies, such as those involving the use of donors.[56] Although numerous writers have examined the regulatory policies of specific countries, the absence of regulation in the United States has gone largely unremarked by Americans because they consider it a right and take it for granted.[57] It has been advantageous for some who may be viewed as socially marginal, such as single women and gay couples. Unfettered by legal restrictions on access to services, anyone who can afford the new reproductive technologies is free to use them regardless of marital status, sexual orientation, or religion, a state of affairs that has resulted in expanded opportunities to create a family as well as contributing to new understandings of what constitutes a family.[58]

ABOUT THE STUDIES

When I began my research on infertility, I wanted to include every major aspect of the social experience of medical treatment. To understand that experience fully, however, I believed I needed to understand everything about infertility treatment. How practitioners thought about infertility and their philosophies of practice were thus important components of the research, as was the relationship between patients and physicians. I felt the inclusion of biomedical perspectives was necessary to understand the "big picture" of infertility and to make sense of people's experiences. For all the years of this research, I therefore carried out a multisited ethnography[59] that included not only repeated in-depth interviews with people undergoing medical treatment for infertility but also interviews and informal discussions with physicians, regular attendance at talks on infertility and reproductive technologies in two hospitals, and frequent attendance at informational workshops and symposia conducted by Resolve, a nationwide support organization for those dealing with infertility.[60]

Seeking treatment for infertility is a middle-class phenomenon. People with low incomes simply cannot afford it because even the most basic medical treatment involves repeated medical appointments and drugs. I was not content to examine infertility treatment only for the middle class, however, and I believed that if we searched for people with low incomes seeking treatment for infertility, we would find them. I was wrong. During all four years of the study we made a concerted effort to locate low-income clinics that treated fertility problems, and the people who utilized them. Unfortunately, these services were almost nonexistent, and our extensive efforts to locate individuals with low incomes who were going through infertility yielded a limited number of people.

Ultimately the ethnographer must choose what to emphasize, and in doing so she shapes the nature of the ethnography. There was never any question in my mind where my own emphasis lay—in people's experiences of infertility. I believe that the multiple and overlapping stories from my research provide a lens onto a series of questions and problems in U.S. society that no other method of inquiry can offer. A comprehensive analysis of reproductive technologies is beyond the scope of this work. What I attempt to do here is to portray in depth the perspectives of people undergoing these treatments in the context of contemporary cultural phenomena. I do not wish to suggest that their experiences are the central ingredient in such an analysis but rather that those experiences are a highly salient piece of a much larger picture.[61]

The majority of women and men in the study had undergone medical treatment for three or more years, although twenty had undergone medical treatment for a year or less. These women and men were recruited from medical practices, adoption counseling services, and a self-help group, and by other participants.

Within this predominantly middle-class sample, 15 percent of whom were members of ethnic minorities, there was a considerable range in income.[62] Although differences in income greatly affected the ability of women and men to pursue costly treatment, they did not affect the richness of respondents' narratives in recounting the disruption caused by infertility or their interpretations of the meaning of infertility for their lives. See the appendix for more details of this research.

I interviewed everyone in the pilot study myself and half of the people in the larger study; the other half of the interviews were done by five other interviewers—three women and two men. Women and men were first interviewed together in detailed interviews lasting two hours or more; follow-up individual interviews took place approximately six to twelve months later, with final follow-up interviews with both partners taking place twelve to twenty-four months later.

The stories in this book illustrate the deep connection between bodily distress and the social order.[63] By this I mean anything pertaining to bodily experience, such as physical and emotional suffering and a person's feelings about his or her body. People's stories express bodily experience. When someone narrates such a story, the story itself can be seen as the enactment, or performance, of bodily experience.[64] Such performances constitute action, a transition from viewing something in one way to viewing it differently. And, as we will see, this process is gendered.

One goal of this work has been to scrutinize people's stories for clues to their bodily distress. I studied all references to the body and bodily distress and examined all reports of medical interventions, as well as all expressions of intense emotion, for their relationship to bodily concerns. I also scrutinized people's stories for links between expressions of bodily distress and discussions of cultural expectations.

When I returned to the homes of people in the infertility study months or even years later, people would frequently say, "Since the last time you were here I have been thinking more about what we talked about, and I have some new ideas about it," or "I am in a different place from when you were here last." The images that people project of themselves and the world through their stories are thus subject to change. Performing one's story to an audience may facilitate that process, especially during times of transition when people viscerally experience their own passage through life.

One of the abiding frustrations of those seeking social change is the resilience of certain dialogues within society that maintain cultural ideologies and thereby impose a limited view on life possibilities. People who repeatedly attempt to live up to cultural ideologies, yet fail to do so, experience acute social discomfort and emotional pain. They may eventually come to see those ideologies as interfering with and delaying their attempts to find alternative ways of regaining a sense of normalcy and thus finding meaning in life. I believe that this is why so many people volunteered to participate in this research: out of a conviction that ideas about fertility and parenthood in United States society need to change and that, collectively, their voices might make a difference. It was not easy for any of them to talk with us. Almost without exception, they would have preferred their pain and their innermost thoughts to remain private. But they believe there is a story to be told, a puzzle so complex that only by adding their singular stories to create a whole can they help others facing the same problems to find better answers—answers that involve society as a whole.

CHAPTER 2

Confronting Notions
of Normalcy

Erin, a forty-three-year-old marketing executive married two years ear-lier, describes how medical treatment affected her: "Infertility has been the damnedest thing, to try to keep myself from letting it take over. I keep telling myself, 'This is part of my life, not the whole of it.' I keep coming back to that whole medical system, which makes it hard. Be-cause you're not allowed to be a whole person. You're a body part." Erin's comments address her sense of bodily disruption. She reflects on a problem common to women who are undergoing intensive medical evaluation for fertility: feeling depersonalized. Seeing herself as an as-semblage of "body parts" reflects Erin's sense of her body being tech-nologized as a machine.[1] She continues,

A bunch of people clucking over your ovaries and the post-luteal phase of your uterus. It's real hard to say, "I am a person. I have friends. I have a husband. I have a job." Why don't you keep it all in perspective? It just takes more fortitude than I've got, and I think part of the stress was because I wasn't able to maintain myself throughout the infertility and the miscarriages. I did it as a patient, not as a full person. I couldn't maintain that balance that I seem to need. I don't know how other women do it.

It is obvious that Erin experienced medical treatment as an assault on her body and that she felt chastised by health professionals for the bodily defects they identified. Indeed, the physicians Erin consulted routinely said she was too old to conceive and that her miscarriages were a manifestation of her age. They thought she should stop trying to conceive with her own eggs; if she wished to pursue further medical treatment, she should try in vitro fertilization, using an egg donated by another woman.[2] Resisting this perspective, Erin is trying to remind herself of who she is, telling herself repeatedly that she is a "real person" and that this is only a part of her life.

Medical treatment heightens women's and men's sense of abnormality and locates it in the body. Although infertility itself is not a disease, the health care system treats it like one. The medical definition of infertility is a functional one: the failure to conceive within twelve months of initiating unprotected intercourse. The term *infertility* is a medical statement that it is abnormal to be unable to reproduce biologically. The medical evaluation analyzes the medical, social, and sexual history, physical examination findings, and laboratory test results to suggest an explanation for a failure to conceive. Often identified in the presence of apparent good health, these factors raise the specter of clinical abnormalities that were previously invisible and unknown.[3]

Although medical treatment for infertility may end in high-technology efforts to bring about a pregnancy, the medical encounter typically begins with a gynecologist or family practitioner performing several months of relatively inexpensive and noninvasive tests. This approach follows the standard medical model of examining for findings on which to base a diagnosis, with diagnosis-specific treatment to follow. In the past, absence of conclusive findings generally led to treatment with oral fertility drugs or artificial insemination, despite little evidence of their clinical efficacy.[4] In the early phases of current treatment the same approach may be taken, but as time passes the urgency of achieving a pregnancy leads to the use of new, more invasive and expensive reproductive technologies that bypass the natural reproductive cycle altogether, regardless of the underlying infertility diagnosis. As I mentioned in chapter 1, infertility treatment, which in the past rarely lasted longer than a few years or cost more than a few thousand dollars, now lasts until the couple's emotional and financial resources are exhausted.

GENDER AND BODILY EXPERIENCE

Because reproductive technologies engage cultural meanings of fertility, they challenge traditional notions about gender, sexuality, and the family. They raise questions about how we view biology and the body. New reproductive technologies not only have drawn us toward a renewed scrutiny of aspects of everyday life that were previously taken for granted, but they have also been a catalyst for analysis of technology as a cultural form and its relationship to social institutions in the United States.

One of the most intriguing aspects of this analysis is the way in which reproductive technologies both affect and are affected by gender. Social scientists have suggested that technologies are shaped by the operation of gender interests and may reinforce traditional gendered patterns of power and authority. We will see from the study how this occurs, but we will also see how gender is enacted, or performed, through technology.[5] For example, repeated cycles of in vitro fertilization may enable a woman to enact her wish to be a biological mother. Examined from this angle, technology can be seen both to perpetuate cultural ideologies and to be used performatively by individuals as a vehicle for living out their goals. Thus, not only is gender identity reaffirmed through the use of technology, but particular cultural dialogues about gender are also maintained and expanded. In focusing on users' experience of these technologies, my research complements studies of technology that focus on its institutional components.

When they discover a problem, people monitor and discuss their bodies. How they talk about their bodies tells us much not only about the nature of bodily experience from a gendered perspective but also about how people connect their bodies to related issues such as kinship, fertility, and age. The portrayal of bodily experience—the connection between how people talk about their bodies and how they experience them—is also closely linked to people's perceptions of societal expectations for parenthood. It is therefore possible to see links between the personal body—the body of experience—and cultural dialogues about normalcy.

The body is a bearer of multiple cultural meanings about gender, and these meanings are enacted, or performed, as people go through their daily lives. Judith Butler differentiates between gender *expression* and gender *enactment* because *expression* conveys that there is something *natural,* or essential, about gender, while gender *enactment* stresses its social and cultural aspects. When culturally derived bodily knowledge is disordered by infertility, women's and men's understandings of themselves and their world are thrown into chaos, affirming Judith Butler's contention that "performing one's gender wrong initiates a set of punishments both obvious and indirect."[6]

It is not my intent to "essentialize" gender. That is, I do not wish to suggest that gender is necessarily expressed only through stereotyped views of women and men as embodiments of motherhood and fatherhood, respectively. Far from it! But in portraying women and men struggling with the problem of not having children when they want them, I explore complex cultural ideas about gender and normalcy.[7] Such ideologies make it more difficult for people to deviate from widespread cultural expectations.

When women and men aspire to parenthood and find themselves unable to live out this deep-seated cultural expectation, they initially cling to traditional notions about what constitutes womanhood and manhood. In the process they may reduce notions of gender into stereotypical ideas. For example, women in this study frequently expressed the idea that having children is women's primary work. Those who do not conceive after an extended effort, however, begin to question the images they find impossible to live up to. When this happens, their ideas about gender change and expand, and their identities in turn are affected. Everyone in this research was asked the question, Has your identity as a woman/man changed as a result of experiencing infertility? All women and most men responded affirmatively and discussed those changes in great detail.[8]

From the time of birth, we see our gendered bodies through a cultural lens.[9] Bodily knowledge informs what we do and say in the course of daily life. The culturally informed order of our bodies shapes the way in which we understand the world. [10] What is more, we carry our gendered histories with us in our bodies, personal histories that are influenced by social history.[11] But our bodily experience not only encompasses the past and present, it also anticipates the future.[12] When women anticipate pregnancy and imagine that each subtle new bodily sensation indicates they are pregnant, for example, they propel themselves into a future that is culturally shaped.

As people tell their stories and as they analyze their life situations, they generate categories of social analysis through their gendered bodies.[13] For example, when men learn they are infertile, they analyze their situation in the context of cultural expectations about manhood. Bodily experience facilitates an examination of human action, including the ways in which action is transformative.[14] When women and men find themselves at odds with the status quo, they take action. In this book, we will see how many women facing infertility, and some men, turn to collective action through Resolve. Bodily experience can be reflected in

communal life and action, and we will see how this process, too, is
gendered, to shape the experience of infertility and to transform it. People's resistance to the power of cultural norms is grounded in bodily
experience.[15]

Angela's story illustrates these connections between gender, bodily
distress, and action. At the beginning of the study, Angela was thirty-
three, a school counselor whose family had immigrated from Belgium
shortly before she was born. I first met her three years earlier, when she
was still in the early stages of seeking to become pregnant. Since that
time she had had a miscarriage and many medical interventions. Our
interviews, some conducted with her husband present and some with
Angela alone, took place over several years. In our third interview she
reflected on her recent, unsuccessful experience with reproductive technologies:

*It really did hit me about Thanksgiving. I was just . . . I was devas-
tated. And I'm still grieving. I don't know if I'll ever lose that feeling
of loss. But I'm really glad we tried it [assisted reproductive technol-
ogy]. And it's not that it's not an option later on, but it's definitely not
an option for me right now. I do feel like my body is just starting to
get back to the same [as before]. I'm starting to exercise five times a
week. It's [body] just starting to become more normal. How I was in
pre-infertility days. And it feels so much better. I just feel better about
that part.*

Angela's comments about her body returning to normal imply that during the treatment her body was *not* normal. She is regaining a feel for
the continuity of her feminine body that transcends the disruption
caused by repeated medical treatment.

Angela reflects on how she sees this time of her life and on her relationships with others:

*It's been a long journey. Very exhausting. I wouldn't want to recom-
mend it to anybody. But I've learned a lot about myself. I've learned a
lot about people in general. You really know who the people are who
really care about you—even though they're fumbling attempts. Their
true attempts still reach you. Because we [self and husband] were really withdrawn. I was and have been for the past couple of years.*

As she tries to put her experience into perspective, Angela is looking
back on her own recent history, using the idea of a journey as a metaphor for medical treatment and the other changes she has experienced.

The metaphor of life as a journey is a central motif in Western societies and may conjure up many images of, for example, hardship and extended travail.[16] Such metaphors enable the narrator to come to a new understanding of her experience and thus transcend it.[17] Rather than regard the past few years as a brief interlude, Angela views this time as a long and wearing trip in which she grew as a person. The journey thus becomes one that transcends the repeated medical procedures and the physical and emotional pain they represent. The notion of transformation is part of the process of integrating disruption and restoring a sense of order, and thus continuity, to life.[18]

Angela makes it clear that the journey did not occur in a vacuum. She connects the journey to the importance of human caring. She realizes, moreover, that she has not completed the journey. She addresses the next phase:

I'm eager to adopt because I'm ready for a family. I'm really ready for that stage. And the thing that scares me is my timeline. I'm a person who likes to operate on a timeline life. And I'll be thirty-four this summer. To me that sounds really old. I know, I know it just sounds like . . . aww. I thought I'd have children by now. It's hard for me to see twenty-six-year-olds in either of our families having what they want and going along with their timeline. And I keep struggling with it.

So I am really much more open to adoption. Just because I think I'm really ready to love the child that comes into my life. Give it our best shot. I'm willing . . . we will try GIFT [gamete intrafallopian transfer] after we adopt, once more. We'd have to do the blood work first. I think that will tell us if we can go on. If we have a chromosomal effect factor, then I think we'll have an adoptive family.[19] So I think that will determine it.

Angela's comment about operating on a timeline makes it clear how disruptive people find it when the anticipated course of life goes askew and expectations are unfulfilled. But, more than this, Angela is talking about a reproductive timeline. Angela has not completely let go of her efforts to have a biological child, but the new information revealed by her latest medical treatment, the presence of a genetic disorder, gives her a concrete, if distressing, medical reason why she has not successfully conceived. Now she can move ahead with decisions about what to do next.

Her experience in infertility treatment has had a profound effect on her view of her body and her bodily knowledge:

What has changed for me is very ironic. It has happened over time. It's that I really don't care to be pregnant. I would pay somebody to carry it and take care of it and go through the labor and all the pain and go to the hospital, and then I just take it home and say, "Thank you very much." I just really have no desire to go through the medical stuff, to get shot, to go through any more pain. I'm done with that. So it's an irony. I would love for us to have a biological child. But I feel like I've gone over and above, in terms of that. Looking back, we went through too many drug cycles, and then the breast lump [a cyst] was just a really good indicator for us to say, "You know what? You're going way too far. You need to redirect yourself."

The full effects of Angela's physical and emotional exhaustion become apparent with this statement. The grieving that she has alluded to emerges here as an abandonment of efforts to become a biological mother. She has been through so much in medical treatment that she no longer wants to experience pregnancy and childbirth. She no longer trusts her body to carry a pregnancy, a view that amounts to a rejection of her bodily knowledge of herself as a woman preparing to have a child. But now she is "listening" to her body in a different way and refocusing her energies. She finds it easier to envision the baby as a package she takes home after someone else has undergone the pain and suffering, thus protecting her body from further onslaughts and additional failures.

The impact of advanced reproductive technologies on Angela's body and on her gender identity has been profound. This process has reshaped how she sees herself, a change that is filled with emotion:

So I don't know what and how I'll feel—when I cross that bridge—is basically what I'm saying. But I feel a lot of sadness. There's still some anger. And yet I've become a real assertive person. In terms of dealing with docs and getting right with them as much as I can. I feel much more compassion for other people who have cancer or handicapped children or other plights in their life. And I'm just much more of a humble person. I really gave up the golden ball. I was a late bloomer, and I gave it up. I think that's what infertility did. I gave up that idealism a little bit. And it made me painfully aware that life is difficult. It's been a long road.

As Angela reflects on the changes she has gone through, she portrays herself as a woman who has aged from this experience, as she describes giving up "the golden ball"—the idealism of youth. The metaphor of the journey returns as Angela comments on the long, difficult road she has traversed. She ascribes her emotional growth to this experience, in all its bittersweet nuances: anger and sadness are balanced against new-found compassion and assertiveness.

Every person we meet in these pages has root concerns about herself or himself as a person because of the insecurity that infertility provokes about gender identity. Cultural dialogues about reproduction are not simply about different means of reproduction: they reflect dominant views in the United States about what constitutes a person.[20] People in this study said repeatedly that their inability to conceive left them feeling "incomplete." It is therefore not surprising that people go to great lengths to conceive a biological child. While people's stories and their actions are ostensibly about reproduction, the underlying issue is about fitting in—about fulfilling society's expectations.

CULTURAL DIALOGUES ABOUT NORMALCY

In her self-portrait, Angela addresses a set of cultural assumptions about what constitutes normal womanhood. As she talks about her losses and the changes in her body, she indirectly refers to cultural dialogues that equate women with nurturance. Throughout the book I refer to shared cultural assumptions about what is considered normal as "normalcy." Women and men strive for normalcy in their daily lives; infertility disrupts that sense of normalcy. When conception does not occur as planned, women and men experience a sense of difference. Feeling different provokes a reexamination of cultural assumptions about fertility, gender, and the family.

I use the phrase *cultural dialogues* to refer to shared cultural assumptions about a given topic, such as fertility.[21] Cultural dialogues carry enormous moral force because they embody social norms, that is, the range of what is considered normal. These dialogues differentiate between what is viewed as normal and what is viewed as different or deviant.[22] Such dialogues shift over time because they are embedded in social, economic, and historical contexts. They also become more or less dominant as time passes, depending on contemporary cultural emphases. Thus the dialogue on body weight, for example, has changed and become more dominant in the late twentieth century, reflecting the intertwining of health and social issues. Previous norms for body weight have been eclipsed by the growing emphasis on thinness, and those who greatly exceed the current standards are viewed as deviant.

Women and men attempting to conceive are trying to realize life plans while negotiating complex cultural dialogues about parenthood, gender, genes, and the like. These dialogues, both verbal and nonverbal, are continual, both among individuals and in the media. Views of normalcy are affected by factors such as ethnicity, gender, age, and income level, as well as by life experience. They are based on ideas about what "most people" do. Ideas about what constitutes normalcy thus lie at the core of all cultural dialogues.[23] People define normalcy in terms of particular images. Although not everyone has the same interpretation of what constitutes normalcy in a given situation, there is a huge overlap in how people in the same society define normalcy.

Normalcy repeatedly defined and portrayed within certain narrow limits, as in the case of biological parenthood, amounts to an ideology. I use the term *cultural ideology* to refer to such dominant, pervasive ways of thinking. To illustrate these ideas, there is a cultural *dialogue* about parenthood that encompasses all forms of parenting, but there is a cultural *ideology* about biological parenthood because that is so closely tied to American notions of what is normal. As Angela Davis points out, such ideologies are affected by racism and class biases, the current ideology surrounding motherhood being a case in point. She suggests that the availability of reproductive technologies mythologizes motherhood as the true vocation of white, middle-class women. She observes that this ideology does not apply to women of color and women outside the middle class, for whom other policies and practices that discriminate against motherhood apply.[24] This differential treatment of women by color and class reflects the moral economy of reproductive technologies, which draws distinctions about who is deserving on the basis of such biases.

Angela's story exemplifies the power of the cultural ideology of motherhood: she was ready to adopt only after years of effort to have a biological child. We will see how people wrestle with cultural ideologies such as biological parenthood as they attempt to fit into society, and as they examine alternatives when they cannot be accommodated within a certain cultural ideology.

Cultural dialogues about what is normal underscore the moral force that cultural ideologies have on people's lives.[25] Cultural ideologies about fertility, womanhood, manhood, motherhood, fatherhood, the importance of having kin, and the meaning of family, for example, are all tapped by the discovery of infertility. Taken for granted by women and men before infertility was identified as a problem, these cultural ideologies become a focus for identifying what is normal and for working through feelings of being different.

Despite strides in the social sciences in reconceptualizing topics such as gender, fertility, and the family, certain cultural motifs remain dominant, such as the equation of women with nature and the related idea that women will produce biological children. Those motifs represent aspects of dominant ideologies in society that are very difficult to dislodge. Cultural dialogues about gender, parenthood, and family are embedded in social institutions such as biomedicine. Those dialogues recur again and again in medical treatment and are entwined with that treatment. This is why social scientists view technology as reproducing cultural ideologies, power relations, and structural inequities.[26] Indeed, women and men become aware of these complexities and their role in them as they encounter reproductive technologies. Power itself can be viewed as a core constitutive element in the makings of technology, a perspective that has become integral to studies of technology.[27]

Technologies are rarely perceived as morally neutral by anyone concerned, whether it is women themselves, health care professionals, or members of other institutions.[28] Angela's decision to seek medical treatment triggered a dialogue about her moral responsibility as a woman to bear children. Women undergoing experiences like Angela's find themselves desiring simultaneously to resist and to avail themselves of new reproductive technologies.

When social change does occur, people reproduce new approaches in known cultural forms.[29] Those who experience difference may align themselves with alternative dialogues that resemble, in part, the dominant dialogue, or cultural ideology. The desire to fit in, and to develop alternative dialogues in order to do so, is not simply a passive acceptance of cultural ideologies. Alternatives to the traditional biological family, for example, generally follow traditional family forms, such as social parenthood of adopted children or children conceived with donor gametes. This phenomenon reflects the tendency of people to build on existing cultural models.[30]

Angela's story is not unusual. Indeed, her response to the failure of intensive medical treatment to bring about a conception is typical of the response of women in this study who tried unrelentingly to conceive, without success. Every one of those women saw her body and her life as permanently changed by their experience. But it is not only women who failed to conceive who felt this way: women who successfully conceived and delivered a child expressed the same need to make sense of this experience, evaluating their bodily knowledge, the changes they saw in themselves, and their entire lives in terms of this unexpected disruption to life.

Men, too, went through an intense reevaluation of their lives whether or not the treatments were successful. Pursuing infertility treatment invariably triggers a life transition, but it is not the treatments themselves that trigger this response: it is the process of having one's gender identity assaulted, of being forced to rethink basic assumptions about life that sets this process in motion.[31] Men's gender identity plays a crucial and complex role in their experience of infertility.[32]

PARENTHOOD AND THE
CHANGING COURSE OF LIFE

As we modify the ways in which we define and structure families, we are also seeing changes in the way people structure the course of their lives. In the late twentieth century we have seen the growth and development of medical technologies that dramatically extend the life span and affect the timing of the course of life, lengthening some life stages, and sometimes altering the potential content of specific life stages. This is a startling turn of events that has received comparatively little attention.

My research is embedded in the anthropological view that each culture has its own expected "life course." This can be viewed as a cultural unit and a powerful collective symbol.[33] People assign meaning and expectations to specific life events. When these expectations are not met, people experience inner chaos and disruption. Angela, for example, called attention to the disruption of her "timeline" in several interviews. The first time I met her, she alluded to deviating from a biological timeline because, according to her family, she was rather old to be starting to have children. Yet other women going through infertility, whom she knew from her involvement with Resolve, apparently considered her young and her problems less urgent than those of older women. Later, when she had become a "veteran" of infertility, having logged several years of medical treatment, her age became unimportant to others.

I have been intrigued by these cultural expectations and by their effects on people whose life courses deviate from them. In postponing parenthood until the point when conception becomes problematic, for example, people's lives are disrupted. Among those we interviewed, including Angela, delayed childbearing and failure to conceive wrought havoc with their life plans. As with Angela's, the shape of those women's and men's lives was unfolding differently from the life they had anticipated.

The timing of parenthood has changed. Women and men wait longer to form long-term partnerships. Unions formed in one's twenties may be unstable and end without either person having considered parenthood. Many women in this study made statements such as "I never wanted to have children until I met [partner]" or "I was married [or in a relationship] before, but I never considered having children with him." Consequently, many women and men are now single as they enter their thirties. More and more women—and men—are not ready to begin having families until they are in their thirties or later. When they eventually meet the person they consider to be a life partner and begin thinking about having children, many women's fertility has already begun to decline.

The later women and men meet, the less time they may feel they have to explore their relationship before having children. Many of the couples in our studies met, married, and began trying to conceive within a very short period. Couples thus often face complex issues about fertility together before they know each other well. Infertility treatment thus becomes the testing ground for the relationship. The stakes are high, for if the relationship comes apart, by the time they pick up the pieces of their lives and meet another partner—*if* they find another partner—it will probably be too late, at least for women, to consider parenthood. Thus fertility treatment involves not only the stress inherent in the procedure but also the effort to keep the relationship afloat. The threat of losing the relationship as well is more disruption than most people are prepared to face.[34]

Throughout this book, we see both women and men making massive efforts to accommodate the needs of their partners. This is one reason why the infertility quest may go on and on, why one expensive treatment after another is sought. The relationship that the couple works so hard to preserve stands for cultural assumptions about romantic love and commitment in the United States.[35] Although blood ties rank above love in the U.S. kinship system, love and marriage are nevertheless part of the American cultural fabric.[36] Once couples embark on a fertility quest and have their assumptions about their reproductive potential altered, they cleave to the marriage. Women and men consequently work very hard to minimize disruption to their relationship. Divorce rates appear to be low among this population.[37] Perhaps women and men work harder to maintain the relationship in midlife than earlier in adulthood because everything they have learned to believe in is at stake. Stable, long-term relationships are an important cultural value.

The current trend toward delayed childbearing in the United States appears to represent an enduring shift in the predominant pattern of middle-class adult life. Because a woman's fertility declines as she ages, delayed childbearing will have long-term effects not only on the current generation of midlifers but on older and younger generations as well: advances in reproductive technology have extended the potential childbearing years into the sixties and child-rearing into the years beyond that. Such changes are creating major shifts in the overall structure of life that will likely extend into advanced old age for both women and men. The long-term effects of delayed childbearing are potentially far-reaching because of increasing childlessness, changes in social and economic conditions in U.S. society, and advances in reproductive technology that extend the childbearing years potentially into the sixties and the child-rearing years beyond that. As we will see, efforts to become parents are being shifted to later and later points in the life cycle. The potential effects of this age shift on society are complex.

CHAPTER 3

The Embattled Body

Marcy, a thirty-three-year-old woman, describes how she felt when she heard about her infertility. After starting an infertility workup to find out why she was not conceiving, she soon learned that her fallopian tubes were blocked.

The effect of finding out about the infertility problems for me was that I felt completely useless. I felt like, basically, a piece of garbage. And I thought, "Wait a second, this is not a time for you to feel worthless. This is a time where you really need every ounce of confidence you have." Your feeling of self-worth just plummets when finding this out because everyone always says, "You can have kids. Everyone can have kids. It's the American dream. Why can't you?" "Snap your fingers and you're pregnant!" But if it doesn't work for you . . . I don't even have the words. It just really throws you.

Marcy's lifelong assumption that she could conceive is typical of many women. When infertility is discovered, her womanhood is challenged and her bodily knowledge of herself is disrupted, resulting in self-denigration and loss of self-esteem.

Marcy's story shows how gender, procreation, and cultural notions about the "American dream" are blended together. The American dream, a metaphor for the good life, was invoked repeatedly by women and men in this study as something they were being denied. This metaphor is a sort of cultural shorthand for cosmic order as people know it.

In *Naturalizing Power,* Sylvia Yanagisako and Carol Delaney trace the idea of cultural order in Western civilization from the order of creation to "natural" order, a key element of which is the dichotomy between nature and culture that emerged in the nineteenth century.[1] They observe that although the term *reproduction* was viewed as a metaphor when it came into use at this time, making human reproduction analogous to that of plants and animals, the process had previously been discussed in terms of procreation, generation, and the biblical terms of "begetting and bearing," which referred to male and female roles. Since that time, men and women have been defined by their contribution to the process of procreation. Women are associated with reproduction as a "natural" activity and constrained by their role, while men's role as procreators remains powerful and more abstract. These categories have resulted in the tenacious view of women as "natural" and men as "cultural."

While feminists have worked to override these cultural assumptions, they persist in cultural dialogues on gender and reproduction.[2] Nowhere is their effect more obvious than among women and men experiencing infertility. These traditional notions exert their power even among many people in this study, some of whom consider themselves feminists and many more of whom consider themselves forward-thinking people who do not follow tradition for tradition's sake. In this chapter I examine women's and men's bodily experiences of infertility in the context of cultural dialogues about reproduction and gender.

THE GENDERED BODY

Gendered ideals of the body profoundly affect women's and men's responses to bodily disorder. For example, cultural ideals about women as naturally fertile affect Marcy's transition from seeing herself as whole and complete to seeing herself as "garbage." Clearly, bodily order is gendered. Bodily order and cultural order are equated with fertility.[3] In seeking medical care to address her failure to conceive, Marcy was acting in accordance with cultural ideals of women as naturally fertile; learning of her infertility made her feel that she had "performed" her gender wrongly.[4]

Although feminists have persuasively destabilized gender, and especially rigid distinctions between women and men, gender ideologies continue to promote such distinctions. People living with infertility who subscribe to heterosexual views of gender experience are sensitive to dominant ideologies of gender. They feel different from others because of their infertility. Thus, while gender has been destabilized, issues of normalcy persist. Those affected react both by attempting to fit into rigid cultural molds and by resisting those molds. Attempts to achieve a state of "gender normalcy" are characterized by inconsistency. The stories that follow illustrate the interaction of gender, sexuality, and feelings about the ability to reproduce in shaping people's ideas about themselves.[5]

When Marisa was eighteen, she was diagnosed with premature ovarian failure (see glossary). Her ovaries had stopped functioning, and she was put on drugs that are usually given to alleviate the symptoms of menopause. Now thirty-one, Marisa has been struggling ever since with cultural meanings of womanhood and her potential for motherhood. For the past four years she has been pursuing the possibility of bearing a child by using a donor egg. At the same time, she has considered both adoption and childlessness. I interviewed her over three years, from the time she had no children until after she had given birth to a baby conceived with a donor egg; this interview took place when she was pregnant. She was, however, having some bleeding and was afraid she would miscarry. She described her feelings about her body:

I feel like my body is . . . there's something very "off" about it. It makes me question my femininity and sexuality, and I thought this experience of pregnancy would kind of confirm in my mind more about being female. I feel like I question my sexuality and femininity. I think having the pregnancy will make me question that less. And if I don't have it [complete the pregnancy], I still have this feeling like being not completely female. That's a hard thing, to feel that way. You know, you're in a world where you want to be one sex or the other and it feels a little different not to be aligned with one side or the other. That's just the way it is. I don't really have any choices. I have to kind of accept it and realize that that's my body and that's the way things are.

Because Marisa's ovaries have stopped releasing the eggs and hormones that produce regular menstrual periods, she takes combinations of hormone medications to mimic the natural menstrual cycle. With donor egg technology she has the chance to become pregnant and give birth because her uterus is still capable of carrying a pregnancy. Nevertheless, because her body is no longer able to perform these tasks on its own, she questions her femininity and her sexuality, and she has confused them both with her fertility.[6] She feels androgynous.

Marisa's feelings are not simply the dramatic reaction of someone who has just received a life-altering medical diagnosis. She has lived with this diagnosis for thirteen years, and at the time of this interview she was pregnant. Nevertheless, the powerful cultural dialogues associated with menopausal bodily changes continue to undermine her gender identity.

The Western image of the androgyne, which represents the fusion of masculine and feminine characteristics, dates back to Greek civilization. In the twentieth century androgyny has become a motif of the late modern era, embodying tensions in the cultural dialogue on what is male and what is female.[7] Marisa is experiencing limbo. Her efforts to conceive are underwritten, in part, by her desire to be able to place herself unambiguously in the gendered world as a woman.

Asked if she felt that she had been experiencing a sense of loss prior to learning of her pregnancy, she says:

Yeah, because I know I spent a fair amount of time feeling sad and realizing that. . . . Some people walk down the street with kids in strollers, and I feel like swearing at them. I think the anger and the sadness are all tied into the whole process of grieving. You have to have both of those. I don't know if you ever get over it. I think to some extent in your life it's always kind of a tender point. From what people talk about [in Resolve groups], it seems like at certain times it's not at the forefront of your consciousness forever, like it is when you're going through the worst part of trying to get pregnant.

And one of the things that they were talking about in the last meeting — there is this place that has some Buddhist ceremony about it — I guess they have different ceremonies, and one of them is a ceremony to grieve all the unborn children. And we talked about that and thought that it would probably be a good idea to go to. Even thinking about it a few times, I just mentally tried to think about what the ceremony would be, and how you would take part in it and how many people would be there. Half of Resolve would be there.

Tears came to my eyes just thinking about physically having a child and bearing it. So there's still a lot of sadness. It's not gone by any means.

Although Marisa does not refer directly to her expectations for normalcy in womanhood, these ideas are implicit in what she says about her femininity and her sense of loss. Asked if the grieving process is both about the infertility specifically and about having been diagnosed with premature ovarian failure as well, she responds:

Yes. I guess if it was something that I could change, I might not be as peaceful about it. But I've lived with it since I was eighteen and I'm thirty-one now. I have a full understanding of it and believe at this point that there is nothing I can do to change this ovarian failure. It's kind of like, this thing has happened, and whatever has happened has happened, and there's no way to change it. So there's no point in fighting it. That's the way it is, and I just need to let it be and try to let myself be who I am with it.

Despite her sadness and residual anger, Marisa is accepting her bodily changes. Transformation is part of the process of integrating disruption and restoring a sense of continuity to life. By looking at things differently, people can reorder experience.[8] The transcendent experience epitomizes Western individualism and symbolizes coming full circle from one's beginnings.

I comment that she seems to have reached a good place in dealing with her situation, to which she responds:

Yeah, I think so. About five years ago—I think of this a lot—I was having dinner with an old friend, a man I had dated before I met my husband. And I was telling him a little about how wonderful my husband is, and we weren't married yet, and I said, "I'm just so scared to get involved in marriage because I don't know if I can have kids." And he said, "Well, you don't get married to have kids. That's not the point of being married." And I realized that I had been so caught up in this not being able to have kids that really, in my mind and at that point, the main goal of getting married was providing somebody with children. So it made me understand and realize different things about picking a partner in your life, and when you get married, the kids are not everything. I think the distinction is lost a lot of times. You really have to rethink the whole thing.

Marisa's conflation of marriage with reproduction was echoed frequently in the research, especially by women.[9] Marisa makes it clear that she views childbearing as one of women's primary functions. The need to "rethink the whole thing" was repeatedly observed in the research as women and men reflected on cultural dialogues about gender, sexuality, reproduction, and marital relationships.

Marisa's story attests to how profoundly gender identity is affected when the known, lived body is suddenly altered. Even though this bodily change was entirely invisible, and even though she was very young when her reproductive cycles ceased, Marisa, attuned to the cyclic nature of her body and everything that cycle symbolized, experienced gender uncertainty. This story also attests that cultural dialogues, while representing a range of views, nevertheless underscore normalcy, and the dominant dialogue is invariably the one that privileges normalcy. When women and men view themselves and their bodies as not reflecting cultural ideals for their gender, their sense of normalcy is shattered.

CULTURAL DIALOGUES AND MEN'S GENDER IDENTITY

Infertility is experienced as an assault on gender identity, and consequently both women and men feel they are in limbo, like Marisa, because they do not fit in with ideal notions about gender. Asked how he felt about his infertility, Ted responded:

It was really hard at first. I just hoped . . . a lot of sadness came with it, and it is what it is. And I felt like there's no choice. What I was really worried about feeling is that when you don't have children you feel pushed out somehow. And I felt that it was really hard to choose to do that [be childless]. So then I felt like what would be right would be that neither of us should have biological kids and that we should adopt. I think it was also, for me, a sense of shame. I actually felt less than a man.

Ted expresses the same loss of gender identity as Marisa. The threat to his potential to be a father makes him feel like an outsider. Ted's preference for adoption over donor insemination is revealing. Were they to choose donor insemination, his wife would be a biological parent, while he would be a social parent—and, according to the cultural ideology of biological parenthood, an inferior parent. If they adopted a child instead, their status would be more "equal." Patriarchal notions of the primacy of the father are thereby upheld. Unlike many men who voiced similar feelings and remained adamant about them, however, Ted subsequently opted to try donor insemination.

So profoundly do cultural ideologies about gender affect men and women that they consistently report feeling marginalized by them. David has known about his infertility for several years. He reflects on how it affects him now:

I see myself as disabled, but it's a hidden disability, I mean, it's kind of hidden from me, too. It's kind of there. It's like that pulse that I said before. It's kind of there and it doesn't often come up. It only comes up when it's on the calendar, you know, in terms of going to a Resolve group, or discontinuing a kind of treatment. At times I have felt that it has affected my self-esteem. That's a lot of what came up for me around IVF. A sense of inferiority around it like this is the only way that I could have children. It's like, "Gee, there must be something wrong with me if this is all I'm left with." To be quite frank, it did feel kind of pathetic to me, and it's a big part of my resistance. Just going into a room with some sleazy magazines and producing a specimen. It just really bugged me, and I felt really degraded the whole time.

Because infertility affects David's gender identity and gives him feelings of inferiority, he keeps it "hidden," not just from others but from himself. He analyzes the prevailing cultural dialogues that feed his sense of shame:

I think I felt ashamed of that, too, in a way. There's something very subtle in this culture that reinforces that sense of shame. And I think I've felt that at times with friends. This is something that's expected. You know, when people joke, "Well, you must be doing something wrong." Or when I told people that I've been married eight years, and they say, "Oh, do you have any kids?" And I say, "No," and they act like, "Well, what have you been doing?" But I think in ways that are very subtle and ways that aren't always subtle. Things I'm not always aware of. Like, I'm not always aware of my glasses but I kind of put them on in the morning. I look for them. There's stuff that we're more aware of in our lives because it's in our face more. And this is something that I found, for me, it's easier when it's not in my face. So when that is . . . that's when it's the pain of not having a child, or "Do I want to go through IVF again?"

David's observations catalogue some of the most commonplace responses to infertility. He is responding to cultural ideologies about masculinity, reproduction, and parenthood, all of which suggest his inadequacy. People in this study repeatedly expressed the deep sense of bodily shame they feel because they cannot live up to dominant cultural ideologies.[10]

Shame is a cultural phenomenon, not simply a psychological one. In the United States people are shamed by others when they do not fit into societal ideologies. Shame is experienced because one believes one is being punished for wrongdoing that everyone else knows or sees.[11] Such beliefs emerge from widespread Protestant religious beliefs in the United States.[12] Audrey, a thirty-two-year-old accountant, surrendered a child for adoption two years before she met her husband:

In the beginning I felt really isolated. Especially before I started building a network of infertile people. I felt thoroughly repulsed and disgusted by my body. I felt totally betrayed by my body. And consequently, it was hard to get too excited about other people's pregnancies and that kind of thing. The beginning was really hard, I have to say. It was really, really hard, and I had a tremendous amount of anger and outrage that this had happened, and I think if I hadn't already had a baby it wouldn't have been as bad. But I just felt like, I just went through this whole phase where I felt like I had been scorned. I had given away my only child, and now I was going to be punished. I went through a lot of stuff about that.

Only a few years after relinquishing a child for adoption. Audrey has now given up infertility treatment to pursue adoption herself. She feels anger and outrage at the irony of this situation. Implicit in her comments is the cultural idea that giving up a child is a monstrous, unnatural act for which she is being punished. Her comment about being "scorned" can be construed as a metaphor for an offense against society, as Hester Prynne was scorned in *The Scarlet Letter*. The term itself, uncommon in contemporary usage, suggests the Puritan wellsprings from which it arose.

Men confuse virility with potency. This view attests to the ways in which cultural dialogues underscore that sexuality is a part of gender. Ed, forty-two years old, discusses his virility. Asked how he felt when he first was given a diagnosis of infertility, he said,

There was a part of me that felt like I wasn't a complete man. Maybe I wasn't all that virile. But that is only a small part because I studied biology in college, and I know enough to know that those kind of things can happen to anyone, and emotionally it didn't affect me as negative as I know that it affects some men. Although I didn't talk about it because I know how other people feel about it and think about it. I work in a fairly blue-collar environment, and I didn't want people to be ribbing me all the time because they might make the assumption that infertility means lack of virility. In fact, I knew one of the men I worked with had taken a long time to have a child, and I

heard some of the jokes that used to be said about him. So I kept
quiet about that at work, but among my friends outside of work I did
talk about it.

In Ed's comments we see the close relationship between bodily distress, cultural dialogues on masculinity, and efforts to control information about gender and sexuality that could be potentially damaging.
As were all the men in this research, Ed is very careful as to whether
and how he shares this information with others. Male infertility is highly
stigmatizing, apparently more so than female infertility.[13]

Although he felt initially that he was not "a complete man," Ed attributes to his education his ability to separate his gender identity from
the diagnosis of infertility. He also suggests that there are class differences associated with cultural dialogues on masculinity: because he
works in a blue-collar environment, he is careful about where he discusses the problem. He is part of the management team at work and
considers himself middle-class, so he reserves any discussion of the problem for his men's group, whom he considers to be his peers.

Men who are diagnosed as being infertile are more strongly affected
by cultural ideologies about the meaning of manhood than men whose
partners who have been diagnosed with infertility. Both studies uncov-
ered specific differences. Men who are diagnosed as having male-factor
infertility have a more negative emotional response to infertility than
men who do not, in three respects: feelings of stigma, sense of loss, and
self-esteem. These differences reflect cultural expectations about male
infertility that profoundly affect men's sense of self, even if their infertility remains hidden from others.[14]

All men in the study reported that they questioned the fulfillment
of their role as a marital partner. Regardless of their own fertility status, men are deeply distressed by conflicts in their relationships with
their partners and by their inability to solve the problem of infertility
quickly.[15] This widespread response reflects cultural dialogues about
men as marital partners that differ from those about male fertility.

Jonathan is a forty-eight-year-old industrial consultant. In assessing
himself and his efforts to conceive with Angela, he mentions his bodily
engagement with the process, but his concerns are very different from
those of men whose fertility has been questioned:

I am missing out on being a father. And I am ready. And I think that
I realized, I think this is important. After the lost pregnancy I realized
that I felt that the detachment that I used was a coping device. Any

coping device is neither good nor bad, it is all a trade-off, and it worked. But the cost of it is that you are out of touch with your feelings because it works in a certain way. It is adaptive. I am beginning to compare my reaction to hers after the miscarriage, and in a way I felt I was missing something in myself. And I am by nature a very strong feeling person. I came to a new consciousness after the lost pregnancy, which is, "I want a baby." That is a conscious want. I want a baby, and I have a yearning, and it is a multisided thing. It is both sad and painful, but it is also affirming. It is directed and it is alive. And it is better to be alive and want something enough so that you know why you are here and what you want. Rather than being too numbed out. So I hurt a little more and I am a little more vulnerable and I will get a tear quicker. I was feeling a little depersonalized. I was a little out of touch. It is okay what I did, and it worked, and it still works, but it was like I am going to make a shift here a little bit. And I connect with her better, and it fits for me now. There is more feeling. I'm alive, and it is all right. Sometimes it's better to hurt than to be numb. At least you are alive.

And now I'm almost fifty, I can feel my body changing. But I am also wiser and happier, and that's all nice.

As Jonathan becomes conscious of the emotions he has been suppressing, he becomes more actively engaged in seeking a conception with his wife. His story is typical of men who do not have a fertility problem. These men are not included in medical treatment to the same extent, and thus for them the process may seem remote, at least until an event such as a miscarriage triggers their own sense of loss and makes the process of trying to conceive seem real, not an abstraction happening to someone else. Nevertheless, because these men do not experience these events in their bodies, they do not usually have the same profound response that women do. Jonathan acknowledges this:

I knew that just because of the nature of things it was much more involving and difficult for a woman, and probably especially if it is a woman's physical problems. But, the bond. The attachment. I can see that in the loss. I wasn't attached. I was starting to get attached to that fetus, but I was also being careful not to get too attached until we were more in the clear with that. I knew these couples who had miscarriages and problem pregnancies, and they were devastated. So I kept a little detached from it. I was thinking of it more in the sense of what it would mean for eventually being a father. And it was very dif-

*ferent for Angela. She was attached to this like it was a living thing, a
being. And it was a living being, but it might as well have been born
in the sense of her loss of it. It became a baby so quickly. So her grief
over that was deeper than mine. I felt helpless and frustrated and
empty. But it really was a death for her. I see that difference and I
have a lot of respect for it.*

Jonathan's observations demonstrate how different the experiences of
men and women are from each other. Whereas for men the idea of a
child remains an abstraction until that child is born, for women the
pregnancy is embodied, part of them.

THE BODY IN MEDICAL TREATMENT

I don't like the word *infertility*. It's really negative. I
wish they would come up with something else. Because
it's like saying your body is bad, in some ways. We
discussed it in my Resolve group.

Diane, age forty-one

During the years I have studied infertility I have repeatedly heard women
react to the implication that their bodies are "bad." It is a common topic
in groups such as Diane's that focus on how to deal with infertility.
Ironically, women and men try to solve the problem of childlessness by
seeking medical treatment, but medical treatment reflects the same attitude they experience in daily life: that childlessness is abnormal. Indeed, it is within medical treatment, through the medical gaze, that these
cultural dialogues about the body have been greatly expanded.[16]

In *Presence in the Flesh*, Katharine Young captures the essence of the
problem of being a patient: from being embodied, "a locus of self, the
body is transformed into an object of scrutiny." Consequently, medical
treatment throws into question the bodily knowledge of both women
and men. The frequent visits to physicians that are almost inevitable in
infertility treatment further undermine that bodily knowledge. People
undergoing this experience sometimes find themselves subsuming their
own bodily knowledge to that of medical knowledge or trying to balance
the two.[17]

Erin, whom we met in chapter 2, describes how medical treatment
eventually overwhelmed her despite her efforts to maintain her perspective:

There aren't many props in the process, as least as I experience it.
There aren't many props that sort of help you get back on cue. Part of
it is just that it encourages this sort of hubris, that "We can make it
happen because we have all these drugs and shots and sonograms, and
you can track it and track it and analyze it and analyze it." You know
what? It doesn't make any difference in the end. But you get so
damned focused on the microscopic level of it that you want to. . . . I
don't have enough serenity of soul to stay in focus. I don't know any-
one who has maintained a good solid sense of themselves through the
whole thing. I really felt neutered by it.

I think Marty was really more aware of how upsetting it was. He
felt it was stressful when people would tell us when to make love, you
know, "Now is the time." He felt that was very violating in a way, in
a much stronger way than I did. For him, that was real intrusive and
violating, to a degree. But he also was just more aware of how it was
darkening my image of myself, or how my view of myself was being
affected. Saying to me, "You know, this doesn't seem to be good for
you." And then I got into therapy, and the therapist said, "You're do-
ing something to yourself that I would never do to myself." And say-
ing that she had a good many female patients who were there, at least
in part, because of the side-effects of fertility therapy.

Erin concluded, "I felt disabled and dysfunctional in a way that was
much more profound than I do now—as a woman, or as a feminist, or
as a human being, and focusing on just one set of organs. The process
is just really cold."

Although Erin is a powerful and dynamic woman in her workday
life, she felt reduced by medical treatment: "disabled, dysfunctional,
neutered." She describes how globally the process affected her—"as a
woman, a feminist, and a human being." But it was only when she went
into therapy that she was able to begin regaining her perspective and to
understand how she had allowed infertility treatment to take over her
body and her sense of self. After this initial response of feeling diminished by medical treatment, Erin became assertive, even aggressive, in
her pursuit of information. Ultimately, she took control of her medical
treatment. She contacted numerous physicians without allowing herself
to be put in the submissive patient role, and she rejected the theories
physicians proposed about her age. Not only did she resist being a patient, she resisted group participation in Resolve because she rejected
the label of infertile.

Erin's perspective is fairly typical of the approach women and men in this study took toward infertility treatment. Driven by cultural ideologies about the importance of children and family, women and men initially entered medical treatment as a practical means to an end. Dismayed by the invasiveness of medical treatment, they gradually came to discover and wield their own power and to resist, in various ways, specific aspects of the medical approach.

Once a woman thinks a problem might exist, she usually seeks medical treatment for herself and her partner. By this point, almost every woman assumes something is wrong with her. At the same time, however, women expect that medical treatment offers the solution and that they will quickly become pregnant once treatment begins.[18]

As people become immersed in the effort to comply with medical treatment, daily life is reoriented around the timing of the reproductive cycle. This effort begins to contaminate the intimate aspects of the relationship. Activities already laden with meaning, such as sexual intercourse, acquire another layer of meaning pertaining to illness, stigma, and failure. Some biomedical tests may intrude into a couple's sexual relationship. For example, the postcoital test, in which a physician removes a sample of mucus from the woman's cervix, is performed within twelve hours of intercourse. The need for sex on cue in infertility treatment adds stress to the sexual relationship.[19]

Michelle, aged thirty-eight, describes how her and her husband's sex life changed:

When we finally decided it was time to make babies, I just thought that it was the best sex in the world. I just thought that it is just more intimate, you throw away all the barriers, there was something about it that was just extra loving and special to me. And you lie back and think that specially wonderful child was going to come out of it. And when it became apparent that there were problems and the first interventions are things like postcoital tests and timing intercourse, I remember going to the doctor with . . . just writing down the days within a week that we had had sex and I had to remember back to some of this stuff, like abstain for two days and then have sex, and you would think, "Okay, I am going to be fertile here, but we can't make love these two days, but you have to make love to me this day."

The idea that sex was something that he is doing for me, I mean, it was just like, "Hey, do me a hell of a favor." And yet he was doing me a favor, and it really put things off kilter. It gets so intrusive when you are having sex in the morning and then running to the doctor for him to examine things, it almost felt like you had been raped and you have to go to the doctor for evidence. It is just brutally invasive. And I remember feeling when I didn't get an adequate number of sperm I was wondering, "Well, maybe if Mitch was more excited, and neither one of us had a really great time before we went to the doctor knowing that we were having sex for medical reasons and for the doctor." Maybe that is part of the failing.

And then you get labeled with "hostile" mucus.[20] That's just the tip of the iceberg. Your sex life is intruded on another time. What happened with us, it was just taken away—the whole process was taken away. I felt horrible about it. We weren't even going to have sex to make a baby anymore. Mitch was going to do his thing into a cup and he had trouble with it, the first time, he is very nearsighted, and it was really uncomfortable for him. It was completely detached from what we were doing. You go the doctor and he inseminates you, and he says, "I hope we got you pregnant this time," and it is like you and the doctor are doing this thing, not your husband. My little brother asked me something about what it was like. And I said, "It is like a guy knocks you up and he doesn't even give you flowers."

Michelle's experience epitomizes that of many couples in this research: sex becomes a clinical process from which the husband is absent. Bodily distress engulfs her, robbing her of feelings of emotional intimacy associated with sex and negatively affecting the relationship. Feeling "raped" and "labeled," Michelle seizes on the crux of the problem: the artificial regulation of sex makes a charade out of a process that is culturally viewed as intrinsic to parenthood and a core part of marriage.[21]

When these initial efforts to conceive with a physician's assistance did not work, Michelle went to a specialist. She describes her experience:

The specialist started finding things wrong with me. This is another bottoming out. I thought, "I can't handle anything being wrong with me." I mean, I'd already lost a tube [in an ectopic pregnancy]. If there's going to be stuff wrong and I'm going to have problems, I almost wanted them to say, "You can't have babies," and take everything away from me. I didn't want to be slowly picked apart. This is wrong, that is wrong. Slowly finding out. And this was what was happening. I couldn't pass any tests. I had hormonal problems. My tube was gone so my ovaries didn't function. My tube didn't function. It turns out my uterus is malformed. I didn't pass my hysterosalpingo-

gram. Oh, I also had a blood test after this miscarriage and that showed some problems.

I didn't take it well. I felt like my body had betrayed me. Finally, the [exploratory] operation showed that my mother had taken DES [see glossary], and I showed very definite signs of this. It was really an unhappy and desperate time for me.

Michelle describes how she progressed from viewing herself as a woman whose body was intact to seeing herself as a collection of bodily problems. She echoes a common theme in the study when she says that she felt betrayed by her body. Few of the women we spoke to had ever had any indication that in attempting to conceive they would encounter such invisible flaws.

Women not only experienced bodily distress when clinical problems were identified; they also experienced a profound sense of loss when body parts were removed in the course of medical treatment. Sarah, forty years old, reflects on her sense of loss some years after her fallopian tubes were surgically removed because they were so damaged:

Even if I'm not thinking about it, I'm conscious that I don't have fallopian tubes and that continues to be a loss, it really does. It doesn't matter that I never got pregnant—never achieved a pregnancy utilizing my tubes. It doesn't matter. They are a body part and a female body part. It's devastating to not have them. The only plus is that I can go into an IVF cycle and with all certainty know that I will not have an ectopic, that's the only plus. In the end, you know, you still feel mutilated in a way and not whole. That's the best way of putting it, not whole.

The sense of loss that Sarah voices attests to the importance of the body's organs to a sense of wholeness. They are embodied, not invisible, to the person in the body.

Marie, a thirty-year-old woman, who agreed to exploratory surgery as a means of diagnosing her infertility, was profoundly affected when an ovary was removed in the course of surgery. She describes an invasive process that took her completely by surprise:

I go in to sign the consent forms. My husband went with me because I knew I wouldn't remember half of what the doctor was telling me. I was really panicked and scared. At the bottom of the consent form there is a line, something about, "You might have to have your ovary removed." It is about one of twenty things. It scared me. I cried in the doctor's office and was incredibly reluctant to get the pre-op. I worried about the worst. But I did all the pre-op stuff.

And the next day they went in and found endometriosis [see glossary] inside that totally encompassed the left ovary, which was interesting, because it was the right ovary that was overstimulated and giving me pain. So they took out the left ovary. They took it out! I had signed that form. I woke up in the recovery room feeling this incredible pain and not knowing what happened. I asked the nurse what happened, "What did they do?" She said, "They took out your left ovary." This was in the recovery room. I panicked because to me . . . I thought they took out the wrong one. There were no explanations in there.

I was pretty drugged up and foggy and incredibly surprised. I felt numb, I guess. I stayed in the hospital a couple of days. I was really sad. It was very, very scary. Because you only have one left, you know? And my luck with that one has never been great.

Women often feel they may be at fault if they fail to go through with the medical care that is offered to them. They may anticipate the worst but proceed, as Marie did, because they see action as their duty. Marie describes the aftermath of her surgery:

I had to stay home for six weeks, probably for the first time in my life. So I'm sitting there feeling really depressed. I'm an active person. The way I get through things is to do stuff, not to sit around. But after abdominal surgery you don't have a choice. I would sit at home and watch TV and there would be a Pampers commercial. I would cry and cry. It was terrible.

I got my records and read the operation notes and questions. I was so sad about losing this body part. What did they do with my ovary? There is a part of me out there. What did they do with it? Did they burn it? Bury it? I'm just very sad about that.

Now I have issues about sexuality and identity. I'm not like the rest of the women in the world anymore. I have half of an ovary, and it's not functioning, and I'm not able to reproduce.

Ovaries are laden with cultural meanings, signifying fertility, motherhood, and nurturance. For Marie, the loss of an ovary has destroyed her knowledge of herself as a woman and everything that designation entails. Marie is mourning the loss of a body part that has always been invisible but known, as part of her. The loss of this missing piece alters her bodily knowledge, encroaching on her feelings of sexuality and her identity as a woman. She laments the incapacitated ovary that remains: it is disabled. Moreover, she is angry: someone took this symbol of her womanhood when she was defenseless, unable to protest, and discarded it. The ovary, disembodied, becomes a symbol of everything she has lost and calls attention to her sense of difference from other women.

THE VULNERABLE PATIENT

These statements are not only about the sense of depersonalization people experience during infertility treatment; they are also about loss of control over the body. This is a perennial issue in infertility treatment. As people move towards more complex technologies in an effort to conceive, issues of control intensify.[22] When people feel that they are ceding control over their bodies to biomedicine, cultural dialogues about personal autonomy and control vie with cultural dialogues about reproduction and gender and biomedical notions about cure. In this complex situation, women and men may initially appear to capitulate to the biomedical process, submitting themselves repeatedly to medical procedures about which they feel ambivalent. But despite the conflict they continue to experience, they learn to exert agency over the process, beginning with the body.

Sarah addresses underlying issues of control and vulnerability that accompany medical treatment: "It takes the control away from a woman. That feeling of vulnerability, that feeling of being on your back and sort of pinned down with your legs up—it's incredible, it's incredible that more women don't leap off of the table with fright." When Sarah asks why women submit to being put in such a helpless position, she provides a view of a part of medical treatment that is usually taken for granted by both patients and practitioners.[23]

It is not only women who feel their bodies to be vulnerable and intruded on. Men report their responses to medical encounters with the same intensity. Richard, forty-three years old, observes:

It was such an awful experience having to go into a public bathroom in a medical building and produce a sample. I mean, there is somebody in the stall next door. Then another time, they sent me to another place that was supposed to be set up better: I walked into this room and it was like, I was just waiting for the manhood to come out. I mean, I am in this room. There are no windows. There are maga-

zines everywhere. From the most tame to the most vulgar. There are lubricants to beat the band. Lubricants to beat . . . I mean, they had a multitude of choices, and all you have to do is create a sample, knock on this little window, a hand comes out and takes the sample. Literally, that's what happened.

Richard finds it depersonalizing and invasive to be expected to masturbate and produce a sperm sample under these conditions. The questionable privacy renders normal bodily functions subject to scrutiny and surveillance.[24] Underlying this concern is one question that arises any time a man has to give a sperm sample: whether the sperm in the ejaculate are normal. This determination calls into question what men see as the tangible product of their manhood.

Men are outsiders to reproductive health. Although between 40 and 50 percent of all infertility can be attributed at least in part to the male partner, there is little, if any, treatment for male infertility per se. Only recently have techniques been developed that can produce pregnancies with very few sperm, such as intracytoplasmic sperm injection (ICSI).[25] Such treatments not only are expensive but also involve invasive procedures that are carried out on women. As a result, men feel left out. Tony commented, "I was never part of the interviews or counseling. 'Hand over the vial,' that's as personal as it got."

When men learn they are infertile, almost invariably they are shocked.[26] Craig reports his reaction to finding out he was completely sterile:

That was a real shocker, but I wasn't as upset as I thought I'd be. You know, like people in Resolve, the men, you know, they want to carry on their line, and it has to be their kid, and they want to adopt, they want to do artificial insemination. . . . It seemed to me that some of them were pushing their wives a lot further than their wives wanted to be pushed. I didn't feel that. I don't feel that I have to carry on my line or that it had to be my kid or something like that. That part didn't get to me. It's just weird that you're like that. It's like, you didn't think you're like that your whole life and you are. So coming to that realization, that's really a shocker.

And right away a decision was presented to me for donor insemination, which I wasn't real crazy about at all. As much as it didn't have to be mine, I didn't want it to be somebody else's.

To Craig the diagnosis is the antithesis of the cultural ideal of manhood, and he is having great difficulty viewing himself in other terms. He tries to differentiate his reaction from that of other men who have the same diagnosis, but it is clear from his statement that he is just as conflicted about it as the other men to whom he refers.

Gus was more than shocked about his diagnosis initially: he did not believe it.

My first reaction was I didn't think that I was infertile. My reaction was, "Well, they probably made some kind of laboratory procedural error or something like that." I've worked around laboratories a little bit and I know that it's possible to screw up and blow the experiment. So I thought that's what happened. Then some more tests were done and they were normal. But then that final test was done, and it was very clear [that he was infertile].

Similarly, although Terry demonstrates some confusion in reporting the medical details of his infertility, he understands that the medical tests say he is, without question, infertile: "So I had a semen analysis and it came back with no sperm. And so they did another one and it was the same or 'less than 1 percent.' Which is less than a million per cc, effectively zero." His partner, Kelsie, interjected: "Which was pretty shocking." Terry went on: "Shock, disbelief, anger, feeling like I failed, something was wrong with me. And then very, very slowly I accepted it." Asked, "Do you feel like you've accepted it?" he said, "Not entirely. It's still painful. Kelsie's been very helpful, and we joined a Resolve support group." Terry describes a progression in his response, a gradual—but not yet complete—coming to terms with the unthinkable.

Some men are completely immobilized by the knowledge of their infertility, and some feel compelled to follow up with further tests and any treatments that are available. Prior to the introduction of ICSI, surgery was one option men considered.[27] While men are sometimes eager to find a solution that allows them to keep reproductive control in their body (and thereby avoid treatments such as donor insemination), they may have second thoughts as they face an operation. Kenny commented on his varicocele surgery: "I had surgery. I was scared to death. I had never had surgery before. If they hadn't put that Valium into my arm . . . I was thinking about how I could wrap that thing around my butt and get out of the hospital before they cut."

Sam, a thirty-five-year-old man who had been identified as infertile, also decided to go through surgery. He wanted to keep reproductive control in his body, and he also wanted to match his wife's efforts:

*Two weeks after the biopsy I went into surgery to correct this block-
age. He told us that there was a 20 percent chance of success. Optimistically, one out of five would achieve success—success being any
kind of sperm count. So he said it wasn't a high-yield thing. It was a
long shot. But we were certainly going to try it. I felt bad because I
was the source of the infertility. I was not at all concerned about
having the operations because the operations come and go. It was something I wanted to get through as soon as I could to find out whether
we could correct the problem. The biggest thing was the disappointment of not being able to have a family. And that far outweighed any
concern about the operation. I did the biopsy in early October and the
surgery two weeks later. I wanted to get it over with.*

*The second operation was tough. The biopsy was done on an out-
patient basis—in the morning and out in the afternoon. So I thought
it [surgery] would be in and out. The guy [physician] said, "Well, you
are going to feel a little discomfort, a little more this time. You will
probably be out [of the hospital] tomorrow—Saturday." Well, tomorrow I wasn't looking so good, so they made it Sunday. And I stayed
home for a week. I recovered pretty rapidly from it. I wasn't concerned about the procedures until after they occurred, especially the
second one. Which I used as a device constantly with my wife to remind her that I had gone the distance.*

Although Sam expected the surgery and its aftermath to be straightforward, they weren't:

*Six months after the operation I developed a case of acute prostatitis.
Which came on like getting hit by a bus. It was three to four hours
from feeling fine to going to the hospital. The prostate just totally
clamped down. I was in the hospital for four days. That was kind of
a bummer because that sort of set us back. That was my third episode
in the hospital in six months. It was very painful.*

*After I was in the hospital the third time I did a series of sperm
counts to find out what the damage was. Within a month or two
things pretty much recovered.*

Asked how he felt about his infertility, he said, "It's a disability. I feel
disabled by it."

Telling this entire story in a controlled, neutral voice, Sam describes
his task-oriented approach to the treatment. His demeanor and approach differ markedly from those of women, who invariably discussed

surgery and unexpected sequelae with emotion and distress. Sam seems very detached from the entire process until I ask him how he feels. Even though his sperm count is now close to the range considered normal, he views his infertility as a disability, thus underscoring the gulf between how men often present their infertility problems and how they actually feel about them. Masking emotions in this way may be an expression of profound bodily distress for men, who must also try to meet the cultural expectations for manhood of being controlled and impassive.

Cultural ideologies about womanhood and manhood shape the bodily distress that infertility provokes in gender-specific ways. Both men and women react negatively to the implication that their bodies are "bad," but their responses are dictated by specific cultural ideals about womanhood and manhood. Their words and images reflect these gendered associations. Subsequent chapters show how women and men take action, wrestling with and often reworking these gendered ideals to find solutions that enable them to go on with their lives.

CHAPTER 4

Genes and Generations

We had this unfortunate thing happen to us. We're not able
to create a family. We're not able to fulfill the second half, or
the third part, of the American dream. It just seems terribly
un-American.   *Tanya, thirty-five years old*

When my sister was alive, my brother-in-law had a vasec-
tomy. And they chose not to have any children. Not an easy
decision. My husband's brother is disabled and very unlikely
to ever marry or have children. Those are the only kids. This
is it. We are it. And so there's this "generations" concern.
You're not only *not* producing another child, but you are the
only one who could possibly produce a grandchild. And you
also feel like there is some terrible sense of not going into the
future. Just this lack of regeneration and new life. A feeling
of going on into your old age and a kind of longing for that
[regeneration of self]. I also think you feel totally isolated. It's
ironic. Everyone's out there: "Family family family!" I think
you have this terrible sense of isolation and loss.
                                          Alicia, forty-three years old

The discovery of infertility leads women and men to question a lifetime
of assumptions about how the world is ordered. Beliefs about biology,
reproductive potential, gender roles, definitions of family and kin, the
meaning of being a person, explanations of how the world works—all
are torn down. Tanya goes to the heart of the matter when she bemoans
the loss of the "American dream." Having children is taken for granted
by most people in the United States, but Tanya and her husband don't
fit in. Her articulation of an "outsider" experience reflects how troubling
unwanted childlessness can be: it creates a profound sense of disorder
in Tanya's life. When women and men engage with new reproductive
technologies in an effort to conceive, they do so in an effort to reestablish

order in their lives, to reclaim their right to be American and to everything that identity signifies.

Although Tanya is African American, in using the metaphor of the American dream she is reaching beyond her specific ethnic group to encompass shared understandings in American culture about the meaning of family. Tanya's generation is the first to have been systematically exposed to television's symbols of mythical American dream families, as in *Ozzie and Harriet* and *The Cosby Show*. In contemporary political life, the slogan *family values* has become not only media shorthand for dominant cultural ideologies but also a political tool. Dialogues about family values in American politics are laden with moral authority: those who are not viewed as upholding family values are looked down on and may even be viewed as "un-American." Being childless does not fit these cultural ideals of family, and consequently, women and men feel the weight of moralizing dialogues about normalcy.[1] Like Tanya, Alicia comments on feeling isolated from others by childlessness. She raises an additional concern, as well, about "the lack of regeneration and new life," which disrupts expectations about the flow of generations.

Values are the ground on which cultural dialogues develop. They give unifying meaning to people's lives and are a primary means through which individuals interpret and explain reality.[2] Through values people are able to make connections between the mundane events of everyday life and broader social, historical, political, and economic arenas. People in chaos cling to values as a means of ordering and making sense out of their experiences. Values may be linked to memories of significant life experiences to form an individual belief system, to life experiences and goals for action, or to the ways in which dominant social ideologies are connected to experience: for example, people may cite their values and life experiences in support of a specific ideology.[3] Values are integral to culturally specific guidance for individual action and are the basis for commonsense ideas about the world. Indeed, values lead to the creation and perpetuation of ideologies, which often encompass and synthesize several related values.[4]

It is necessary to understand the force of values in a society to understand both the paralyzing grip that infertility can have on people and the effect of reproductive technologies on society. This is a complex task, however, because U.S. society is remarkably heterogeneous, encompassing multiple ethnic groups, religions, age groups, sexual orientations, social classes, and political persuasions. Discussions of values may seem to have a leveling effect, assuming that everyone subscribes to the same ones. This is far from the case. However, there are dominant cultural ideologies with which people must contend whether they subscribe to them or not. These have roots in Western thought, religion, and historical practices.[5]

I have discussed disruption and the expectation of continuity in life at length elsewhere.[6] The tendency in the United States to focus on continuity in life rather than on disruption can be seen as a cultural ideology that informs people's efforts to ameliorate infertility: these are attempts to restore order to their lives.[7] People have clear ideas about what constitutes order in a wide variety of contexts, and they create order in culturally specific ways. The tendency to view life as a predictable, continuous flow heightens people's sense of disruption when something unexpected occurs.[8]

Many people's lives are anchored by a belief in a cosmic order.[9] Narratives about origins describe the order of things and the relationship between things and different kinds of people; origin stories thus have a sacred quality. The discovery of infertility challenges people's identities because it strikes at the origin stories in which they believe. Such assaults on fundamental beliefs may contribute to an erosion of faith in explanatory schemes, to renewed efforts to shore up those perspectives, or to both.[10] Women and men facing infertility are bewildered by the threat to their gender identity and to their explanations of how the world works, but they usually renew their efforts to have children, taking action for themselves individually as well as sometimes joining a self-help group.

Expectations about continuity permeate responses to disruption as well as efforts to create continuity after the disruption. A particular cultural view of order enables people to believe that it will eventually be regained. Steven, forty-two-years old, compares his previously orderly life with the incongruity of having a problem such as infertility:

I think of myself as a "good person." It [infertility] goes against the way I've interpreted life so far. In a way it's been easy for me to interpret life so far because I've led a—I don't want to say a charmed life—but I've gotten off pretty okay. Haven't had physical problems, never been sick, very loving parents, of means, you know, middle-class, done well in school, gotten by, had good jobs, all that stuff. I don't want to say that I haven't struggled, because I always worked hard to

*get what I want, but I haven't had troubles with a capital T. So this is
for me a profound period of deep struggle.*

*I'm not sure how it fits into my life, which is new to me. I'm sus-
pecting it's one of those things that's so intensely difficult it will help
me build character. Because by and large, although I've worked for
what I wanted and received, I haven't had things taken from me. I
haven't not been able to get what I want. This is the first time that I
haven't been able to get what I want and may not be able to get what
I want. It feels like a story that hasn't played itself out yet, and I don't
like being this far away from knowing the outcome.*

Steven's sense of coherence has been disturbed because this event does
not fit the context of his life—"a charmed life"—and his sense of who
he is, "a good person." Steven is Jewish, but his invocation of an element
of the so-called Protestant ethic, hard work, to explain his past success
illustrates how dominant ideologies in the United States that were formerly attributed to religion are instead class-based (Steven identifies with
the middle class).[11] Steven's new uncertainty about the future is playing
havoc with his sense of coherence. In trying to explain this disruption,
Steven uses the rationale that misfortune will help him to build character, a perspective that is embedded in the U.S. cultural ideology of self-
determination.[12] Unable to make sense of his dilemma through traditional explanatory systems of understanding, Steven identifies this
period of his life as one of "deep struggle."

The engagement with new reproductive technologies, a decision replete with physical and emotional challenges, can be seen as an expression of the cultural ethos of perseverance.[13] Fighting disorder by pursuing difficult infertility treatment is a culturally sanctioned way to
overcome the problem. Turning disorder back into order is a central
theme of people's efforts to "undo" infertility. In this chapter I explore
cultural ideas about natural order, biology, genes, and kinship and examine some of the associated dialogues that emerge when expectations
about fertility are disordered.

REPRODUCTION AS NATURAL ORDER

The families I am concerned with in this book are heterosexual couples
who intend to have children, a model that continues to dominate cultural dialogues on the family in the United States and that represents

the cultural norm. As Jane Collier and Sylvia Yanagisako observe, the U.S. folk model of reproduction contains the underlying "assumption that 'male' and 'female' are two natural categories of human beings whose relationships are everywhere structured by their biological difference."[14] Biologically driven kinship continues to dominate the view of families in the United States despite anthropological analyses that demonstrate that kinship is a symbolic system, not a natural system.[15] Kinship with others is based either on blood ties or on marital ties. Of the two, blood ties are seen as more binding. Yet the idea of what constitutes a family has recently undergone major expansion, as increased numbers of families are headed by gay couples, single parents, and grandparents and other relatives.[16] And families are no longer defined simply by the presence of children. Large numbers of childless couples have led to increased recognition that families come in many forms.

Meanings of male and female reflect culturally imposed differences that have their basis in the structures of a society. They are not simply "natural" differences. But American views of reproduction are so focused on biology that many people find other ways of seeing reproduction implausible.[17] This makes it very difficult for people who are unsuccessful in conceiving. Other cultures regard reproduction differently, for example as a cultural achievement rather than a biological process. Annette Weiner, in studying Trobriand Islanders, concluded that biological reproduction was sufficient to produce a biological human being but not a Trobriander. Among Trobrianders, reproduction brings together social, cosmological (religious), material, and physical dimensions of culture to create a child's cultural identity, the most significant component of which is kinship—the person's relationship to ancestors, parents, siblings, and extended kin.[18]

This biological focus in the United States is misplaced. When we hear what people think is really important about having a child, it is not biology but having a child who is emotionally connected with the family, who develops a strong identity, and who is integrated into his or her community—indeed, the very qualities that make up a Trobriander! New reproductive technologies reinforce the cultural ideology of biological parenthood, diverting people from their primary goal to become parents and greatly lengthening the process.

Assisted reproductive technologies provide an endless array of medical treatments designed to produce a biological child. But these technologies have also introduced treatments that result in children being born who may not be biologically linked to their parents, such as technologies using donor gametes. The use of these technologies is sometimes kept confidential so that only the parents know if one or both parents are not the biological, or biogenetic, parents. Such practices perpetuate the dominance of the biological model.

Women and men in this study expressed the need to persevere with infertility treatment because they felt entitled to fulfill the norm of biological parenthood. People place the struggle to conceive within Western conceptions of culture and biology, as Jana, a seven-time IVF user, attests. She epitomizes attitudes expressed by study participants: "The need to reproduce is probably next after survival. It's even wrapped up in survival, I'm sure. Are people entitled to be treated for infertility when children are starving? Everybody is entitled to have their needs met. We can do without bombers and stuff like that. Those resources should be reallocated, not infertile people's money, or the chance to have children." Jana paints a dramatic picture of entitlement on moral grounds and juxtaposes bombers against it, which she considers to be wasteful of life and superfluous. Underlying these images is a belief in "natural" order, that goodness will prevail over evil. Jana's comment about the need to reproduce illustrates the cultural belief in the primacy of biology in parenthood. Her comment also attests to the moral authority of her position. It is one indication of the power of the cultural ideology of biological parenthood that so permeates people's approach to parenthood.

This dominant cultural model of biological reproduction is based on the Western theory of natural order. Media portrayals of natural order abound, especially in science programs about biological phenomena among different species. Such programs powerfully reinforce cultural beliefs.[19] Jo Ann, a forty-five-year-old woman who had finally abandoned efforts to conceive, discussed how one of these programs affected her: "This TV program I watched made a point of saying that the end point of all biological systems is reproduction, and that in many species the adults die but biology doesn't care what happens to parents after the point of conception, that the force of life is about reproducing." The idea that the purpose of life is reproduction suggests to those who are unable to have a biological child that they are superfluous. Jo Ann's husband, Brad, interjected, "Biologically, you're reduced because you're infertile." Jo Ann went on, "That's right, so you don't realize the throwback. This gets back to the purpose of life. So in the universe you just have to make more of yourself. And you're lucky if you have different dimensions."

Jo Ann had been addressing these very issues for the past several years. Each time I interviewed her she had questioned her purpose in life and her efforts to make more of herself to make up for not having children. Brad's remark underscores this sentiment.

Jo Ann and Brad take this biological generalization from a TV program and personalize it, underscoring the pervasiveness of such messages about the primacy of biology. They are forced to ponder deep philosophical issues about themselves in relation to the world, as Brad does:

I've been going back to that experience at the infertility workshop we told you about. There's a spiritual omen to that: what is the meaning of life? What are we doing here? Are we just animals that are reproducing our DNA? Or are there other things that are as important, if not maybe more important, in life? These are multifaceted and complex questions, and most people never get past it. . . . A lot of people don't get past being intelligent animals. It's sort of sad to see. I saw three men who doubted their masculinity because they were not able to father their child. I've never been in a group of men where there's been more raw emotion expressed than in that workshop. Men are usually reserved and reasonable and stuff, but I saw more pain openly demonstrated, talked about, and more tears in that experience with men than in any other experience I've ever had with other men. A man thinks that because his sperm doesn't have active flagella that he's not a human being? Not a man? Incredible! Others think he must not have a soul? He must not think he has any meaning beyond that. That's pretty sad.

This discussion illustrates how science-based models alter explanations and meanings of things. Brad suggests that the acceptance of science models has confused how people think about natural order and about themselves. He then unwittingly demonstrates this mixture of models. He questions the science metaphor of people as animals, yet he then applies the metaphor to his fellow workshop participants. He pits the science model against the meaning of life and suggests there is a "spiritual omen" about biological reductionism. He also addresses the assault of components of the science model (sperm with active flagella) on men's sense of masculinity, and ultimately, on their humanness. In doing so, he demonstrates that cultural notions of order in the universe are implicit.

In a discussion with Hank, a forty-year-old man, and his wife about the possibility that they might either use a donated egg or adopt, Hank raised the notion of natural selection and related issues about biological lineage:

Trained as an evolutionary biologist, I feel like I wouldn't date just anyone. You know, I dated women that I really liked, and respected, and admired. But I wouldn't want to just throw my sperm in with any old egg, either. I believe in not just selection and people, but animals, plants, all choosing their mates, and so picking an anonymous mate sort of goes against this long-term scholastic training. And more than that, it's a personal philosophy. It's really how I think. So it's part of the reason why I have trouble with adoption. It's this same sort of issue. You know, I want that lineage.

Although he attributes his ideas about natural selection to scholastic training, Hank also acknowledges them as a "personal philosophy." Natural selection is part of his explanation of how the world works. His desire for "lineage" and everything it signifies is related to this belief. This stance upholds a patriarchal perspective on reproduction, although that is not Hank's intent. His stance does not augur well for the couple's becoming parents. He acknowledges that he and his wife are approaching the problem from different perspectives:

But we're at a different place here because I'm not having the fertility problem right now. I'm approaching it and probably feeling about it differently. . . . I have different issues than she does, who is facing her own infertility. And I think that colors it a bit, how we look at this, and the way we approach it. It really does shade how you approach it. As far as we know, I'm fertile right now and I have an infinite number of possibilities ahead of me, whereas she doesn't. So that's one thing. The other thing that we talked about is that we came to the recognition that everything we've done up to this point has been really easy. That has been the stuff that we always wanted, which was her egg, my sperm.

For Hank the early stages of medical treatment for infertility have been "easy" because they involved the couple's own biological material. Egg and sperm are cultural icons that signify manhood and womanhood.[20] Joining them together signifies the conjunction of cultural ideals. In the face of declining hopes of having a biological child, Hank clings to these ideals because they represent more than the "facts of life"— they represent culture as he knows it, a way of life. What remains unspoken in Hank's comments is whether he would prefer to stand by these cultural ideals, and forgo parenthood altogether than to raise a child he might not view as truly "his."

EMBODIED GENES

Biological determinism in the United States has expressed itself in a wide range of contexts. It has been the basis of justifications for racist views, rationales for intelligence testing, and arguments against adoption.[21] In particular, these ideas have been represented in eugenics movements. The emphasis on "parental worthiness" at the beginning of the twentieth century led to a campaign for mandatory sterilization of those who were thought to be unfit. Views of African Americans and other people of color as inferior fueled this movement through much of the century.[22]

Dorothy Nelkin and Susan Lindee observe that biological determinism is now being embraced in a new form, genetic essentialism, which "reduces the self to a molecular entity, equating human beings, in all their social, historical, and moral complexity, with their genes."[23] Tracing the history of this trend through the eugenics movement of the early twentieth century, to a reaction against eugenics because of the rise of Hitler in Germany in the mid-1930s, to a subsequent shift to the primacy of "nurture" in the nature-nurture debate, they now see a new development: a swing back to an emphasis on "nature" through the "molecular family." They note that the idea of the molecular family is based on the cultural expectation that a biological entity can determine emotional connections and social bonds—that genetics can link people to each other and preserve a reliable model for a family.[24] The effects of these social and historical shifts on families and on people who contemplate starting a family have been complex.

In this study women and men expressed a wide range of opinions about the importance of genes, and those opinions could often be directly related to the extent of their experience with infertility. That is, opinions changed over time as many eventually relinquished the goal of biological parenthood. Even early in their efforts to conceive, some people felt genes were unimportant and were eloquent about the importance of social parenthood. The majority, however, initially felt that biological parenthood *was* important. Everyone in the study agreed that cultural ideas about biological parenthood had to be reckoned with, regardless of an individual's own beliefs, because of the attitudes that their children would confront. David, thirty-seven years old, comments:

There are milestones [in life]. I mean, marriage was a milestone, being in the Army, university, traveling. Different things were milestones. But there is no kind of societal milestone, like, you know, you're finally grown up. Someone gives you this certificate. But I think I've had a sense somehow that when I will be a father I will have a sense of that connection, that kind of lineage through the generations. Coming from my father, my grandfather, my mother, her side of the family kind of coming through me. And the sense of "Well, now I'm the parent." And I'm responsible, rather than this kind of, uh, it's almost this kind of limbo thing that I'm not . . . I'm no longer a child. That is very obvious to me, and, at the same time, there's something tangible that's missing. I don't know if it's a manifestation through a child. But that's part of it.

It's part of an adopted responsibility. It's one of the expectations, a mark of an adult, of someone who works, someone who is married, raises a family.

David voices several cultural expectations about family creation and parenting that are widely shared among people experiencing infertility: first, the idea that a series of milestones lead up to parenthood; second, the feeling of limbo when parenthood does not occur, and David feels that he is neither a child any longer nor yet a full-fledged adult;[25] and third, the loss of generational continuity, of passing on traditions from one's forebears to the next generation. David's feeling that something tangible is missing, the manifestation of these experiences through a child, was expressed in one way or another by everyone in this study. His conclusion that parenting is an "adopted" responsibility underscores the essence of his statement: parenthood, along with other cultural expectations, gives definition to adulthood.

At the end of his interview, an hour later, David is asked if infertility affects his sense of purpose in life. He returns to the same themes:

I have this feeling that when I become a parent things will fall into place. I have this desire to connect with others in community, and that comes from a place that would normally go to a child, if a child were there. It's not like I don't have a purpose. But I'm really aware of not feeling . . . I grew up feeling unconnected to my father but I somehow feel that by having a child I will somehow feel more grounded and somehow feel that lineage that came through my great-grandfather, my grandfather, my father, kind of through me, and goes on through

*the child. And somehow now I'm on the end of this sword. Like a
fencing sword, so it's like I'm on the tip of it and it's kind of moving
around, and I'm kind of moving around. I'm in this kind of limbo
space. And there's nothing forcing the end of the sword to stand still.
And if I had a child I guess I would feel like that would stabilize. But
it's not like I walk around saying, "Woe is me, I don't have a purpose
in life because I don't have a child."*

David again expresses his sense of limbo and a desire to feel "grounded."
His image of a wavering sword is a powerful metaphor for limbo. He
juxtaposes this image with a desire for stability, which he equates with
community and assumes that a child would provide.

David then returns to comments about generations and lineage, questioning himself in the process:

*I notice every time I say it, the linkage of the generations, that I say
my father and his father and my dad, and maybe I'm making an assumption that I'm going to have a male child. But I don't know if it's
as a man or as a human being. I mean, it's hard for me to differentiate
between the two. I've never been a locker room kind of guy. I can't
say that there's any kind of thing that goes into that that makes it difficult. But out in society, and oh, just being at a point where I would
like to be a father, I think.*

*I have felt a sense of jealousy around men that I know that have
kids. There's a bond there that I don't have, you know. I know that I
don't belong to that club. So I feel like, as a man, maybe on that level
I'm left out of something.*

Although David is unsure about what he thinks specifically about a male
child, it is clear that parenting has a definite set of cultural meanings in
connecting him to other men—both to his father and the male line in
his family and to other men his own age. When he reports feeling jealous
and left out, he echoes another dominant theme among women and men
who are dealing with infertility.

Angela, whom we first met in chapter 2, expresses this theme from a
woman's perspective:

*I think that another issue that has come up for me since the miscar-
riage, the fact that I'm a woman in his [husband's] family and I'm not
productive, and he's a male, and "What if no one can carry on the
line?" You know, the lineage and the name that goes with it. His sister-*

in-law's baby, it was another girl, so now there's two girls in the family.

And my cousins — all younger than me, having babies. Young eggs. I'm thinking, "Am I old?" Then I start thinking, "How do the aunts see me?" I still can't get pregnant, and I had a miscarriage, and I think about it in the back of my mind. Like, "So how do I fit in with the whole scheme of things? Do I belong?" And I didn't realize how powerful my aunts and uncles were when I was growing up, because we had that kind of tight-knit family where you see them every Sunday and everyone looked out for one another. So their opinions of me have a lasting effect, and it reinforces my feeling that I'm different in the family. I have to disregard their perceptions of me.

Angela raises the same concerns as David did about lineage and the family line, and particularly about continuing the male line. David himself acknowledges that his thoughts keep returning to his *male* forebears. He never mentions carrying on his wife's line: his concerns relate solely to his own family. And although Angela uses the women in her own family as the measure of her gender performance, it is carrying on her husband's line that concerns her. Patriarchal imperatives underlie both women's and men's efforts to conceive a biological child. While David's feelings of being an outsider are based on comparisons to other men, Angela raises the same questions with respect to other women. Dialogues about gender and dialogues about kinship are inextricably connected.

Ashley and Scott, a couple in their late thirties, are also thrashing out these issues as they continue trying to conceive. They agree on only some of them. They have different ideas about the importance of biology. Although Ashley maintains that biology is not important to her, she contradicts herself:

I am not the kind of person that really romanticizes pregnancy. With my surgical history and my age, I already know that it will be a C-section. My doctor has told me. But I don't romanticize the physical discomfort. In our support group we have met women where carrying the baby is so important to them and going through the birth process. And for me, I want to be a parent, that is what excites me, so I can give that up, the pregnancy part, easily. The genetic part, I actually can give that up too, in a way, because first of all, I don't think that I have such great genes, and I think when I fantasize of a child, I don't think of a little Ashley. I think of a little Scott, and I kind of fantasize all of his great qualities and I hope it has red hair and I hope that it is good in math, and I hope that it has this easy-going disposition, so I kind of imagine a little Scott.

I don't really want it to have my qualities, I want it to have his qualities. Probably because with this infertility thing, my self-esteem has just plummeted, and I have lost touch with what I even like about myself. So I feel like if it takes after me, it will be compulsive and anxious, and terrible in math, and I guess I really don't want to reproduce myself. But I would like to reproduce him; so that does seem like a lot [to wish for]. But when I am being really realistic about it, I know you usually don't get what you want, anyway. It is a roll of the dice that I would have just as good a chance [of] reproducing the worst qualities in me or the worst qualities in him. You can't cherry-pick for quality.

As she tries to enumerate what is important to her, it emerges that the biological connection is important to Ashley, but it is her husband's genes she is concerned with, not hers. But Ashley, like many other women in this study who were unsuccessful in becoming pregnant, mourned the loss of being able to see her partner in a child, thus asserting the connection between patriarchy and biology. This tendency could be viewed as a desire simply to reproduce the partner. Men in this study, however, did not make the same comment. Men who were considering donor insemination hoped that the child would at least look like one of them or stated a wish for the wife to experience a pregnancy, but they did not talk about the wish to see specific physical features of the partner reproduced. Maintaining the biological lineage through a child that is not only biologically related but that visibly resembles the father may reinforce patriarchy.

When Ashley likens the genetic makeup of a child to a dice game, she uses a gambling metaphor that arose repeatedly in this study. A second metaphor, about "cherry-picking" the qualities of a child, reinforces her feelings about gambling and her anxieties about not being able to control the process. These metaphors help Ashley to deal with the uncertainty she experiences and also are part of a shift in her attitudes about the importance of genetics, in which she is coming to see nonbiological parenthood as equally valid.

The negative feelings that Ashley expresses about herself and her own genes were common among women. The effects of repeated medical treatment and the necessity of a cesarean section also contribute to her portrayal of herself and her body as defective. Cultural ideologies about womanhood and the capacity for motherhood profoundly affect women's gender identity.

As Ashley talks, she continues to register ambivalence about giving up the idea of a biological child:

So I think that whole genetic thing is really a bunch of crap. You get what you get, and in terms of the bonding, I have known friends where it was their own child and they had trouble bonding with it. And so I think that instant bonding is a myth. And I think that if you want to be a parent and you have longed for a child the way adoptive parents have, I think that maybe you even have a greater chance, if not as good a chance, of bonding with just a concept. So I don't worry about the bonding. I can give up the genes easily. I worry so about the child being accepted into the family in terms of the grand-parents. You know, not having that link of heritage. Of feeling this is our little line carrying on. So that seems like a little bit of a rough spot, but it feels far enough away that I am not too worried about it now.

But I do think about how when you have your own children, and everybody is always saying, "Oh, that expression is just like your grandfather's, or just like your mother's." That in some way that is very enjoyable and quaint and bonding with the whole family, but in some ways I think it is not the best thing for children because it gets turned around, too. We have all grown up with the parents saying, "You have a temper just like your father," so I think that even though it can be played out in a positive way, it can also be played out in a negative way and maybe more commonly is. In some ways not being able to do that because you know the child doesn't have your genes— in some ways I think it may be to their advantage that the child—I am sure you can still screw up your child in all the ways that you can screw up, but that is one particular way that we probably won't have open to us. Because the child will have to sort of stand on its own genetics, or something, on its own genes.

So I guess I am sort of . . . maybe because it is more an intellectual thing, I am intrigued by the possibilities and also the personal growth challenges and opportunities of not having our own genetic children. But I don't think that extends as far as taking in a special needs child or some of the classic issues. And, like Scott, I think that this is per-

*fectly legitimate, worrying about the health of the child. And the
health of the birth mother and all those sorts of very legitimate concerns. But all this sort of stuff with heritage and genes, I think that is
kind of . . . I don't know.*

Ashley firmly rejects the "myth" of instant bonding with a biological
child, thus voicing a widespread assumption that is insidiously reinforced in the child-rearing literature read by the general public. Many
women and men expressed fears that they would not be able to bond
with a child who was not biologically "theirs," whether that child was
adopted or was conceived with donor gametes. This concern was subsequently dismissed by everyone in our study who became parents of
nonbiological children.

Ashley sees adoption as "an intellectual" thing from which she would
benefit, a possibility for self-growth. This is an effective, middle-class
way of rationalizing not getting her first choice, a biological child, and
it enables her to begin considering adoption as an alternative.

At this point, Scott, who has been listening quietly, interjects his
views:

*I don't feel all the things that Ashley does, so I just want to get that
out. [To Ashley:] I thought what you said, you said very well, and a
lot of the things that you did say I agree with. [Turning to interviewer:]
Clearly whether I adopt a child or not, I am not going to go through,
personally, the pregnancy, but I will not have any opportunity of going through the pregnancy with Ashley. And that, to me, does mean
something to me. It will be a loss to me that I am going to have to
deal with. I said in our discussion group at Resolve a couple of weeks
ago, when I heard of my brother's first child being born, and the party
they had, how powerful it was for me. And again, this was the first
grandchild in our family, so that had special significance for my father
and mother. But the whole process of bringing the child into the
world was something. It was a journey. Not that there isn't a similar —
or different — kind of adoption journey that you go through, and depending on your relationship with your birth mother, you can be present at the birth and all these things. I am learning all these things, and
this excites me, too. But I am going to feel that loss if we don't do
that [conceive themselves].*

*Secondly, genes, heritage, it doesn't quite capture my feelings about
it. But, it is not like — I guess it is in some ways — the selfish feeling
that I want to have my genes and Ashley's genes regardless of how*

good they are. I think that is what it is. It is my gift. To me, it is one of the greatest gifts I can give to the world, is giving of myself through my genetics.

Scott's statement captures the cultural significance with which a birth is greeted, not only by the parents but by extended family members as well. Such experiences reinforce the cultural ideology of biological parenthood, which is symbolized by genes. Scott reaffirms his desire for his own and Ashley's genes, regardless of their quality. For Scott, his genes are embodied. He sees them as a way of sharing himself with the world, a form of community. This statement can be interpreted as a belief in his genetic superiority, or as communal feeling, or both these things.[26] However he intends it, Ashley takes issue with him:

ASHLEY: *I just think that is bullshit.*

SCOTT: *But the bullshit means something to me. I feel it. All right, discount it for you, but I am saying for me.*

ASHLEY: *I think that the greatest gift we can give is to bring up a child, and to me that is the gift.*

SCOTT: *To me that is the gift to the world. I agree with that, but there is something powerful. I can't explain it, but there is something very powerful.*

ASHLEY: *But it is just an accident, parenting.*

SCOTT: *You are being very rational. I am just telling you that is something powerful for me.*

ASHLEY: *I can't agree.*

SCOTT: *Well, maybe you can't. Okay. All I am saying is that is how I feel about it.*

ASHLEY: *Well, really, you should give to a sperm bank. I always thought, "Who would give to a sperm bank?" I guess maybe that is how they feel.*

SCOTT: *That doesn't mean much to me. What means a lot to me is the mutual creation of another person.*

To Scott, using his own genes to create a child has deeply rooted cultural meanings. Ashley, on the other hand, has detached herself from the cultural significance of parenting a biological child to focus on parenting without biology. Scott disagrees with Ashley's implication that this desire represents male egotism about the value of his genes.

Ashley, responding positively to his statement, continues the discussion, but in a more conciliatory vein:

I think the miracle of life, that is high. And that is what you heard at your brother's party. But that is what we hear from adoptive parents when they are witnessing the birth of their child because it is a miracle of life, and it is feeling some emotion attached to that miracle. It is not something that you are watching on TV. It is something that you have a relationship with.

So, I think that the feelings are as intensive, and I guess for pregnancy—given that I feel like every bad thing that could have happened has happened—getting pregnant is just the beginning of a whole bunch of more risks. That you have to make it to the three months, then at my age you know you have to make it, and hope that it doesn't have Down's and get through the birth, which would be harder. I would be forty years old. And I guess to me it just seems so perilous, and I probably would be anxious through the whole thing. Having a twenty-five-year-old carry the pregnancy seems a lot safer, even though, of course, there are other control issues with that.

Ashley delineates the critical *social* significance of the birth of a child, regardless of whether it is biological: having a relationship with the child, experiencing intense emotions about it. But once she has imagined the birth of a child, her bodily knowledge momentarily takes over, as she remembers the perils of unsuccessful pregnancies, both real and imagined. Scared by all the problems she foresees, she quickly rejects this possibility once again.

Asked by the interviewer if she has thought of using a surrogate, she said, "Yes, I want his genes. I don't care about my genes. That's interesting. I think I would if it was easy to do."

With no hesitation, Scott said, "If it was easy to do, I would consider it."

Ashley, forgetting her fears about pregnancy, begins to recant her willingness to use a surrogate: "And then we could do donor egg, which is basically the same thing."

Donor egg is not the same thing, as Ashley knows, having explored this medical option thoroughly. Having toyed with surrogacy for just a moment, but long enough for Scott to state his willingness to consider it, she moves to another technology, donor egg, that would give her more "control" over the pregnancy, even though the only worry it would alleviate, in her case, is the fear of Down's syndrome.[27]

They spent a few more minutes exploring this possibility and then, asked how their parents would feel if they adopted, Ashley began talking about adoption again:

I am concerned about that. I think that my mom could love the child instantly whatever it was. My dad, I think, maybe intellectually could talk himself into it but might have some trouble on the emotional level. We talk about adoption, it is not like they . . . I haven't actually said to them, "What do you think about adoption?" But they supplied me with names of people they know, and they seem to be supportive of all that, and so I imagine that maybe their longing, just like our longing, kind of changes you and kind of breaks down some of those biases. But I do have some concerns because my dad can certainly be prejudiced, and I am not sure about a child of another race. I am not sure for us, but I am sure my dad would not accept that.

Scott, too, has concerns:

I am not sure if my parents would accept that, too. But I sort of let my parents know that we are considering adoption. I have not asked them, "What do you think?"

Ashley continues,

I think for me, I don't want to know. I feel like I am dealing with so much. I don't want the kibosh put on it early in the process.

Scott adds: "I feel the same way."

Uncertain about how their parents will feel about an adoption, they are not providing any openings for the parents to voice an opinion. In this respect they echo the majority of people in this study, who feared that parental resistance to adoption would undermine their efforts to proceed. The cultural ideology of the biological child has such power that even when couples have worked through and reconciled many aspects of this ideology for themselves, they fear derailment of their plans by family members.

The cultural ideology of biological parenthood powerfully underscores issues about the potential parent being a full person. There is a strong relationship between living out one's gender identity and subscribing to biological determinism. When David discusses how definitions of family are connected to definitions of adulthood, he is connecting these cultural dialogues with issues of being a person and gender identity. Similarly, when Brad reflects on the anguish of men who cannot fulfill cultural expectations about potency, he is addressing gender identity and personhood. Indeed, everyone in this chapter has addressed what it means to be a person, and everyone has addressed the turmoil of having their bodily and social identities overturned. Some are rehearsing alternative possibilities, such as adoption and surrogacy, to find another way to fit into the cultural ideology of reproduction. At the same time, they are resisting the conclusions they reach about not belonging.

These stories reveal that the cultural ideology of biological parenthood is first and foremost about the self and not about the child. The assault women and men experience on their gender identity comes about because cultural ideologies support the assumption that biological performance—reproduction—is central to being a person. The goal of parenting a child is therefore completely displaced while people grapple with the relationship of the self to biology. These stories are not concerned with what would be best for the child; that question comes much later, after the initial impact of infertility on people's gender identity begins to abate and they begin to ask themselves what is really important. First, they must move beyond the cultural impasse of equating selfhood with biological functions. This is no small task. Understandings of self encompass the self as a biological entity, attesting to the ways in which cultural conceptions of the person as a biological being are lived out. The careful dissection of cultural dialogues on genes and generations is a first step in people's efforts to scrutinize these relationships.

CHAPTER 5

Experiencing Risks

During medical treatment for infertility, women and men are engaged in an ongoing assessment of the risks of various therapies. Polly's efforts to maintain control of her reproductive system have entailed a series of different risks. Looking back, she belatedly identifies the risks associated with the use of a particular IUD and looks ahead with irony to the next medical encounter, which she views as risk-laden:

I had a Dalkon Shield [an IUD associated with an increased incidence of pelvic infections]. I used the perfect form of birth control, it seems: permanent and forever. I had no idea. I was twenty-two. The doctor who was putting it in said, "You're crazy to get this thing. Nobody knows what it could do to you." And I just thought he was obnoxious. I was married to a guy I just knew I didn't want to be the father of my children, and I just said, "I don't care, just do it. I'm willing to take the risk." You know, big smile. I had it for about a year and a half, and then I started experiencing some discomfort when I had relations and things just didn't feel right down there, so I went to a doctor and he removed it. I went on the pill at that point, and later I did have an IUD for ten years, I had a Lippe's Loop put in. Which had a good track record, and I never had any problems with it. So because of all that, I'm doing IVF, which is full of risks.

The notion of risk is generally defined as the likelihood or probability of some adverse outcome. Notions of risk are embodied in complex cultural configurations of beliefs and ideals, and they reflect the historical era as well as the political and economic climate.[1] Mary Douglas suggests that the meaning of risk has changed from its nineteenth-century inception; formerly a neutral idea that took account of the probability of both losses and gains, the notion of risk now has primarily negative connotations. As the cultural dialogue on risk has evolved, so have opinions about what constitutes a risk to health.[2]

For women in this study, fears about putting themselves and their bodies at risk with new reproductive technologies were overruled by their desire for a child. They frequently expressed the philosophy, "If you want a child, you have to take risks." At the outset of treatment, they weighed the benefits of action against those of inaction and perceived the medical risks as small compared with the problem of childlessness. In this chapter I trace the development of ideas about risk in women's and men's decisions about infertility treatment.

TAKING RISKS IN INFERTILITY TREATMENT

Although public and professional debate about the appropriate use and safety of various drugs that have been used to aid reproduction may raise concern in women's and men's minds about the risks they are taking in the pursuit of fertility, the scale of the risks is not always clear—or even known. The primary medical risks are drug-related: the side-effects of fertility drugs, medical complications such as hyperstimulation of ovaries and tubes, multiple births, and unknown long-term risks, such as cancer of reproductive organs.[3]

People's notions of risk may differ considerably from medical definitions of risk, which are based largely on statistical estimates.[4] Yet, until recently, the public's notions of risk have been viewed as unimportant by scientists. Individual ideas about risk may be shaped by cultural assumptions, bodily knowledge, people's life experiences, experiences as patients in the health care system, and stress, discomfort, and financial burden. People's understanding of risk depends on the circumstances and constraints of their everyday lives as well as of specific situations.[5]

Karen's concerns about risk in undertaking medical treatment for infertility emanate from her early life and her family history. Karen, who is thirty-seven, is very concerned about risks associated with a range of medical interventions, from surgery to drugs.

He [physician] wouldn't even discuss the risks of hMG at all, and he was mumbling about the sperm count and not even looking at us in

*the eye to talk to about it. It was very disconcerting. So I've been try-
ing to find someone that's not threatened by my questions. And she's
[new physician] willing to try insemination first without hormones.
I'm very leery of what hormones are going to do to me.*

*I haven't had a laparoscopy yet.[6] I actually have a lot of fears
about that. I wonder what they're going to learn. If it's a good idea, if
the surgery will . . . who knows what? I just don't like the idea of being cut up unless there is some real reason. Or if there is something
they're going to be able to do for me. But mostly what everyone has
told me is they just want to know what's in there. Not that they can
necessarily do anything.*

*I don't know where my fears of doctors comes from. I don't know
how much she [mother] understands that. I don't think she is as worried as I am about taking the drugs. I think that she probably thinks
that it's not as big a deal as I think it is. But she is generally aware
that I have to make the decision.*

Although Karen has not been in infertility treatment long, almost everything about it makes her nervous. Her fears are related to her family
history:

*A lot of my fears come from fears of cancer. There's a lot of cancer in
my father's family at a very young age. And I sort of look at my life
and think that taking in as little strange things as you can will help
protect you. Nobody that I've read says that any of these things or
hormones are going to give you cancer. But I just sort of found this
general pulse that you're not supposed to take weird substances, if
possible.*

*My father died at forty-seven of multiple myeloma, and his sister is
now forty-seven and she's dying of a brain tumor. My mother is looking into whether there is any kind of cluster where they lived or if this
is just a family thing or what's going on. I don't know. But it certainly
affects my way of looking at my life. And it scares me too, wondering
when I . . . when you start with the assumption that you're going to
get pregnant and it's going to go along. But then when it doesn't and
you have to go to all these external, sort of extra needs to make it
happen, then you begin to wonder if this is the right thing to do or
not. And I worry that I don't know what my life span is going to be.
I worry about that. And I worry about having a child at this late age
and how long I'll be around. My father died young, and my two
younger siblings were only toddlers [at the time]. So it [father's death]*

*had a major effect on all of this. I was twenty-one but they were four
and six. So I sort of ask myself all these questions. I don't really know
the answers to any of them. And I really don't know how far I'm going to go with trying to have a kid. I question myself about it all the
time.*

Karen's way of trying to control the threat of cancer she perceives is
to limit all medical intervention. She is weighing the risks as she sees
them: the desire for a child versus the need to maximize her own chances.
She views each medical possibility as having certain risks. Because of
her uncertainty, she postpones taking any action.

Several conflicting problems lie at the heart of Karen's dilemma. First,
she is faced with the question, What is the right thing to do? Working
from the initial assumption that she would conceive naturally, she wants
to pursue the responsible course of action in trying to have children.
When her father developed cancer and died, with small children still at
home, it was a shock to everyone. But now that her aunt is dying and
it appears that there may be some familial connection to cancer, Karen's
efforts to conceive take on a moral dimension. What if she pursues a
treatment, only to be diagnosed with cancer while she has small children? Because of her own family's experience, she is reluctant to expose
her husband to such a risk, especially since her desire for children is
greater than his. Although Karen does not discuss expectations about
motherhood here, her concerns are directly related to these cultural expectations, and her own. The cultural dialogue on reproduction and on
motherhood affects her efforts and her fears. She speaks from her position as a woman with the moral responsibility to conceive.

The notion of living with risk is very different from biomedical definitions of risk. Women's and men's perceptions of risk are also affected
by specific health issues, and these views may differ considerably from
practitioners' views.[7] As contemporary societies become increasingly
medicalized, it may be difficult for people facing risks in medical treatment to resist such treatment. Indeed, Karen was unusual among women
in this study in her resistance to taking risks, but her family history of
cancer was also more daunting than the family histories of most women
in the study.

Most medical treatments for infertility are carried out on women,
even some procedures designed to compensate for their partner's infertility. For example, intracytoplasmic sperm injection (ICSI), although it
addresses male infertility, involves procedures performed on women.

Therefore men in this study seldom faced medical risks themselves. But men were concerned about risks to their partners at all stages of medical treatment, especially those associated with surgery and with the drugs given to stimulate the reproductive cycle. While women were preoccupied with trying to conceive, men were concerned about possible danger for their partner.

Because women's involvement in infertility treatment is greater than that of men and because they are often more intent on treatment, women become the final arbiters of risk. Men defer to their judgment. Overall, women identify more risks and are more willing to take risks than men. At the outset of treatment, they perceive the risks as small compared to the potential benefit. As time passes without a successful conception, they view the risks they take as a necessary byproduct of persistence.

Nevertheless, people's notions about risk focus on both gains and losses. Women and men in this study evaluated risk by its overall effect on their lives. They weighed the danger of taking action against the danger of inaction, concluding in most cases that the risks did not outweigh the potential benefits. Their decisions about taking risks invariably entailed a series of trade-offs. Their views were further shaped by negotiations with health professionals.

RISK AS ROUTINE

Women and men entered infertility treatment with the one preconceived idea that seeking medical treatment would lead to a pregnancy. Medical treatment appeared to hold little risk initially, as women and their partners underwent a series of tests to determine the causes of their infertility. The question of taking risks was not raised unless one partner had a preexisting medical condition.

Women who had preexisting reproductive health conditions, such as problems associated with DES, pelvic inflammatory disease, endometriosis, polycystic ovaries, or premature ovarian failure (see glossary), raised questions about risk taking earlier than other women. Women who had life-threatening chronic illnesses and men whose infertility was attributed to previous medical treatment, such as radiation therapy for cancer, also raised questions about risk taking early in treatment. Their prior experiences with medical care socialized them to think in such terms.

Although the fertility of these women and men had, in some cases, already been affected by medical treatment, they nevertheless proceeded.

Marcy, whose story appears in chapter 3, described how she learned she had blocked tubes as a result of using an IUD:

I had been told at one point in the regular annual pelvic exam that because I had had an IUD, that if I ever had problems conceiving, that it might be related to that. So that kind of planted a seed in my mind. I had an inkling there might be something not right. So then when she [physician] did the HSG [hysterosalpingogram — see glossary], it turned out to be a fairly dreadful experience because the dye did not go through the way it is supposed to [causing severe pain]. Instead it was blocked. They didn't know whether that was because I had blocked tubes or because I had a muscle spasm. They weren't sure. So they scheduled me for a laparoscopy. We found out pretty quickly that I do indeed have two blocked tubes at both ends. So the bottom line was, "You won't get pregnant as things stand right now. There are some options for you, including further surgery, in vitro, childfree, or adoption." So that's how it was presented to us. It was a lot to emotionally digest all at once.

This experience, and the assumption both she and her physicians have made that her blocked tubes are related to the IUD, has affected how Marcy views IVF, the one medical option that now remains:

It's really frightening to me. It's very frightening. Both personally now and for the future because I don't trust it [science/medicine] anymore. I just don't. I mean, I feel like I was victimized by it once and I'm . . . very skeptical now. I was betrayed by science.

The money I can even deal with, okay. You can always make money again, somehow. But you can't repair someone's health if it has been altered. Without the ability to repair it. That scares me more. I mean, not only mine, necessarily, but, you know, our child born out of this technology. And I don't think there's any way to answer that question particularly. I guess it's just something that you have to put into your risk equation.

Marcy abruptly learned about risks and reproductive health when she found out that her IUD might have increased the risk of damage to her fallopian tubes, which her physicians now considered irreparable. She feels "betrayed by science." She mourns the loss of her reproductive health and is reluctant to expose either herself or the child she has yet to conceive to more risks. Once unaware of risks, she now talks about having a personal "risk equation," a term she has borrowed from biomedical terminology. The moral authority with which she speaks reflects her position as a woman who tried to become a parent, only to find that medicine itself has hampered her efforts.

If an infertility factor is identified during the infertility workup, that diagnosis often points to a specific treatment pathway. But if no specific diagnosis is made, empirical therapy is still offered: a progression of therapies that physicians have found by experience to be successful, with minor adjustments for individual circumstances.[8] The reliance on empirical therapy affects the speed with which people move from one treatment to another. Infertility specialists who recommend trying less invasive treatments first may begin by prescribing drug therapy. But cost is also a consideration. Clomiphene, an inexpensive drug that is taken orally, is usually prescribed first, although physicians believe it has more side effects and is less effective than more expensive, injectable fertility drugs. Since assisted reproductive technologies have become widespread, some physicians suggest that IVF be attempted almost immediately, thus skipping low-technology and less costly procedures in anticipation of achieving a successful pregnancy sooner.

Despite the preference for starting with less invasive options, treatment often escalates relatively quickly, raising questions for women about immediate rather than long-term risks. Women may soon realize that more may be at stake than their fertility. Once activated, fears of risk taking are not easily assuaged. The cultural dialogue on reproduction does not highlight risks to women's health that may arise from fertility treatment, such as the potential dangers to both mother and fetuses in multiple births.

CHANGING VIEWS OF MEDICAL TREATMENT

As women and men in the study proceeded through medical treatment, their notions about risk evolved. A new awareness of risk was often reported following physicians' presentation of treatment plans that involved fertility drugs. Awareness of risk was also linked to people's specific experiences of infertility treatment, pregnancy, and childbirth, and it reflected the extent of their medical treatment as well as their concerns at the time of the interview.

Although some degree of risk may be acknowledged by a practitioner, it may be minimized by both patient and practitioner in their eagerness to find a solution to their problem. But when specific questions arise about the risks of particular medical procedures, women and men become engaged in an ongoing dialogue about risk. If pregnancy does not readily occur, the disappointment may create conflict, uncertainty, and a reevaluation of the emotional, physical, and economic risks of further treatment. For example, Tracy, a thirty-one-year-old woman, described her previous surgeries for endometriosis (see glossary):

When I woke up [from the anesthetic], they told me that I definitely had endometriosis and that unfortunately, the laser equipment malfunctioned and the doctor was unable to do anything, except with an electrical needle. I was left with the impression that they used the laser for a while before it stopped working. When we sent for the operative report from the hospital, it became clear that, really, next to nothing had been done. With the second surgery, I got some kind of infection. And both times I was sick and nauseated for a long time afterward. It affects my willingness to consider a third surgery.

As infertility treatments progressed to the more advanced reproductive technologies, fertility drugs were used more aggressively and in combinations. Women and men were concerned about both short-term issues, such as side-effects and ovarian hyperstimulation, and long-term consequences, including multiple births and cancer. Fertility drugs that require intramuscular or subcutaneous injection, such as hMG, engendered specific, immediate risks: they had to be carefully monitored by ultrasound to avoid hyperstimulation of the ovaries. People viewed hMG therapy as riskier than oral medications such as clomiphene (see glossary). Carolyn, thirty-eight, became concerned in the middle of an IVF cycle when she began reacting to the drugs:

After we had the tests and found out the results, I was getting all these real funky symptoms. Definitely, we were both real emotional through the whole thing. And going off the hMG and having all the other shots. The hCG and then you have the withdrawal from the hMG probably, and getting all bummed out. But I started having all these physical symptoms, and that's what really bothered me. Like my eggs [ovaries] would get real painful and hurt at night. I had some surgical stockings and I put them on my legs, but it was like, "What's happening to me?" And so I started freaking out, thinking about what the hormones were doing to my body. You know, what's going to happen to me in twenty years because I took this junk? Do they know the long-term effects? No. Have they done any studies? No. You know, we don't know what this is going to do to people in twenty years.

And I'm starting to think, "Well, suppose we do get lucky, get pregnant, have a kid and he's twenty years old and mommy dies, you know from . . ." God, is this worth it? I started getting a real bad attitude about it during that period of time. It's just like anything else. Sometimes you go through it and you're real optimistic. You think, I can do this. But then you have no idea how bad it is and how tough it is on you until you actually go through it.

So, then we got the test results that were negative. That we hadn't gotten a pregnancy. And then we kind of hit bottom. That was a year ago. That was a real tough summer because what happened after the in vitro failed, then I started having to deal with losing that [previous ectopic] pregnancy. Then it all started to really hit. It really hadn't gotten to me before. Before, I had something I was focusing on.

Like many women who stay buoyed up by the hope that IVF will work, only to have it fail, Carolyn was suddenly hit by a backlog of grieving, for both the failure of the IVF and a previous ectopic pregnancy, which necessitated IVF in the first place. She began to imagine the worst: that she would die prematurely from her efforts to conceive. Since that time, a year ago, she has taken no further action. She is rethinking the risks she took and the losses she sustained and wondering why she pursued medical treatment for so long. She is at last questioning the cultural ideology of reproduction.

Because hMG and GnRH agonists, such as Lupron (see glossary), are routinely administered in IVF treatment, women who elected to try this technology required daily injections, usually given by their partner or another person. Women and men were concerned about the potential effects of hMG, but they were even more concerned about drugs they considered experimental. Cynthia, who was reluctant to take powerful drugs because of her history as a DES daughter, nevertheless decided to try a new drug regimen when she went through IVF:

After the first hMG cycle, they [physicians] were concerned about a cyst that had developed during the first cycle, and so we skipped a month, and they suggested Lupron. Lupron was designed to inhibit cancer growth in men's prostates. It has the function of totally shutting the hormones down—it suppresses the hormone production and that somehow keeps the prostate from swelling up. I had some doubts about taking this drug for infertility but I did it.

Women are often frightened by the ability of such drugs to alter their natural cycle. They also sometimes experience unexpected symptoms that throw their bodily knowledge into disarray. Margaret, a thirty-eight-year-old woman who was preparing to start an IVF cycle using a donor egg, describes her reaction to Lupron:

Lupron is like going into madness. I get on the Lupron and I get this agitated depression, really severe. I have never felt suicidal in my life, and during the test cycle [to see how her body responded to the drugs], I actually had thoughts, and it is so unlike me. You kind of know at some level it is just the chemicals. I am not looking forward to it, especially with the agitation on top of it. For me that is the worst part—that combination is just deadly. I also get migraines, and I get a lot of hot flashes, so it is just going to be a real difficult few weeks. I guess whatever you get or you are going to get in menopause is what it's like. Another woman in my group who was taking it found this out. She asked around in her family, and sure enough, the women had started losing their hair when they had menopause, and that was what was happening to her. So whatever is going to come out then, you are getting a preview now.

So in some ways, the Lupron is just this little shot in your thigh, it seems so benign. But it's not. The depression seems like such a common response to the Lupron.

Despite the severity of Margaret's reactions to Lupron, she is focused on enduring the cycle rather than giving up the potential to have a child. Enduring the side effects rather than questioning the wisdom of taking such drugs is widespread among women.

One of the greatest risks in trying to conceive is ectopic pregnancy, a pregnancy that develops in a fallopian tube rather than in the uterus. A history of fallopian tube damage not only increases the chances of infertility but also raises the risk of ectopic pregnancy, even when infertility treatment is "successful." Colleen, forty years old, and her husband, Russ, tell the story of a disastrous ectopic pregnancy as they prepare to undergo an IVF cycle. After learning about her pregnancy, they scheduled a weekend at a remote country inn to celebrate. Awakened in the middle of the night in acute pain, Colleen assumed that she was having a miscarriage:

I woke up because of this terrible pain, and I think it must have taken me about fifteen seconds to realize that something awful was happen-

ing. And I think I knew almost immediately that it was life-threatening. It's like I could almost feel that my blood was being drained away. I noticed I was having trouble breathing. I think that it was mostly that the pain was awful. And I woke Russ up—I was thrashing and groaning. I said, "Something terrible is happening—go call an ambulance," and he did. And the funny thing about it was that he seemed to be so slow going downstairs to get the ambulance. He was saying, "Let me put my pants on first," and I was saying, "Don't worry about your pants. Go call the ambulance. Something terrible is happening," and he went downstairs and I thought, "Maybe we should be calling out to see if there's a doctor in the house." But we didn't do that. And he came back upstairs and held my hand. They were there really fast.

Russ interrupts, telling his wife, "They could tell you were in shock immediately." Colleen then continues:

Right away, they put me on oxygen. I think Russ told them over the phone that I was pregnant and it was the seventh week or whatever it was, and the ambulance drivers were telling him as they were driving us to the hospital that they thought it was a painful miscarriage.

I don't remember the ride too much. I just know I was in terrible pain, and getting into the emergency room, and the different doctors come in and out. They did this very, very painful procedure. They kept wanting me to sit up so they could do this procedure where they stuck something up inside of me so that they could see if there was blood up inside my abdomen. And they made me sit up. And it was so painful sitting up. I think it was at that point where the doctor starting saying that they had to do this test, to see whether they had to do surgery. And so they did get what they thought confirmed, which was that I was having internal bleeding and they explained to us that I would need to have surgery. And I don't remember too much after that.

In surgery, Colleen was found to have an ectopic pregnancy. Her other tube was damaged as well, and both tubes were removed. Russ concludes, "So we were no longer pregnant. But we were quite thoroughly traumatized."

COLLEEN: *Russ was in tears. He isn't talking about this part but he was absolutely terrified during the whole thing.*

RUSS: *Colleen was in the hospital for a week. We came home and went back to her doctor, and she looked at the charts and said, "You know, you had a pretty bad experience there, didn't you?"*

COLLEEN: *We were freaked out about it and we just could not imagine being pregnant again. It took a long time for me to be ready again [to try to conceive] after that.*

Because Colleen's tubes had been removed in the surgery, the only medical treatment left to them was IVF, which represented a major emotional and economic hurdle. They decided to go ahead. Given the danger they experienced, Russ and Colleen's perseverance in seeking further medical treatment may be surprising, but it is typical of many couples' actions.

CHANGING VIEWS
OF BIOMEDICAL INTERVENTION

Once a woman has been identified as being at high risk for an ectopic pregnancy, she may be subjected to intensified scrutiny, which has its own dangers. Physicians may become overzealous in their attention to risks. Kate, a thirty-five-year-old woman who had recently delivered a baby after several years of infertility, discusses her subsequent experience:

We just had another miscarriage just in the last couple of weeks. It wasn't a planned-for pregnancy. We actually conceived, so something was working, and it was a very strange situation. Given my history of ectopic pregnancies, they started monitoring this pregnancy right away and treating everything that might be a "potential ectopic." So we started doing ultrasounds at seven weeks. And they didn't see a sac in my uterus, so we just pulled back for four days and watched my hCG levels, and they kept skyrocketing [indicating a pregnancy]. And they did another ultrasound, still no embryo. No sac, no nothing. So, finally by the end of the week, my doctor said we have to go in and see what's going on. They found an ovarian cyst [previously], and he said, "It looks like a cyst but it also could be a fallopian tube being stretched to the max." You can't tell on the ultrasound. You have to go in. So about two and a half weeks ago they did a laparoscopy. He said, "We better go in [do diagnostic surgery] and do absolutely nothing. Just an exploratory [operation], or you may end up with a lapa-

*rotomy and you might lose a tube. We just don't know." So they
ended up doing a laparoscopy but they couldn't find anything. The
tubes were pulsing and pink and it was just an ovarian cyst, which
they drained, which came back again a couple of days later. It was
fluid-filled or something.*

*And so then the doctor said, "Because of your hCG levels, they're
still soaring and skyrocketing, it's acting like a normal pregnancy and
even with an ectopic, the embryo somehow implanted somewhere on
the organ. So I'm afraid we're going to have to consider a rare form
of cancer that mimics pregnancies because we can't find the embryo in
the uterus and we can't find it in the tubes or anywhere in that area."[9]
So that's the next step to determine that. And he said that the only
thing we have to do before we go see the endocrinologist is just see
if we can find a cancer cell in the womb.*

As the interviewer began to interject sounds of alarm, Kate said, "By
the way, I don't have cancer." She continued,

*It's just terrible. Just awful thinking that you might die after all the
years of trying to have this baby, and then getting cancer because I
was pregnant. Talk about unfair!*

*So this went on for another week, and in the end they found it was
it just a normal miscarriage. If I was just a normal person out there in
a normal world, it would have ended up just a normal miscarriage. I
would have had the miscarriage and it would have been sad. But you
know, I would have gotten over it, and I wouldn't have had surgery,
and I wouldn't have been told that I had cancer. It just seems so crazy
that here I am with this as a special patient, and I guess they just
don't think that anything easy could happen to me like a normal miscarriage. They were going for all the exotic things. It was just a placenta left over, and that's why they couldn't see it in the ultrasound,
and that's why my uterus was empty, because sometimes it doesn't
show up on an ultrasound. It was the most horrible thing to happen
in my whole life. It was the most horrible thing. I wouldn't wish it on
anybody.*

The interviewer interjected: "More horrible than the years of infertility
treatment?"

*It was more horrible than that. All those years rolled into one. I was
absolutely devastated. I thought that I was going to die, and I felt that
I would never see my child grow up. It's just funny how your perspec-*

tive changes because here I am thanking God that I didn't have can-
cer. I had a miscarriage and I almost feel like having to cry to cele-
brate it, "Yeah, I'm not going to die!" It was absolutely devastating.
To conceive this baby, I had several miscarriages and two ectopic
pregnancies. And this baby is the only one that stayed in the uterus.

Personally, I'm thrilled [to have a miscarriage]. I don't want to give
up the chance [to have another baby]. Maybe there is just a limited
time chance at conceiving again without drugs and everything. I don't
know. I guess I don't want to wait too long, plus my endometriosis.
You never know when that's going to come back.

Simply because Kate was not viewed as a normal pregnant woman
by her physician, she was subjected to surgery and emotional turmoil.
Her paradoxical response to having another miscarriage is to be
"thrilled" because it means she may be able to conceive again and
have the fetus implant in the uterus, where it belongs. Although it
has only been a matter of weeks since she contemplated dying and not
seeing her child grow up, her fears of dying of cancer are already assuaged. She is once again looking ahead to trying to conceive a second
child.

As treatment progresses, people understand risk to be an extremely
complex issue. Taking risks can encompass a deep sense of loss and
represent a threat to life for a woman or her child. Yet perceptions of
risk are seldom factors in decisions to stop treatment.[10] Women's willingness to continue to take risks is a testament to the power of the
cultural dialogues about biological parenthood. Those dialogues drown
out competing dialogues about risk taking.

SURVIVING CHILDBIRTH

Women going through infertility treatment often think conception is the
only hurdle and do not think about potential problems in pregnancy
and childbirth. Yet these risks include miscarriages, ectopic pregnancies,
stillbirths, and birth defects resulting in therapeutic abortion of a fetus.
While all pregnant women are at risk of having a medical complication
in pregnancy or delivery, such as gestational diabetes or preeclampsia,
pregnancies conceived through IVF may have increased risks for ectopic
pregnancy, preterm labor, multiple gestation, and infants small for their
gestational age. Sherry tells of the complications during her pregnancy:

I had preterm labor. I went into labor at twenty-five weeks. I had been feeling that something wasn't right, and I had an appointment in two days, and it was like, "Should I wait until Friday, or should I call?" So I called, and they said, "Come into the hospital now." I didn't know what it was. I just knew that I was having too many contractions. So I did have preterm labor, and I had to control it just by having to come home for a couple of days. And I started to dilate. So they put me back into the hospital and sent me home after two days in the hospital on a drug used to reduce contractions in premature labor. And I was home in bed for ten weeks. I left work in the middle of the day and never went back.

I had this planned and that planned and vacations planned. Our whole lives just stopped. It was very scary because the baby was only twenty-five weeks gestation. She probably wouldn't have survived at that point. So that was pretty anxious and was a very traumatic experience, and the drugs that they give you . . . this drug causes panic attacks. It makes your heart race and so it makes your mind think that you are in a state of panic because your whole body runs up. Plus you are already in a state of panic because you are in the hospital unexpectedly.

I was thinking about what we had talked about before, about this sense of lack of control over infertility and what it can do to your life. And that was sort of the same thing happening all over again. Being told that I could get up ten minutes out of every hour to go to the bathroom and that was it. So I was on bed rest for almost four months.

And then, a month into it [bed rest], I developed gestational diabetes. So that was a clincher. I am at high risk to develop it later, but I don't have it now. It was one of those things. After a month of being on bed rest, I felt like I had adjusted to it [bed rest]. It was terrible and it was very depressing, but I was managing. And friends came over and cooked for me and brought me food. One of our friends is a chef. We were eating very well. People were great. And then I became a diabetic. And then they took food away from me. That was the second nightmare. I was on insulin and I was on this very controlled diet. Because she was growing much too fast and I was gaining weight really rapidly. After they tested me, they sent me to the diabetes clinic and a woman was telling me that if my blood sugar level continued for three more days, it could kill the baby. And I had al-

ready had it for at least two weeks before they diagnosed it. I was just
hysterical.

Although Sherry had a long history of reproductive health problems, including polycystic ovaries, and had had several surgeries for those problems, once pregnant she expected, like other women in this study, that the pregnancy would be problem-free. Already consumed by her efforts to conceive, Sherry found that the problems she faced in maintaining the pregnancy took over her life.

The baby's survival depended on Sherry's staying in bed and eating very restricted foods. The responsibility for its well-being lay solely with her. This sense of responsibility forged women's determination to endure all kinds of deprivation. Biomedical perspectives on giving and enhancing life complement women's desire to bring new life into the world. Medical risks and discomforts may be viewed by both practitioners and patients as minimal compared with the possibility of a "take-home baby," as successful pregnancies are called in infertility treatment. By reaffirming cultural meanings associated with risk and the reasons for taking them, biomedical perspectives provide legitimation for action and reinforce patients' views about the danger of inaction.

Sherry, who identified herself as a high-risk patient during her pregnancy, had great difficulty during the birth of her child:

I had a terrible labor. By the time I got to the hospital, I was just
screaming in pain, and they said, "You're not even dilated. Wait until
you're really in labor!" But fortunately they admitted me because I
was considered a high-risk patient because of the diabetes, and they
gave me tons and tons of morphine, and I was in labor for twenty-
seven hours. And then the baby wasn't coming down. I was almost
nine and a half centimeters, and I guess I stayed there for a couple of
hours.

They thought she was a ten-pound baby, and in fact, her shoulder
was stuck, so they decided to do a C-section. She was going into dis-
tress and they had an oxygen mask on me and all that kind of scary
stuff. So they went into to do a C-section, and the cord was around
her neck, and when they went in, they found all these adhesions from
the ectopic I had last year, and had an ovary removed the year before,
so I had had two abdominal surgeries already. And I guess they cut in
to take the baby and there was all this junk in the way and the adhe-
sions had wrapped around my bowels and my bladder and they were

tucked into different places. So that was why my labor was so bad. Because every time I had a contraction, it was my uterus contracting. Everything was being pulled all over the place. Afterward, they apologized for giving me a bad time.

I was awake for the C-section. I did want to be awake, but what did I know? You're not supposed to feel anything, and yet you feel plenty. They say it's not pain, but my anesthesiologist friend tells me that if you perceive it as pain, it's pain. That's what pain is. And you hear a lot, and you feel a lot of pushing and tugging and stuff. It felt like pain to me but I was so . . . it was a very strange experience because when I went into the operating room, I kind of went somewhat psychotic and was aware of it, and it was a very strange experience. My husband and my sister thought that I had already been given some drugs because I was just crazy. And the anesthesiologist told them that I hadn't been given anything yet. I had a lot of morphine but I hadn't been given anything that would make me psychotic.

I don't remember seeing her [baby], but they said they offered her to me, and I remember her crying, and they told me it was a girl. I was already going out at that point. But she was healthy and she was very small. She was only six and a half pounds. Not very small but considering they thought I was having a ten-pound baby, it was much smaller than they expected. Apparently, what they had been feeling were my bladder and my bowels in the wrong place.

Then later my doctor came in and explained the surgery to me, and the bottom line was that she felt that I would never be able to get pregnant again. That this was it. Because of the way they had to cut into my uterus to get the baby out. It was not the normal way you do a C-section. They had to kind of go around. And apparently my sister and my husband already knew this. I think this was discussed in the operating room. And the doctor had called my husband that morning and said that she was going to come in and talk to me, and I guess he didn't want me to know, but he knew that I had a right to know. I'm not stupid, and I knew that this was very complicated, and that my body had already been through a lot. So I wasn't shocked to hear this. But at the same time, hearing you're never going to have another child again! It was very difficult. It's still very difficult.

I've gone back to see my doctor twice since the surgery, and she's really almost changed her mind. She said I had sort of a miracle recovery. I'm supposed to have an MRI in six months to see how well the healing was. Her feeling now is if that if this looks okay, then I could probably get pregnant again, but I'd have to have a cervical cerclage and I'd probably be in bed for six months.

So that's where I'm at right now. I'm adding a new chapter to this infertility chapter of mine. If we do this again, I'd have to wait a year and a half or two years to try and get pregnant again. We wanted a big family to begin with, and now I feel like, "How can I complain?" I got this beautiful, one, perfect baby. But you want what other people have. You want what you feel like you're entitled to have. So it's not over for us by any means.

Sherry, trying to place this experience in perspective, is using the metaphor of her life as a book in order to make sense of these unexpected difficulties. Even though this was a very dangerous delivery for both her and her child, she is not ready to conclude this "chapter," and consequently she and her husband have experienced conflict over issues of risk. She concluded: "This pregnancy was a tremendous strain on my husband. I talked to him about having another child. He thinks I'm crazy. As dramatic as this pregnancy and delivery was for me, I think it was as bad, if not worse, for him. Particularly the delivery. I wasn't that aware of what was going on, and he was quite terrified. So we've had a lot of fights about whether to try again."

Sherry's persistence in the face of a life-threatening experience is impressive, yet she couches this experience in terms of entitlement: she always wanted a large family, and she believes she is entitled to one. The amount of stress her determination places on the marital relationship may be the deciding factor in whether or not she tries to have another child. Sherry believes the risks are worth taking.

Notions of risk are apparently informed, first and foremost, by societal values to which both patients and physicians subscribe. Specific cultural values dictate how people identify risk in medical treatment as well as the actions they take. The infusion of biomedical concepts into everyday life promotes the notion of risk as routine. When efforts to live up to cultural norms are embedded in people's biographies and are reflected in the health care system through well-delineated patterns of medical treatment, risks inherent in medical treatment may be denigrated, and women's experiences of treatment may become medically intensive. Infertility treatment epitomizes this process. When initial efforts to conceive are unsuccessful, the decision to proceed may be viewed by both women and their physicians as a risk-benefit trade-off; and if a baby is a priceless benefit, then almost any risk is worth taking.

NONMEDICAL RISKS

In addition to holding a wide range of medical risks, new reproductive technologies pose nonmedical risks as well. These include severe emotional stress for individual partners and for the relationship, a heavy financial burden, and the potential for multiple births, which in turn carry their own medical, emotional, and financial risks. Although well aware of these risks, people often discounted them in light of the alternatives of childlessness or adoption. Colleen reflects this ambivalence as she looks back on her ectopic pregnancy and forward, toward the unknown:

The idea of IVF just felt very depressing and full of risk, scary, and that we faced too much of a chance of lawsuits [referring back to traumatic ectopic pregnancy, over which they later felt they should have sued], and that I was going to have to go through all this physical stuff. There was this tiny bit of lightness when I would think about adoption, but we only kind of touched on that. And then we were having to make this decision really fast, of whether to go to the April cycle. So I decided to.

Colleen, as the person who would bodily go through this process, made the final decision. The stress she experienced escalated even before the cycle began:

So Russ went on his business trip, and I totaled the car. Then I really knew I was under a lot of stress. And that was the sign that I really needed to start cutting back, and I did pretty good. People in the support group said they knew friends that had quit their jobs while they were going through IVF. But it was very hard to ask for time off from work for IVF. I had a lot of issues about telling people what I was doing. And I didn't tell many people.

During the cycle, Colleen suddenly found herself focused on a new set of issues she had not thought about before:

So then it was the IVF weekend. Everything went beautifully. They took out sixteen eggs. I was so thrilled, the entire team was there—all

three doctors. . . . And the recovery was fine. And I went home, and
they called us the next morning—I went home on bed rest—and said
we had ten embryos, and he hoped at least six were good embryos
and maybe seven. And I should think about it if I wanted all seven to
be put in. I wanted to ask about selective reduction [see glossary], and
what's that all about? How do we make those kinds of decisions?
How do we decide how many embryos to put in? It was hard to ask
those questions. He said they recommended six. He said that most
couples decide to have six put in, and most couples really focus on
getting pregnant and they really don't worry about how many are go-
ing to implant. They worry about that later. It seemed like a really
important issue. He would give me the statistics, about 75 percent of
singletons and 25 percent chance of a multiple, and you know, 20
percent chance of twins and 5 percent of multiples. So he gave me the
statistics, but it was like I felt brushed off. Whenever I brought up
these questions, the response was, "Think about that later, don't
worry too much about that now." I'm the kind of person who likes to
have lots of information real early on and have lots of time to think
about it and then make a decision. I don't like being told how to do
things and that I have to make a decision quickly.

So we went back to the doctor's office, and I told the nurse, I think
he wants to talk with us before we go over to the hospital to talk
about how many embryos, and she said, "Oh, no, go on over to the
hospital and he will be over." So she sent us out to the elevator, and
we're standing in the hallway and the doctor comes running after us,
saying, "Oh, we have to talk about the embryos, you've got six good
embryos and six four-cell embryos and one two-cell, and how many
do you want to put in?" We're standing by the elevators, and I
wanted to say, "Could we go into your office and talk about this?"
but it seemed silly for me to say, "I need to sit down in a chair, I want
you as the doctor to be behind the desk and I want to talk about this
in a formal setting." So I sort of stifled that and asked if we could talk
about it more at the hospital and give us a little time to think about it.
So when he came over, we did talk about how many to put back in
and we decided to put seven in.

Colleen and Russ had not considered one of the central questions that
arises when people undergo IVF: how many embryos to use. According
to them, their physician denigrated the importance of this issue, and
they proceeded without time to think it through.

Then I went in for the blood test, and my period never came, and the next morning came, and my period didn't start yet, and the next morning came, and still no period, and I was starting to feel optimistic. Then we got the phone call, and the nurse said that we were pregnant. I was kind of excited, and I said, "What was our score [hCG levels]?" and she told us what the numbers would be, that if we were definitely pregnant, it would be thirty to fifty. So I said, what was our number? She said, "182." I said, "What does that mean?" She said, "Well, you probably have twins or you might have a multiple." I freaked out. I was so upset. I was very anxious, and so the next couple of days, I was so sure I was going to have triplets, and I was so overwhelmed with that idea and how was I going to cope and we were going to go bankrupt, and I would never be able to go back to my career again. I would spend the rest of my life raising triplets, and I just couldn't see how I was going to cope. I was having fantasies that I was pregnant with six, and I would have to go through selective reduction, and was like this freak who had all these babies inside of me. And I was sort of imagining what it would be like to carry triplets. I've seen really premature babies, and I didn't want premature babies that were really sick and might have all kinds of problems later, I was freaked. Russ wasn't that upset about the idea of having triplets. But I was sure we were going to have triplets.

We were guarded about whether we were really going to term, and he was telling people the numbers. Then we got the second test back and the level had almost doubled, and the nurse's response was, "It's a good sign. I means that you're definitely pregnant, it's going up the right amount." But the fact that it wasn't going up in astronomical numbers meant that probably I didn't have super high multiples but that I probably had one or two. So I might have twins. Who knows? I feel ambivalent. I'm not sure how I feel about being pregnant yet. When everyone in my group burst into applause, it was very overwhelming. And we don't know where our pregnancy is going to go yet. I'm trying to focus on feeling good. [Loudly:] Whatever happens, we are pregnant right now!

So we are talking to the little embryos, you know, making up all these silly little nicknames for them. Russ talks to them, and I enjoy that. They [friends in Resolve] are always talking about this guarded optimism. And I think we're both very guarded optimists. But I think we also need to enjoy the pregnancy right now. And if we lose the pregnancy, then we lose it. I want to get as many bits of pleasure out of it as I can. So that's kind of my focus for the next few months.

Colleen's feelings at this stage are fairly typical of women who have experienced many setbacks in trying to conceive. She is ambivalent, overwhelmed, excited, and fearful all at once. Indeed, Colleen turned out to be pregnant with twins.[11] At four months, she was diagnosed with gestational diabetes and developed severe liver disease. She was put on bed rest for the duration of the pregnancy.

After the delivery of the babies, her health restored, she returned to work. She and Russ found parenting twins to be a task for which they felt poorly equipped emotionally or financially. Colleen became chronically depressed, and their relationship was affected. One year after the twins' birth, she reported: "I was thrilled to go back to work. When I went back I could feel my sense of depression lifting up from me. Because I was somewhat depressed staying home and was really exhausted." Russ interjected: "And never getting a break from them is just too much." Colleen agreed:

I was watching them by myself from seven A.M. until 7:30 at night. It was very, very hard. So when I was at work, even though I went back under bad conditions, my boss believed I was incapable of doing my job now that I was a mother of twins. But it was restful, and I was happy to be working. But then my boss started hassling me, and it got really hard, and I had to deal with a very difficult situation with her. And then she left—she moved away. So now I'm working thirty-four hours a week, which is too much, and my new boss won't let me cut my hours back. My days are long.

The stress of raising twins was compounded by her work situation, but Colleen could not afford to quit her job.

It's still difficult. I look forward to being with them, and I say to myself that I'm going to have a nice day and relax and have a nice time. But no matter how much I vow that the day never goes quite the way I wanted. I can't get them to take a nap at the same time, and I don't get a break. And by the time it's six I'm just absolutely exhausted again. Even though I'm only doing it one day a week by myself, it's still just like all those months where I did it every day, where by five I would be in tears on the floor trying to figure out how to cope with two screaming babies. That still happens. I think that taking care of twins for that many hours straight is just too hard for one person to do and have it be in any way fun. I think ideally to have twins you should have lots of money, and you just really need to have a lot of relatives.

When Colleen and Russ had twins, they exhausted their personal resources as well as their limited financial resources. So intent are women and men on conceiving that they seldom consider the possible long-term consequences of using the new reproductive technologies. As time passes without a successful conception, women come to view the risks they take as necessary. They experiment with their bodies out of a sense of responsibility to produce a pregnancy and their sense of entitlement to one.[12] They often sacrifice their well-being to achieve this goal, facing unknown risks to their health. Their gender identity is permanently altered as their view of themselves as infertile takes hold during the course of medical treatment.

CHAPTER 6

Taking Action

[Resolve] is wonderful. I volunteer now on the telephone.
It has been the best thing for me. It is really good because
you learn a lot, and it is like you are helping other people,
and there are all kinds of good things about it.

Carla, thirty-seven years old

One of the central themes of this book is women's and men's actions as
they encounter and undergo new reproductive technologies. By actions
I mean not simply deciding to undertake such treatment and going
through with it, but *all* the actions they take on their own behalf. These
take a wide range of forms. Women and men in this study sought psychotherapy, professional counseling, and alternative forms of healing,
but they also joined self-help groups and became advocates for infertility
awareness.[1]

In other work I have emphasized the power and transformative qualities of people's actions in dealing with infertility.[2] While acknowledging
that there are significant constraints on people's actions, I consider action, or agency, to be a critical, and often overlooked, component of
social change.[3] In this chapter I emphasize how taking action not only
can be personally beneficial but can also lead to large-scale collective
action and to social movements that can penetrate social institutions
and alter social policy. Collective forms of resistance to the status quo
have the power to influence cultural practices, to shift and broaden cultural dialogues, and to introduce new cultural themes.[4]

Rooted in ideals and moral aspirations, contemporary social movements are a form of identity politics and a means of struggling for power.
Such movements are political because they involve refusing, diminishing,
or displacing identities that others may impose on them. These social
movements reflect a shift to a politics of difference.[5] Specific interest

groups may want to change the way they are viewed by society or call attention to themselves as a collective engaged in action to create social change, such as the civil rights movement of the 1960s, the women's movement, and the many health-related social movements of the 1980s. Not only are these groups shaped by cultural phenomena, but they also in turn shape these phenomena and usher in social change.[6]

I focus here on one example of this phenomenon, the groundswell of action related to infertility over the last twenty years. The idea that gender is performed, or enacted, through women's and men's actions is salient to an understanding of such action. Feminists view gender practices as sites of critical agency.[7] Examining such actions can enlighten our understanding of gender practices as well as our understanding of collective action. Judith Butler connects such actions to the theatrical sense of "act": as part of a performance, acts are a shared experience and a collective action.[8] We will see how such collective acts are socially, culturally, and historically grounded and how they are experienced and expressed both personally and collectively by participation in the self-help group Resolve.

THE GROWTH OF A SELF-HELP ORGANIZATION

Many years ago, when I was making the transition from being an infertility patient to studying infertility, I attended a workshop in a classroom of a local community college. About fifteen people were present. It was one of the fledgling outreach meetings of the Northern California chapter of Resolve, a self-help group for people dealing with infertility. The purpose was education, and the emphasis was on coping emotionally with infertility. As I watched with interest the interactions of the panelists and the audience, I saw the capacity of this kind of educational program to ameliorate suffering. Fifteen years later, this organization has a large membership and holds educational workshops that hundreds of people attend.

I did not become closely involved with Resolve subsequently, because as a social scientist I had been trained to keep my distance from self-help groups. Social scientists then believed, and still believe, that self-help groups develop and reflect a particular perspective, one that is not necessarily shared by everyone who shares the problem. To become part of a self-help group or to study one may lead to an exclusive focus on that group that might exclude the study of people outside the group who have other perspectives. The risk of such an exclusive focus is thought to be greatest for social scientists like myself who conduct research up close, that is, in repeated face-to-face encounters.

Staying on the sidelines made my job both easier and harder. It was easier to observe the workings of Resolve when I was not absorbed by them. But Resolve was a major source of potential recruits for my studies, and my peripheral stance made it difficult to talk with them. Also, it was hard for me to remain a semi-outsider when I shared so much personal experience with others. I often felt left out, through no one's actions but my own.

It was not until ten years later that I began to relax about keeping the organization and its members separate from my research. I realized from my interviews that the majority of people undergoing infertility treatment in my geographic area knew about Resolve, and many attended its meetings. From a small organization with a handful of people, Resolve had become a fixture on the local infertility scene. Many of the people I interviewed referred to Resolve frequently. Midway through writing this book, I realized I couldn't leave out Resolve because its role in people's use of reproductive technologies forms part of the story.

Over the years I have seen Resolve's emphasis shift as a result of the availability of reproductive technologies. Although its goal has always been to provide information and to enable people to feel control over their bodies, with the burgeoning of infertility services it has taken on an additional focus: policing the field of reproductive technology, with respect to both evaluating individual practitioners and influencing national policy and legislation.

Self-help groups such as Resolve have their roots in the voluntary organizations that have played an important role in U.S. society. With their emphasis on community and collective action, they provide an important counterpoint to the cultural ideology of individualism and self-determination.[9] Barbara Eck Menning gave the name "Resolve" to the self-help organization she started to highlight the centrality of bringing unwanted childlessness to a successful conclusion. The name not only reflects the goal of the organization to take individual and collective action in the interest of self-determination; it also underscores culturally sanctioned ways of dealing with problems and differences in the United States. As various social conditions such as infertility have become medicalized, self-help groups have offered an antidote to the sense of difference that medicalization may foster.[10]

There are over fifty local chapters of Resolve, and in the geographic locale of this study the chapter was extremely active. As in other voluntary organizations, local chapters of Resolve have officers and a board, as well as various committees and subgroups that work on its various projects and pursuits. As a local chapter grows, those entities proliferate. This particular Resolve chapter grew over the fifteen years of the research from very small to extremely large. Nationwide, Resolve sponsors support groups, informational meetings, and telephone hot-lines, works on and lobbies for legislation, evaluates physicians' per-formances, and disseminates information about infertility and repro-ductive technologies. This chapter has a regular newsletter, an advisory group of physicians, a central office (staffed part-time), and committees and subgroups to run programs such as semiannual symposia and meet-ings of support group leaders. Informational literature about Resolve and its services can be found in the waiting rooms of every local prac-titioner treating infertility.

Resolve is a predominantly white, middle-class organization.[11] Al-though members working on outreach have reported their efforts to reach people in other ethnic and income groups over the years, no one I spoke with feels they have been very successful. When I mentioned my problems recruiting nonwhite and low-income people into my study, Roseann observed, "I think it's really servicing the needs of the com-munity. The upper middle- and upper-class white community, that is. We're not reaching the Latino community and we're not reaching Af-rican Americans. Although we have made efforts, it's probably the same problems that you're having." Her husband, Burt, joined in: "It's reach-ing to the upper middle-class Asian community. There are Asian people involved." But Roseann responded, "Not very many. Not that many. It's pretty Caucasian. I would say 90 percent white."

This problem is linked, in part, to the issue of who seeks and receives medical treatment. Those who cannot afford to pursue medical treat-ment or private adoption are unlikely to learn of Resolve, and the kind of information Resolve disseminates is minimally useful to those who cannot afford these services. Consequently, Resolve represents the pri-orities of the middle class.

INFORMATION AND SUPPORT

The primary goal of Resolve is to provide information and support to people going through infertility. Not every such person joins Resolve, and, of those who do join, only a proportion become actively involved. But most people who learn about Resolve attend some of its informational meetings sooner or later. No other single source offers such comprehensive information on reproductive technologies available locally. For example, a sample of three of the evening meetings, held monthly, might include discussions of IVF, the use of donors, and how to adopt.[12] For each topic, medical, legal, and psychosocial practitioners are on hand to discuss pros and cons and philosophies of practice and to address medical and technical details of various procedures. One annual symposium addresses the entire gamut of issues, including new reproductive technologies, adoption, surrogacy, and childlessness, and another focuses solely on adoption.

People who find their bodies under long-term assault in infertility treatment are empowered through Resolve. The majority of people interviewed for this study, especially women, stated that participation in Resolve was a major source of support, and even a catalyst, in their lives. Through Resolve they found reassurance for their bodily concerns, gained the courage to question physicians and insurance companies, and expanded their knowledge of the issues and of their options. Eddie reported:

So you want to reduce as much stress as you can. We tried meditating. We both tried different avenues of minimizing stress. . . . Joining Resolve initially, and also trying to get into a support group. I called them and I said, "Do you know who is putting together support groups?" My idea was to get into a support group. We had no idea about the symposium. We had no idea that this would be a real knowledge thing. We just thought we're going to be able to network, we're going to be able to get into a support group. That looks good for your statistics. It helps you get pregnant. So that was the motivation. Everything at the symposium was gravy. It was the most incredible experience for me. It's like, I want to hear it all.

Eddie is describing a contemporary middle-class pattern of seeking help in the United States: networking, and joining a support group as a way of managing a health-related problem. Resolve offers something more, however, that solidifies involvement with the group: education, or, as Eddie puts it, "a real knowledge thing." This gives people the potential to become lay experts in a confusing and intimidating medical field. Resolve thus not only extends the opportunity for personal empowerment to people, it also provides an opportunity for collective empowerment to which many people are quick to respond.

Resolve's support groups are very popular, and people may eventually join more than one. Some groups last the agreed-on time of eight weeks, whereas others go on for months and sometimes years. A group is led by a Resolve volunteer who usually has been professionally trained in psychotherapy or in running therapeutic groups. Nora and Walt describe their response to joining a group:

WALT: *We went to the first group together.*

NORA: *Did you want to go or did I drag you?*

WALT: *No, I was willing to go.*

NORA: *Did you want to? I mean, I needed to go.*

WALTER: *I wanted to go because I wanted to go for us. No. I wanted to go for us. It was important that we do this together, so because it was important, yes, I wanted to do it. I didn't go screaming, kicking and screaming or anything. And the first group I felt was worthwhile. Made some friends from it. Some friendships that have endured. Then after the first group, Nora did another group. I went to the first meeting. I just wasn't interested. The second group, I just didn't like the people, I didn't care for them. Two people dominated the first evening's conversation.*

NORA: *The whole thing was just so funny. Because here you are with a bunch of strangers and you're talking about the most intimate details of your life. "Yeah, we had to have sex four times last night, and I just wanted to sleep through it because . . ." [laughter]. I mean, things that you don't want to talk about. "Yeah, I took that sperm sample while I was on the bus . . ." [laughter]. It's pretty comical. But it's true there are a lot of people out there that I don't have anything in common with, other than the fact that I'm infertile. Even though you're talking infertility, if you don't click in other ways, then you don't get that support, at least for me. So that's why some groups work and some don't. Just like every group in psychotherapy doesn't work.*

Nora is describing some of the key dynamics in these support groups: a group of strangers come together and talk about the intimate details of their lives, creating close bonds with people who may well become long-term friends. The intimacy is created not simply by talking about sex, but by talking about all of the frustrations of infertility, which people may be keeping secret from others in their social world. The group thus becomes a place where people can talk about a wide range of specialized issues that they seldom discuss otherwise. Successful groups often make a verbal contract to stick together until everyone has a child. This is difficult to do, however, because with the first pregnancy or adoption in the group, other members are faced with the same dilemma they face in the rest of their lives: feeling like outsiders. Group members may work through this difficulty collectively and stay together for years, or they may eject new parents from the group. Most groups end their formal work before the majority become parents, and those people, ideally, leave the disbanded group with a greater sense of how to manage their infertility.

Resolve is a catalyst in the reworking of gender identity and the personal resolution of cultural ideologies about biological parenthood. While Resolve subscribes to the cultural ideology of parenthood, it takes issue with the dominant ideology of biological parenthood. Resolve views adoption, for example, as an acceptable means of living up to this cultural ideology, and many opportunities exist for people to address how they feel about this possibility and to listen to the perspectives of others.

For those who become involved with Resolve, the peer pressure of friends who had children without difficulty is replaced by the peer pressure of others who are experiencing the same problems. The bonds created between those who feel marginalized and turn, as an antidote, to Resolve, are in many ways more powerful than bonds with other friends, and they may develop into long-term friendships. Peer influence plays an important role in keeping people in treatment, especially in the later stages of treatment. When "everyone" in the group is considering using the donor egg technology, for example, rejecting this possibility may be more difficult.

Although it does not espouse resolution solely through having children, Resolve is not an easy organization in which to opt for childlessness. The momentum created by the organization's participants is toward resolution by having a child. From one angle, Resolve can be seen as abetting the work of biomedicine. At the same time that Resolve stands for resolution of infertility through all available means, the peer pressure it exerts to persist in efforts to have a child may be a major factor in keeping women in treatment. By making it more difficult for couples to consider the alternative of not having a child, membership in Resolve may have a significant influence on women's and men's conceptualization of the situation.

THE PROFESSIONALIZATION PROCESS

The local chapter of Resolve is run almost exclusively by volunteers, most of whom are women. Women became involved in Resolve during the course of our study independently of our contacts with them. Growing involvement with Resolve often indicated that people were becoming more deeply immersed in medical treatment. Women often stated they needed something to balance medical treatment, and Resolve frequently offered the antidote. At the time of the latest study, the local organization still had no paid staff members.

Volunteering for Resolve gives women a sense of purpose and direction during a time that many view as stagnant, in which they are caught in limbo, waiting to conceive. Carla explained how her involvement with Resolve pulled her out of a clinical depression:

The first two years I took it [infertility] real hard, and I didn't even know about Resolve. I didn't have any support except for my family, and that wasn't the best support because they always kept telling me, "Just relax, it [conception] will happen." So the first two years were bad. So now I'm involved with Resolve. Bill will occasionally go to an awareness meeting, but that's about it. He doesn't like talking about the infertility with men. I help out on the phones. I've been doing that for a year now. I really enjoy it because I can talk about infertility for three hours every two weeks. And once I get that out of my system, I'll talk out [meaning she won't need to talk about it anymore].

Bill agreed on the benefits of Carla's involvement with Resolve:

I'm glad she got involved with Resolve. Because if she hadn't . . . she was in really bad shape. And when she got into that and started doing the phones . . . she was just a different person after a while, a couple of months. Three months. She got much stronger. It was like a 360-degree change in direction, because it was bad there for a while. I was getting very worried. It would tear me up just seeing her that way, in this great depression. The windows and everything were all closed. She was always in her robe. Didn't want to go outside and stuff like that.

CARLA: *Yeah. I wouldn't answer the phone for days. Or answer the door.*

BILL: *Resolve was the best thing that happened to her.*

CARLA: *Yeah, once I contacted Resolve that was the beginning of my getting better. And then when I started volunteering to do the phones, then I really got better. Now I'm almost my old self.*

Carla's experience is one of many testaments I have heard to the benefits of involvement in Resolve. Self-help organizations serve many functions, but their core purpose is to help people to deal with their sense of difference through community. Shared experience is a powerful tool in helping people to restore a sense of normalcy. Carla enjoys extending to others the sense of community that was extended to her:

On my shift I get a lot of people who are calling for the first time — since I started going back to school. Most of them are calling to find out, "What's Resolve? I heard about Resolve from . . ." And they're delighted when you tell them that we're a nonprofit organization for the infertile. And we'll talk on the phone. I'll share with them what we've been through. They just really appreciate that. It makes them much more comfortable, and then they start opening up. I try to spend at least twenty minutes with each caller, and then I mail their packets out.

This combination of personally connecting through shared experience, information, and education has affected Carla so greatly that she is considering a career shift:

When I started talking with people over the phone, so many people said, "I feel so much better after talking with you." And I go, "Well, this is a really good feeling." It was like a high. I had already taken classes in drafting because I thought I wanted to be an engineer. And it just wasn't exciting me anymore. So I signed up for classes in psychology.

Carla's experience is not unusual. Women frequently shift their career plans after involvement with Resolve. Their activities in the organization often give them a newfound focus. Those already established in a related profession, such as psychotherapy, may become more focused on infertility in their work lives. Frances, a psychotherapist who adopted a child shortly before this interview, describes the transition she is in:

I am really trying to think about what do I want to do now. I have always done agency work along with my private practice, so this is the first time that I am thinking I am going to try just to do my private practice. After I talked to you last year I got on the Resolve referral list. So now I am on the referral list, plus I did a support group. I loved running the group. I had a great time. A lot of the people in the group were moving toward adoption, so that also was very fun for me. It was terrific. So that was real great, and so I am trying to think about this. I don't know how much I want to deal with people who are just dealing with medical treatment, because that is not what I am doing now, although it is interesting to me. But I am not as up on that as I am interested in adoption and the issues that come up with adoption, so I am trying to think how I am going to capitalize on that. How I am going to use Resolve and use these people and make something work for myself that I really like. So I don't know exactly what I want to do and how I want to expand this, but it is very interesting to me. It is very important in my life.

Frances's story is a good example of how women consolidate their roles with Resolve, enhancing their own work at the same time that they participate in community and political action. Having begun her connection with Resolve as a recipient of their services, she now has become a provider of services, running a support group. She has already made the decision to shift her private practice away from general psychotherapy to specialize in infertility; now she is considering whether to focus her work specifically on adoption or on all aspects of infertility. Now that she is on Resolve's referral list, she is likely to have a steady stream of clients whose concerns are familiar and interesting to her.

One of the dilemmas that Resolve faces is that its members spend more time as recipients of services than as volunteers because of their personal needs. Nora comments on this:

It's always been a volunteer organization, but volunteers really were not spending very much time volunteering, so it's tough to get into a support group. Six months later they call you, which is not really servicing the program. Now [a few years later] I don't know how that end of it is working, but I know the parts I'm involved in, people volunteer a lot of hours for a long time. It's very professional.

For those who do volunteer their services for Resolve, the work often resembles a paid job. Women often view their participation as a form of reciprocity: giving back time to the organization, after they have conceived or adopted a child, in return for the help they have received. Women often stay in Resolve as active volunteers for several years. Women like Frances, whose professional careers become tied to the organization, stay with Resolve and develop a mutually beneficial arrangement. These women form the stable base for the organization that has enabled it to survive the turnover of volunteers and become increasingly powerful over time.

Women who do not have children, or a professional interest in infertility, drop out, however, usually at the point when they decide to give up trying to have a child. They find it too painful to be childless and remain in an organization in which almost everyone eventually becomes a parent. The membership of such an organization is therefore in a continuous state of change.

BECOMING POWERFUL

New social movements have distinctive forms of engagement with science.[13] Although Resolve's priorities may shift over time, a current focus is to influence the way in which medical care is delivered.[14] Resolve is concerned with issues such as ethics, how treatment is represented to patients, the cost of treatment, and other aspects of treatment. Pauline describes one way in which Resolve tries to influence the delivery of care:

Now I'm volunteering for Resolve, setting up panels with these other women. What our goal is, putting doctors on a panel so they can't hide behind their credentials. You know, "Let the buyer beware." Like, in an IVF panel with four competitive doctors together, we will structure it so they cannot just list their statistics. We will give them the questions beforehand, and they will be very specific. Like, "How many cycles did you start?" And, "Of those cycles, how many reached retrieval?" And, "Of those retrievals, how many reached pregnancy?" And, "Of those pregnancies, how many had a baby?" . . .

It's really interesting. Because usually they'll give you statistics. And the other doctors on the panel will call them on things. They'll have questions, "What is that you're looking for?" "Who's a candidate for IVF?" One doctor will have his opinion and another doctor will say. . . . But physician sensitivity is also something that we're acutely aware of. Because all of us have gone through infertility, and all of us know what it was like. We know which doctors are frauds or jerks, and which ones are nice. Notes are compared. We are in a position where we hold them up [physicians] in front of people and let them display their true colors, and we don't have to spread the gossip. We let them show the audience themselves, and so it's a wonderful opportunity. I really enjoy it . . . the awareness meetings.

I really enjoy taking part in it because it is done from that position. We want to educate the public in something that we're very interested in. Because we want people to not have to go through what we went through. So it's really neat. I think community service is so important.

Pauline emphasizes that these undertakings represent more than a community service: they constitute a political process, a concerted attempt to reshape medical treatment to make it more responsive to patients. They raise questions about who controls the treatment process. Resolve clearly does not control the activities of physicians, but consumer action in this particular geographic area has strongly influenced reproductive health services. Because the organization has grown so large, its power is considerable. Because it is a primary source of physician referrals for people seeking medical treatment, it has the power effectively to censure physicians whose practices do not meet with its approval by leaving them off the referral lists and not inviting them to participate in meetings and symposia. Physicians therefore make efforts to comply with Resolve's standards. Physicians may also be sanctioned informally, by word of mouth, as Resolve members have literally hundreds of contacts with whom they can discuss the pros and cons of specific practices. This kind of information can have a significant effect on the number of people seeking the services of a particular health professional in a competitive marketplace.

Resolve takes the same stance with others who provide services, such as those working in the adoption industry. Adoption services have expanded enormously in the last ten years in this geographic area, resulting in increased competition and, occasionally, questionable practices. Persons working in this industry are subject to sanctions by Resolve in the same way that physicians are. The majority of those working in the adoption industry in this geographic locale worked closely with Resolve and made efforts to conform to Resolve's principles, and consequently they had not only a forum for demonstrating their abilities but a steady stream of referrals as well. Many people in this study stated that they had selected a particular adoption professional because that person was recommended by Resolve. But when couples heard of people in this industry who got results despite questionable practices, they would sometimes enlist such a person to find them a child. Lois described working with an adoption counselor who had been sanctioned by Resolve: "It was a great adoption. It was really very, very easy. [Name] was a great birth mother. We found her through [Name], who was certainly on the shit list at Resolve. Resolve won't use her. Our attorney referred us to her. There was considerable unhappy stuff with her, but she did ultimately find us a child."

Lois's comment indicates not only how Resolve may influence referrals but also the limitations of their censure. Lois and her husband used a particular adoption counselor because of their attorney's referral, and they experienced some of the problems that others complained about. But they persisted with her even after they learned about Resolve's stance. Although the desire for the chosen outcome often overrides the organization's judgments about a particular service provider, most people are responsive to these efforts to control service delivery.

Eddie and Phyllis, interviewed shortly after their first attendance at a large-scale symposium, were enthusiastic about this kind of educational experience. Eddie commented:

You pay $100 to look into an infertility specialist's eyes and hear him talk. You go to the symposium, and on different panels you get to see all the Who's Who. We had heard all their names, and we had seen some of them, but they were the Who's Who. In fact, three of them were on one panel and they started fencing with each other about their statistics. So you got to see how they interacted and stuff. It really helped us jell our ideas about things.

Phyllis continued, "About what kind of a doctor we wanted and everything. What we want. . . . After the symposium Eddie is more open to adoption than he ever was before. Just working through some of his emotional stuff." Resolve's ability to bring about changes through education illustrate how resistance can be creative and transformative on a group level as well as an individual level.[15]

Advocacy efforts in Resolve are undertaken in response to current policy issues. Efforts to influence local, state, and federal legislation and policies range from letter-writing to lobbying and may include occasional appearances by national representatives of Resolve at congressional hearings. At one point in the study, national health care reform was under serious consideration. Lois reported her indecision about writing a letter on this topic:

They keep telling us in Resolve to write letters to Hillary Clinton and I haven't. And the reason I haven't is that I am very ambivalent about saying, "Make this part of national health care." To me it is not a priority, as a general policy to be spending money, for the federal government to be spending money on infertility to me is like . . . I have not written to her and said, "Please cover this." I am very mixed about that, but I haven't written because I just . . . it is not what I think this health care coverage should be covering for people. I think it should cover basic care. For me, this is luxury care in some ways, at least some of it. For me, it certainly was. I don't feel comfortable with IVF. I think there are certain diagnostic procedures that it should cover, but for IVF I don't really think it should. What about those people who just need basic medical care? If that is going to take away from people's basic medical care, then I think that can't be . . . I don't know.

Although Lois remained indecisive about this particular issue, many people are prepared to participate in letter-writing campaigns for Resolve. Increased national attention to "family building," including the endorsement of adoption by the Clinton family, is one indication of the success of Resolve's lobbying efforts to make adoption better accepted.

Organizations such as Resolve illustrate the importance of identity politics in contemporary U.S. society as a vehicle for action and as a way to resist institutional forces. Resolve provides people with a collective focus and offers a collective way of working on issues of individual difference. Resolve also represents ideological concerns and frames its policies around those concerns, seeking to modify cultural dialogues to better accommodate its members. As we have seen, however, women and men do not necessarily subscribe to all the principles the organization supports. While people sometimes reframe their views to reflect those of the organization, they may remain resistant to social pressure to do so.

CHAPTER 7

Selling Hope

Women and men equate new reproductive technologies with hope. As this message is the cornerstone of marketing new reproductive technologies, it is quickly appropriated and absorbed. Polly describes the intensity of its effect:

To go through in vitro to start with, you have to believe in miracles. You really do. Your chances are this much in this much space [indicating a limited space with her hand], so each time I go through that. And then I've talked to my girlfriends who were in my personal support group about this, my Resolve support group, and we've become friends and we really talk about this a lot. We agree that each time [each IVF cycle] you pretend, you know, "I could be in that 15 percent, I could be in that 20 percent, it's going to be me this time," and it's such a bunch of bullshit. But you have to do that or you wouldn't . . . you have to lie to yourself or you have to hope for the best or imagine that possibility or you wouldn't even be wasting your thousands and thousands of dollars to try, so it's just a wretched combination of trying to find the balance between fantasies and dreams and reality and wanting to be positive thinking. But not wanting to get your hopes up so that the crash is really hard.

There is a widespread belief in the United States in the power of technology to cure. Its failures undermine the explanations by which people make sense of the world. Cultural assumptions that life is orderly are thrown into disarray.[1] When this happens, people are challenged to search for answers to situations they never imagined, situations that are out of synchrony with their expectations and previous experiences. The people in this study believed, like Polly, in the importance of maintaining a hopeful attitude. Hope is closely associated with American notions of individualism and responsibility for health. Both lay and medical literature attests to the importance of maintaining a hopeful attitude in taking charge of one's illness, and the propensity for optimism is reflected in medical practice.[2] In the field of reproductive technology, hope has become part of the process of commodification, a marketing tool.

Persistence, too, has been appropriated in this way. It has been emphasized by the biomedical science establishment and the medical technology industry.[3] Persistence, one means by which people attempt to control their environment, is demonstrated by those seeking medical solutions for a wide range of conditions.[4] In the United States, doing nothing is equated with a failure to take responsible action, whereas doing *something* is viewed as taking action to better one's own situation. Losses tend to loom larger than gains in most people's decision making, and, consequently, the prevention of regret through persistence is central to decisions to use medical technology, suggesting that people want to prevent negative feelings later on that may result from a wrong choice.[5] Indeed, the themes of hope and persistence appear in a wide range of marketing techniques, from drug advertisements aimed at infertility specialists to the ways in which success rates are represented.

Although socialization to being an infertility patient begins slowly, it soon picks up speed. Preceding the decision to try IVF, a woman may have spent three months to a year undergoing a relatively noninvasive office procedure, intrauterine insemination, or IUI (see glossary). Her last several cycles of IUI may have been accompanied by treatment with human menopausal gonadotropins (hMG), which requires daily intramuscular injections and costs between $1,000 and $3,000 per cycle. A laparoscopy, outpatient surgery to look at the condition of the pelvis and fallopian tubes, may be performed along the way. IVF becomes the final step by default, because other, less invasive, less expensive treatments have not worked. Primed by exploratory surgery and by exposure to these drugs, women and men may take the shift to IVF in stride, especially now that ultrasound-aided egg retrieval precludes the need for surgery. A long period of acclimatization to the idea usually precedes couples undertaking IVF: typically, they weigh the pros and cons of these treatments as they count down the number of cycles remaining in their pre-IVF treatment plan and assess their financial resources.

Polly comments:

No matter what happens, after they do that embryo transfer, I mean, you can't help but hope. I mean, the second time we did it, I remember going in saying, "I'm totally cool about this. I'm just going to assume the worst, I'm going to assume I'm not pregnant. I'm just going to kill some time until I can take my pregnancy test and I'm going to go about my life as though there's nothing happening." But I'll tell you, the week before, I was getting my pregnancy test on a Friday and we started that Monday. It was like this countdown that took place without my even having any control over it. And everyday I got closer, I just got more and more anxious over it, and it just, that kind of subconscious stuff has a mind of its own, literally. I mean, it just keeps going on without you, no matter how much you want to say, "No, no, no, stay down there, I don't want to believe." You go through it, and it's just an emotional nightmare. Just an emotional nightmare.

Polly's entire account is dominated by her efforts to temper hope, yet her discussions with her friends who are going through the same process demonstrate how talking with other women may help to keep hope alive. She juxtaposes the belief in miracles with her initial attempts at detachment, trying to balance her fantasies and dreams with reality, while trying to remain positive.

Polly has done four cycles of IVF. Without her mother's help, she would not have been able to afford IVF at all. She describes the emotional toll it has taken:

We did two successful [cycles where she went through entire process but did not conceive]. I had two cycles where I ovulated before he could retrieve the egg, which was very upsetting, very upsetting.[6] And then I did two cycles where he did retrieve an egg. One time totally nonstimulated and one time with Clomid. Which was an interesting experience. It just made me crazy. You know, and it was Christmas time. It was the holidays. He [physician] just could not have picked a worse time. I was just driven to do this. I could have said, "Okay. Let's wait a few months." But, I didn't. "No, no, no. I've got to do this. I'll get it done. I've got to go." You know, so I did, literally, I

*think I did—in five months I did four cycles! In five months! I just
didn't want to stop until it was done.*

Polly is so socialized into this process that she refers to completed
cycles as successful even though they did not result in a pregnancy. This
measurement of success is one indication of the insidious nature of patient professionalization.[7] Women's expectations become skewed; the
mere completion of a cycle becomes a positive and encouraging achievement. Indeed, plans for subsequent cycles of IVF often hinge on completed cycles because women are spurred on by having experienced a
measure of success. The completed cycle leads people to hope that the
next cycle will result in a pregnancy. Polly continues:

*I think it came to about $12,000. Each cycle . . . For the whole thing.
But my insurance, I lied to my insurance company and they paid for
some of it. They paid for certain parts of it and my mom has actually
been paying . . . I mean, she kind of gave us an allowance and . . .
I spent it wisely and got as much reimbursement as I could and cut
back wherever I could, you know, with medical costs. She basically
sprung for it, so it hasn't cost us anything, yet. And right now we've
got $5,000 on deposit with [physician] towards the final cycle, which
is the donor cycle, which is the final cycle.*

Her husband, Colin, interjects, "That's the last time we'll do it." Polly
concludes, "And that's it."

Asked how they came to that decision, Colin replied, "Enough's
enough. You could go on and on and on. It's also money. I mean, it cost
a lot."

Polly concluded, "For me it's, um, the decision was all that, plus a
limit to the emotional stress I could put myself under. For what I'm
not sure is a payoff I'm willing to continue putting myself through hell
for."

It emerges that Polly weighs the emotional stress of undergoing IVF
at least as heavily as she weighs the cost. Although Colin points to the
limitless nature of IVF, Polly realizes she is reaching her emotional limit
and needs to stop. That Polly's mother pays for her treatment demonstrates a trend in reproductive medicine: potential grandparents are as
much consumers of these technologies as are their children. They are
purchasing the hope of future generations to succeed them.

Waiting endlessly for a pregnancy while trying to remain hopeful
takes its toll. Despite the emotional exhaustion they reported, women

stayed in treatment because it continued to symbolize hope. Each new treatment or physician brought renewed hope.[8] Because of their deep sense of responsibility for a pregnancy, the majority of women were unable to seriously consider nonmedical options, such as adoption or childless living, until they had exhausted the medical possibilities. IVF was thus viewed as a last-ditch effort to conceive, into which couples put great emotional energy. IVF offered their last hope for a biological child.[9]

Jennifer, a DES daughter, has patiently gone through years of infertility treatment. She took her time in opting for IVF. Indeed, each time I had previously visited her, she recounted failed cycles and ended by saying, "If nothing else works, we will do IVF." Now, on my last visit, she had done one cycle of IVF: "I think all along it has been IVF, IVF, IVF. Although each time when things have not worked, and as I got closer to having to do IVF, it was like IVF is still only 20 percent [effective]. That is certainly better than these others [treatments] that are 2 percent, or 10 percent, or whatever they say. But 20 percent is not a guarantee, or a 50 percent, or anything."

Like many others, Jennifer reports how she has rationalized trying IVF—by looking at the odds.[10] Even though the odds are only 20 percent that she will conceive, she compares them with other, unidentified treatments that have poorer odds. This view of IVF, as a possibility not to be ignored, has kept her going.

Some practitioners attempt to regulate use of new reproductive technologies by limiting them to those in whom they are most likely to succeed. The majority of practitioners in this geographic area are viewed as maintaining a measured approach to the use of such technologies: their programs test and evaluate patients extensively before admitting them to an IVF program, offering less expensive options when they are seen as appropriate. Practitioners attempt both to provide patients with appropriate care by offering IVF only to those who will not succeed with less expensive treatment and to keep their IVF success rates high by discouraging patients with a poor prognosis.

Hope escalates as couples wait to see if they have qualified for an IVF program.[11] Assessments of the odds escalate as well. Leslie's comments suggest that people err on the side of optimism in considering IVF. She says of her discussions of IVF with her husband: "My husband, being male, was more statistical about it than I was and kept bringing up the fact that 70 percent [of IVF cycles] don't work, and I kept thinking, 'But somebody's got to be in the other 30 percent. Why not us?' " In fact,

Leslie's estimate is high. The national average percentage of IVF cycles that produce a viable pregnancy is closer to 20 percent than 30 percent.[12]

The very inaccessibility of new reproductive technologies helps to create their allure. Leslie reported, "When we finally passed all the tests and jumped through all the hoops to be able to enter the IVF program, we joked about it, "You mean, I get to give you my money?" I was so excited. Although it didn't work, it gives such hope for a short period of time." Her husband, Stan, concurred. Having borrowed money to undergo this cycle of IVF, which subsequently failed, he remarked, "What they're really in the business of doing is selling hope to people, people who otherwise wouldn't have had the dream of having a biological child." Leslie agreed: "It's hard not to get caught up in it—each little thing that happens, each little test that you do well on, you get sucked into this hope. You've never seen two people happier about writing a $7,500 check than we were." The cultural ideology of biological parenthood drives such last-ditch efforts. Leslie delineates how the entire process thus becomes skewed as she talks about her excitement about being permitted to write a check with borrowed funds when the tests indicate she and her husband qualify for the program. Thus, the very inaccessibility of IVF helps to create its attraction. The harder it is to undertake, the more desirable it becomes.

When the time actually arrived and she went through the procedures, however, Leslie began to see IVF in a different light.

I met another woman who was one day behind me on all the procedures, so I kept seeing her and we started talking. We went through a lot of the process together. And then I went back for my embryo transfer, to have them put back. Actually, it was exciting because you still had hope at that point. We had embryos and we were putting them back, and, you know, you want to name them as they go in, so that day was kind of an upbeat day for us.

But the staff was upset, and because they knew this woman was a friend of mine, they told me they had retrieved fourteen eggs and they didn't have a single one that fertilized. And when the nurse told me this, she said, "The worst part is, this is her second IVF attempt." She got pregnant with a set of twins the first time, had an amnio [amniocentesis], got an infection from the amnio, and lost the twins at twenty weeks.[13]

And when I heard that, I thought, "This is like a house of horror chambers." I mean, I felt like this is insane, and I don't want to do

*this again. I've had friends tell me that they wouldn't want to be in
my position because medical science can almost offer you too many
options. That it gave you . . . that the hope was there, and it was hard
to let go of all those things they can offer you. I had heard of women
who did IVF nine times. I mean, you're talking a minimum of
$10,000 each time, and God knows how many years that takes.
I think it gets almost unhealthy.*

In recounting her experience with IVF, Leslie recounts how upbeat
she initially felt about it: making a friend, then having viable embryos
to place back inside her, embryos she wanted to name because they had
become real children to her. Gradually, though, she came to see IVF
differently, first when she learned that her friend had lost twins, and
subsequently when she herself did not conceive. Referring to IVF as a
"house of horror chambers," her metaphor reveals the dark side of IVF,
when something initially thought to be wonderful is revealed to be complex and problematic. At that point she begins to view IVF as "insane"
because it offers too many options for her to make rational decisions
about it.

UNDERLYING CULTURAL ASSUMPTIONS ABOUT MEDICAL TREATMENT

At the outset, women and men seldom grasp the complexities of using
assisted reproductive technologies. They begin this phase of treatment
by expecting a straightforward course of treatment, starting with their
relationship to the physician. Roberta, thirty-seven years old, reflecting
on her own medical treatment, identified the general public's lack of
familiarity with intensive medical care as a factor contributing to the
difficulties involved:

*My experience with doctors . . . Dr. [name] was a very nice man, and
I appreciated his gentleness and his sincerity. I liked him a lot. What
happened is sort of the evolution of infertility. I realized that our experience with doctors is very limited. Usually, we consider them for
healing, and as the people that are going to take care of us when we're
sick. Because we haven't had a lifetime of illness or have been faced
with the fact that doctors can't always cure you, so I think most of us
go to doctors thinking they are going to cure us, and that's our usual
feeling when we go for infertility treatment. Through the evolution of
the process we realize that they may not be able to cure us. I think*

from my experience, by the time I was finished with my first episode
[of GIFT], I had a complete view of what a doctor's role was, and I
realized that with infertility, the science of infertility was really a
mark, and it was a fudge line mark and really didn't live up to what
I considered a doctor should do.

Roberta acknowledges a common phenomenon: patients expect medical care to cure them, and it is only over time that people realize a cure
may not occur. She is reflecting the disillusionment that becomes common as hopeful couples gradually realize the limitations of reproductive
medicine—and of medicine in general. People in the United States and
other industrialized countries have come to expect that medicine will
work miracles, a belief fostered by the medical profession, the media,
and supporting corporate interests. Physicians note that within the profession there is a tendency to rush new technologies into practice without
caution and discrimination and, consequently, a tendency to replace
proven conventional approaches with more expensive and technological
approaches that may not necessarily be more effective, such as replacing
CT scans with MRIs.[14] Paul McDonough notes that increasing competition for patients, demands for financial performance, and the need for
a "market edge" tempt even the most conscientious health practitioners
to select highly technological modes of diagnosis and therapy. These
modes may seem more legitimate to the public than to scientific peers,
raising the question of the extent to which the marketplace determines
practice patterns and may ultimately affect the direction of medicine.[15]
Once therapies receive public acceptance and become medically fashionable, they are difficult to pass over.[16]

Roberta has her own view of why the disparity is so great between
patients' expectations and the outcome: "The thing that was most striking to me was that they don't inform their patients. When they walk in
the door, they don't say, 'This might not work, and this isn't normal
practice, and really, even though you think this is a science, this is really
an art. There's a real good chance this is not going to work.' " Roberta
differentiates between the science of medicine and the art of medicine,
between "normal" practices and those that are not normal. She concludes that infertility treatment is more experimental than she had previously realized, a judgment with which many practitioners would concur. Infertility treatment is, if not in its infancy, perhaps in its
adolescence. The question of how much to explain to patients about the
experimental nature of fertility medicine is a perennial one, which is

made more complex by the strong desire of both patients and practitioners for these technologies to work.

Brian counters Roberta's statements with support for physicians' approach:

Well, the way they tell you that is by telling you what the success rate is, but that's sort of an indirect way of telling you. Because I think what they want to do is to fill you with as much optimism as possible so you can approach it with the kind of enthusiasm I think you need to approach it with. Because it's hard to get through. And if you approached it thinking, "Oh, it's probably not going to work, it's not going to work . . . ," I mean, it's hard enough to do anyway.

Brian, rationalizing the need for optimism on both sides, goes on to talk about why it is so important and how he views the procedure:

The first time [they did the GIFT procedure] I went into it with very high hopes. I went in with really high hopes, because I really wanted the problem to be resolved then and there. I really wanted it to be over with. At the time I was not sold on the idea of adoption. It seemed very foreign, and I thought, "God, I really want this to work so we don't have to adopt." I wanted the GIFT to work so I didn't have to become acclimated to the whole wide wonderful world of adoption, which meant dealing with a lot of unknowns, basically, and really sort of throwing the dice. When you have a biological child, you feel that you have some sort of control over the product because it contains your genes, your wife's genes, that's a certain extent of unknown quantity. You're going to have a kid kind of like you. But in the adoption process, you don't have a kid kind of like you because you don't have that link, so you don't really know what you're getting.

In expressing his preference for having a biological child, Brian is expressing another trend in the marketplace of reproductive medicine: the commodification of the biological child. This tendency is not surprising, given the expense of medical treatment. But treating the child as a product has powerful implications. Things have a social life. Even children, treated as things, can have a commodity phase. In some societies young women are treated as commodities that fetch a certain bride price. The potential child, with a price tag of $10,000 or more, may be treated as a commodity in medical treatment, especially because it remains an abstraction.[17] The treatment of the child as a commodity is made more complex still because of the inference that the child is a gift.

In Brian and Roberta's case, the use of a procedure referred to as GIFT (gamete intrafallopian transfer) renders the situation somewhat ambiguous, as the acronym accurately describes the medical procedure. The dual meaning of the letters is probably a coincidence that certainly didn't hurt when advertising the procedure, however. Gifts are a form of commodity.[18]

Brian's statement illustrates why new reproductive technologies have so much appeal in the United States. First, they provide consumers, at least initially, with a semblance of control over their situation.[19] Second, these technologies uphold the cultural ideology of the biological child and promise to replicate one's genetic makeup. Adoption is a less desirable option. Third, these technologies facilitate commodification, which provides people with a language for understanding and engaging with them: the language of consumer culture.

Although women and men may become caught up in the commodification process, ultimately they recognize what is most important—that if their goal is to become parents, they need to look at things differently. Roberta, returning to the central issue of how to become parents, concluded, "It took going through this process for us to realize that it doesn't matter where this child comes from." Interjecting their ultimate conclusion into this discussion brings it back to earth: going through this process enabled them to sort out what was and wasn't important to them. Biology stopped being important. After their unsuccessful effort to conceive, they turned to adoption.

PAYING FOR TREATMENT AND GAMBLING WITH IVF

New reproductive technologies, and indeed most infertility treatments, are usually excluded from insurance coverage. Despite the consumer pressure on insurance companies to cover these procedures, the insurance industry has in fact worked to reduce coverage for infertility treatment. The insurance industry maintains a low profile in social analyses of new reproductive technologies, even though it plays a significant role.

Consumers attempt to maximize the benefits of the insurance coverage they do have, and those efforts take time. Chuck describes how attitudes of infertility specialists may compound the problem:

What I think is really important for us to discuss is about the insurance industry practice towards this, acceptance or denial of it. We have found that first of all, doctors take a very gingerly approach to this, and they are a little bit standoffish, whereas the better doctors you get [referring to subspecialists for infertility treatment] won't even deal with the insurance. You have to pay before the services are rendered and that is it. Which is a little different from the way most doctors operate. So we have to submit these claims to the insurance company, and sometimes the doctors write it up so that the insurance company will take it, and sometimes they don't. It is like they are trying to hide from this, when that is just plain stupid. So when it really came to a head was when we switched over to [physician] and he is giving us advice about dealing with insurance. He said, "What you really need to do is get a copy of your company's policy, and if it is not specifically excluded, then it is included." That made a big difference, but no one ever suggested it before.

Lack of insurance coverage for IVF technologies limits use of these technologies to those who can pay for them and those few whose insurance does cover them. Because of the out-of-pocket expense, gambling metaphors, which are repeatedly used to characterize infertility treatment, pervade discussions of IVF, especially among people who borrow money to undertake it.

Nobody in this study considered in vitro fertilization affordable. No one had ready access to the funds needed to employ this technology. Thus IVF always entailed a sacrifice, such as constraining the couple's existing lifestyle, giving up contingency plans to adopt, or assuming large debts. That people repeatedly found ways around the financial constraints is a testament to the strength of the cultural ideology of biological parenthood and the related cultural imperative to use available technology.

Those who underwent IVF were primarily two-career couples who made over $60,000 per year. They cited various methods for raising the money, including saving, mortgaging homes, using credit cards, taking out bank loans, and borrowing money from friends and family members. For example, Eileen, forty years old, said,

Getting ready for IVF, we started living on my salary and saving John's in order to be able to pay for it. It was better for us psychologically to have the money and pay it off, and then if it didn't work, that money's gone. But some friends of ours put it on their credit cards. I said, "You guys are crazy!" They just didn't get the papers together soon enough for the credit line. They were working on it and they ran out of time. So they put it on their credit cards. I said, "You are out of your mind!" And she said, "Well, we thought about it and it's just easier to put it on the credit cards."

They were lucky it worked. Can you imagine paying off an IVF cycle that failed every month?

John and Eileen, preparing to try IVF again, this time with a donor egg, addressed their own situation:

EILEEN: *John says this is the first time we've ever been on the game board. We've been rolling the dice for four years and pretty intensively for me. I mean, all the tubal surgeries, all the invasive testing. Really [to husband], you haven't had to do that much. I mean, you had to support me, but for the physical stuff, and my job at risk, there's no question that I've borne the brunt of it. And I really want it to work.*

JOHN: *People that do this just roll the dice. We all do.*

EILEEN: *You would never do this in a business situation. You would never put down this much money on a 30 percent chance. Never. I mean!*

JOHN: *Not unless you had megabucks.*

EILEEN: *And you can't afford to lose it. But that's another thing with infertility and what it does to you. It does strange things to your perspective on what's worth spending money on and what's not.*

Eileen and John are attesting to their lack of control over the process and their feelings. They feel an obligation to make rational decisions, and the gambling metaphor gives them a context within which to rationalize their behavior.

Money for a single cycle of IVF often comes from multiple sources, as Russ explained: "I borrowed the money. This friend, many times over, has offered to loan us money. So when we didn't have enough money on our credit card, I asked her, and she said, 'I could do $3,000. Would that be enough?' That took a load off. And we went to the bank and filled out the forms for another credit line, just in case." Going to such lengths exacerbated women's and men's feelings of vulnerability because of the economic risks they were taking, and it heightened their sense that they were gambling. Julie, a forty-three-year-old woman, felt she had no other options because her partner did not want to adopt:

From what I can glean from the statistics, I have about a 5 to 10
percent chance of it working because of my age. It feels like we are
throwing away money, a lot of money, because we have no insurance
to pay for it. But I thought, "If I can't have a child, I won't look back
on this whole thing and say, 'Well, I didn't try that.'" So I felt good
about doing it, but I don't know where to set the limits. Here I am,
gambling with a very bad situation.

Sources of available funds also included family trust funds, outright gifts
from parents that were specified for IVF treatments, and inheritances.
One woman said, "My parents both died last year. Spending the money
I inherited on IVF to create a new generation feels like the right thing
to do."

EFFECTS OF MARKETING
ON CONSUMERS' ATTITUDES

Although programs in the study locale demonstrated a wide range of
approaches in their presentation of IVF as a potential treatment, when
one new practice began aggressively marketing new reproductive technologies, people's views of infertility treatment began to change. Although few people in the first study raised the issue of the financial gain
to practitioners engaged in medical treatment, attitudes shifted during
the second study from a view of IVF as part of medical treatment to IVF
as a business.

Those who utilize new reproductive technologies frequently question
whether practitioners' motives are primarily medical or financial. For
example, Leslie said, "I felt he was there to fulfill whatever wishes we
had, and yet I also felt in the beginning he was somewhat trying . . . I
mean, it's a business for them and they make money off it, and I felt he
was trying to sell us something." She revised her opinion after she did
one cycle of IVF:

At the post–in vitro session, after it failed, his final words to us were,
"You're the perfect couple for in vitro. If IVF were free and if it were
an easy process, I'd say keep doing it because sooner or later you're
going to get pregnant. But it's not, and that being the case, only you
can decide what to do next. I can't say that it would be a good thing
to do. Only you know that." So I didn't get the feeling, after all, that
he was trying to sell us.

As the market-oriented practice gained momentum during the first eighteen months of the study, all comparable programs in the area were affected. Increasing competition was demonstrated in an effort to maintain numbers of patients seen. Consumers in turn became increasingly uneasy and were often irate about the cost of care. Trust between physicians and patients was sometimes undermined as patients questioned whether money was being made at their expense. Consumers began to view medical practice as a business that profited from their hopes. For example, Jordan and Rebecca described how they scrutinized medical practices as they planned IVF:

JORDAN: *We got really smart. The IVF stuff makes you really smart, and you go through it. We got really demanding with our doctors, you know, asking them, "What's your gross profit?"*

REBECCA: *I don't know how smart that is. It's just that I'm mad they were making so much money. I mean, we became really smart consumers.*

JORDAN: *We're smart coming out of that thing, so we're smart consumers, but also because this is so newfangled that we checked out different ones [medical practices].*

When large amounts of money were at stake, men and women believed it was their responsibility to make informed choices rather than passively allow medical decisions to be made for them. Julie attested: "We're not being good consumers unless we check everything out. We're going to spend a lot of money. If it were anything else, we would ask questions, and shop around, and get a second opinion. And we should do the same for this."

People's views shift when they begin to see themselves primarily as consumers rather than as patients. Being a "good" or "smart" consumer emerges as a social responsibility. Being a consumer thus has a moral stance attached to it, and when consumer-patients address their positions as smart shoppers, their remarks are imbued with moral authority: in their own eyes, they are doing their part of the job by questioning the providers who supply the services.

Consumer choice is a private act that is ideologically out of bounds to public intervention. Don Slater observes that the privacy of individual choice seems to contradict social order, solidarity, and authority, and that this is a main preoccupation of critics of consumer culture.[20] But here we see consumers upholding what they consider to be their individual moral responsibility for the collective social good: challenging health professionals is one way to keep prices in check and get a quality product. This is an expression of individualism at work.[21] It is expressed in diverse spheres, such as individual values and social institutions that reinforce the importance of new reproductive technologies as well as the individual's right to exert pressure on them.

Viewing medical practice as a business had significant consequences for interactions between patients and physicians. People became mistrustful of physicians and were angered by what they viewed as the "salesmanship" of IVF and its underlying profit motive. For example, when the market-oriented program expanded into a nearby county, half-page advertisements appeared in local newspapers offering free consultations to persons seeking fertility services. One couple who responded to this ad reported that they became increasingly cynical during their interview with a physician when he asked them few questions about their medical history and instead talked about his IVF program. They referred to him as "Doc Hollywood."

People who experienced what they considered to be a "hard sell" expressed indignation and outrage, as Samantha did:

I brought my medical records with me. I knew that when I had a laparoscopy, my tubes were open. But his opinion was that my tubes were gnarly from abscess. Then he brought up IVF. I knew there was this baby in England, but I didn't know this procedure was available to us. I knew nothing about the infertile world. He gave me a tour of the clinic and set me up to get started for IVF, all in one hour. My head was spinning. I got to the front desk and she says, "That will be $75 for today's tests and $3,000 for the down payment for the IVF." I said, "Enough! I never heard of this technology before. Hold it! I will pay you for the blood work done today and I am out of here. I want to talk to my husband."

As time passed in exploration of IVF technologies, the hope for a pregnancy was offset by cynicism about physicians' intent. People's feelings of vulnerability intensified their anger and sense of desperation. Nevertheless, they remained hopeful, and sometimes returned for more information. Samantha did: "So we went back together and asked our questions. But I was thinking, 'He needs that money. He just opened this office. He has to pay his rent, his secretaries. This is a brand new building, a high rent district. This guy wants me in here.' I felt like I was at a used car dealership."

Once people experienced information about reproductive technologies as a sales pitch, they became suspicious of all practitioners. Not only did women and men become wary of the way information was presented, they also became suspicious of what was *not* said. Julie noted:

If we go to an egg donor clinic and ask them, "Should we do IVF again or should we do egg donor?" I know what they're going to say: they are going to say, "Do egg donor. We have a great program. We have a 50 percent success rate." They're not going to explain that that's out of a total of ten women. The only reason they did at this one clinic was because I asked specifically, "How many women? Could you tell me their ages?" The nurse told me, but she never once said, "This is a very low number, so statistically . . ." She never put it together for me. I still had to do it, so to me, it's like they are used car salesmen out there. You have to use your head and read and think to put it together.

When a competitive market has been created and abundant medical services are in place, generating enough patients to maintain a profit may lead to wholesale profiteering in the guise of medical treatment. Although women and men often lamented their lack of insurance coverage, the following example from the first study, of a rare instance where IVF coverage was mandated without adequate regulation in one state, suggests that the profit motive might still affect the quality of medical care should the insurance industry ease its stance on IVF. Noreen said, "My regular gynecologist said, 'You've got insurance; you are never going to have insurance like this again. Do it!' The IVF doctor we went to said, 'The more times you do it, the better your chances.' There were women in his office who were cycling nine or ten times, and I think that is unethical. But they bought into this thing. I bought into it, too. I really did." Jim, her husband commented,

The quality of care was deplorable. We weren't treated as patients at all but as consumers. We chose them because their statistics were the best, but they had this terrible way of showing it. They had this number in the waiting room of the number of pregnancies they had. Every time they had a pregnancy they came in and changed the number. I thought it was in terrible taste. In retrospect, I thought the whole

*treatment protocol was deplorable, that they should be shut down,
but that was hindsight. It was not a medical clinic. They were selling
a procedure. There was no concern for patients, like you expect to get
from a doctor. They were filling slots. Once all the slots were filled,
they brought in more folding chairs. After two cycles, we called this
place the "Cattle Farm."*

Although women and men expressed distrust and loss of respect for
some practitioners, they often persisted anyway. They continued to hope
that they would conceive if only they persevered. Noreen observed, "After acknowledging that it was the worst experience of my life, I decided
to do it again."

When we ask why new reproductive technologies are so compelling
and how they have captured the imagination of so many people, the
answer becomes clear: a wealth of cultural phenomena coalesce to create
and foster a desire for the new reproductive technologies. The dominant
cultural ideology of biological parenthood provides the underlying rationale for their use and is a mainstay of the moral economy surrounding
the new reproductive technologies. Although these technologies are tar-
geted at middle-class women and men who are viewed as productive
members of society, and thus as deserving of them, these consumers
express frustration and anger that they must nevertheless endure economic hardship and prove themselves economically worthy. They express dissatisfaction with a system that treats what they consider to be
a basic human right—the right to create a family—as an opportunity
for some to profit at others' expense.

At the same time that they demonstrate opposition to this system and
resist it, however, they feel compelled to utilize it in the quest for a child.
United States consumer culture emphasizes the privacy and rights of the
individual, giving primacy to issues of autonomy, choice, and freedom.
The cultural imperative to make use of available technologies in biomedical treatment draws on these same cultural tenets, specifically organized around notions of responsibility for health and control over the
environment (the body). These technologies are marketed primarily
through the cultural imperative to overcome adversity, the cultural
shorthand for which is "hope." Permeating these concerns are issues of
gender and patriarchal imperatives that shape the specific use of these
technologies. In the next chapter I show how gendered interests are central to the new reproductive technologies.

CHAPTER 8

Decisions about Donors

We were going to have these great kids, right? Why did it
have to be us? His sperm and my egg?

Judith, thirty-five years old

Of all the disruptions to bodily order that are posed by infertility treatment, the intimation that the sperm or egg is faulty is the most acute.
These are cultural icons of gender and fertility, symbols that epitomize
cultural ideals of manhood and womanhood.[1] When these symbols are
challenged, bodily knowledge is assaulted.

The proposal that a couple use an egg or sperm donor strikes at the
cultural meanings women and men attach to gender. The question arises
of how to enact gender when one of the key functions of biological
reproduction is being enacted for a person by someone else.

Until recently, donor gametes were used only in cases of male infertility, but in the mid-1980s a technique was developed in Australia that
enables specialists to remove eggs from a female donor, fertilize them,
and transfer the embryos to another woman. This procedure, commonly
referred to as "donor egg," has extended the potential for women to
conceive at later ages, even after menopause. A highly successful (and
very expensive) technique, donor egg has come into widespread use. In
contrast to donor insemination, in which the identity of the donor is
usually strictly concealed, the use of a donated egg is often characterized
by considerable openness.[2]

The use of donors illustrates how new reproductive technologies are
ideologically shaped by gender interests and how gendered patterns of
power and authority are reproduced through those technologies and the
policies that surround them. Everything germane to donor usage is in-

variably linked to gender-specific assumptions and expectations about what is considered natural. Helen, who conceived using a donated egg, explains why, in her view, donor egg and donor insemination are not equivalent and what underlying gender forces propel these differences:

With donor egg, while it's not my eggs, I get to be pregnant. Whereas with donor insemination, not only is it not his gamete but he doesn't have that "something else" to balance it out. So it creates the need to protect the man against his losses—it's even greater. I think these gender issues operate with ways of conception and the need to protect men from the stigma of infertility. If you look at the way infertility is talked about among average people, it is always talked about as if the woman can't get pregnant. She can't get pregnant. The defect is always ascribed to her regardless of the actual biological source of the infertility. Culturally, we've always been set up to protect men from the stigma of infertility.

As Helen observes, because infertility has traditionally been ascribed to women regardless of the actual source, men are protected from the stigma of infertility.[3] Cultural ideals about manhood revolve around assumptions of potency, and hence the need to protect men from such a stigma shapes the way in which sperm donation is handled. In societies in which descent is traced through both parents but children usually take the father's name, as in the United States, the use of a donor poses a cultural threat to patriarchal traditions.[4]

Helen also points out another distinction between the use of male and female donor gametes: she bears the child, even if it is not her egg, whereas the man contributes only through his sperm, and thus there is no other biological "cement" between male partner and child in the case of donor insemination. The issue of the male contribution to a pregnancy is indeed emotionally important to men who consider this option, but the main disincentive is the cultural expectation that men uphold the patriarchal status quo through their biological contribution to the creation of a child.

Because cultural ideals about manhood and womanhood are so entrenched in U.S. society, those ideals inevitably are reflected in the medical management of donor-assisted conceptions. Women and men receive different cultural messages about the use of donors, which are driven by patriarchal assumptions about nature. In a revealing study of Great Britain's Warnock Report (which established national regulations for the use of reproductive technologies), including interviews with its committee members, Erica Haimes found that assumptions about gender were embedded in the report itself and affirmed in committee members' interviews: semen donation was associated with "deviant" sexuality, while egg donation was associated with altruism. These characterizations symbolized deep-seated assumptions about what is natural, which became embedded in policy and lived out in practice.[5]

The use of donor gametes presents a challenge for men and women and the practitioners who provide these services. Moreover, it represents a challenge for society. Rethinking cultural dialogues surrounding donor gametes poses a threat to the status quo and destabilizes underlying cultural ideologies about gender.

CONSIDERING DONOR INSEMINATION

Until recently, donor insemination was the only medical procedure that allowed couples with male infertility to conceive.[6] This treatment, in use for over forty years, is relatively inexpensive and straightforward, and is one of the most common infertility treatments currently available (see glossary, "Male infertility").[7] Insemination typically occurs in a practitioner's office, although it can also be done at home. If the procedure takes place in a medical setting, the donor is usually anonymous.

Because this treatment uses donor sperm, it challenges cultural ideals about manhood, fatherhood, and genetic continuity. Many men are completely unwilling to use a donor because they consider it unnatural. Asked how he felt about it, David said:

I didn't really know why it bothered me. I still don't know completely why. But it just felt wrong at a gut level base. An emotionally negative response. Like, "You don't like spinach but you don't know why you don't like spinach. Because it doesn't taste good in your mouth." So I think that part of it has to do with just feeling disconnected from the experience. Our relationship is based on equality, and I really felt like if she went with donor, then it would have been much more her experience than mine. Whereas with [the daughter they adopted], we've got a strong, equal relationship. Just like, genetically, she's neither of ours.

And part of it also is just, when I projected my family image into the future and how I relate to my child, I could deal better with it emotionally, for adoption maybe, because I understood it better and I was thinking that when she's a teenager, how will I relate to her?

I could think about the ways I could relate to an adopted baby, but as a donor child, it'd be real hard. It was just a blank. It was like I couldn't imagine what it would be like. So I didn't want that option. But at the beginning I hadn't really analyzed why I was so negative about it. It was like, "NO, NO, NO."

In this emotional statement David is expressing not only his distaste for substituting another man's genetic material for his own but also the issue raised by Helen, that of inequality of the male contribution. Believing that his relationship with his wife is based on equality, he assumes that a child conceived through donor insemination would not be equally "theirs"; it would be more his wife's child than his. Unable to be the genetic father, David opts for adoption so that the child will not belong genetically to either of them. When he looks into the future, he cannot imagine how to relate to a donor child, even as a teenager, so deep are his negative feelings about using a donor. The attitude that an adopted child would belong more equally to both parents than a child conceived through donor insemination was espoused by a number of women and men in this study. Women often stated they would prefer the use of a donor to adoption because they could experience pregnancy and childbirth. When men favored adoption over donor insemination, however, women usually deferred to their husband's feelings because they wanted above all to parent a child.[8]

Geraldine, David's wife, agreed to adoption because she wanted a child, but she had not yet relinquished her desire to experience pregnancy and childbirth by using a donor. Somewhat angrily she responded to David's comments:

I was real frustrated with that. Real frustrated, because I needed an explanation because I felt like he was just arbitrarily deciding on not paying attention to my needs at all. And just sort of arbitrarily saying, "I can't do this," when it seemed to me that it [using a donor] was the cheapest and easiest way to go and it was also a way in which I was able to have a pregnancy. Which is still very important to me.

Geraldine went on to say that although she felt positively about adoption and their adopted child, she eventually plans to experience pregnancy. Using a donor will be the only way unless they attempt IVF using intracytoplasmic sperm injection (ICSI—see glossary). Men in this study who reacted as strongly to donor insemination as David did were unlikely to change their minds and agree to use donor insemination. David and Geraldine's decision against using a donor is one example of how patriarchal ideologies are upheld. David avoids dealing with the issues faced by men who decide to use a donor and thus protects himself from the stigma of infertility.[9]

For men who are trying to avoid using a donor, ICSI now offers an alternative, albeit an expensive one. Successful treatment enables men to uphold cultural ideologies about manhood and fatherhood by using their own genetic material. Since this procedure was first introduced in the United States, there are indications that the rate of donor insemination has dropped off dramatically for couples in which the man has a low sperm count.[10] Its popularity is one example of how new reproductive technologies challenge more straightforward, simpler technologies that have good success rates, such as donor insemination, at the same time that they maintain the status quo by emphasizing the cultural importance of biology.

Steven reported on his attempt to conceive a biological child using micromanipulation (a direct microscopic fertilization technique used prior to the development of ICSI):

The doctor had mentioned to me in passing something called micromanipulation, and just about the same time I saw a little article in the paper about micromanipulation. They manipulate the woman's eggs by drilling in the zona to facilitate the sperm penetrating, and there actually are experiments with microinjection. Where they put the sperm in the egg. So one of my ways of coping with it was just to get it to work, you know, figuring out what can we do about this, and there aren't a lot of places to do micromanipulation. So if there was a micromanipulation program interested in taking us, we were interested in trying one more time. We have health insurance which actually covers two IVF cycles. Very generous. So we clearly wanted to take advantage of that. Even before we did the first IVF, we knew that I had bilateral varicoceles [see glossary]. The doctor felt that they had no factor on my fertility and advised against wasting the time and money and psychic energy to have the surgery. But after the failed fertilization I did have a varicoelectomy or whatever it's called to remove them in the hope that would improve my sperm quality. It was not bad. Really. It's a fairly innocuous surgery. It's done on an outpatient basis.

So we went ahead with the IVF. Anne provided very nice eggs. Twelve of them. And on top of that the doctor said that her endome-

trial lining is really nice. He said that the welcome mat was out. So that was nice, and twelve eggs is a good number, and I gave my sperm sample, and when the call came we had agreed that I would take the call. We didn't really expect very much. You know, you always hope against hope, but we didn't expect very much. And on Friday the doc called to say that none of the eggs had fertilized, that there was zero fertilization. And that what they do is leave the eggs and the sperm together, and there is a slight chance that there would be delayed fertilization. Even though I had really expected that call, I was just really knocked for a loop. Because it was more final than the first time. I crawled over there and just wept, and then I went upstairs and told Anne. And she didn't have a lot of emotional response at the time. With the first news she was beside herself. This time she was . . . stoic is not the right word. I think numb is probably the more correct word.

So with that failed fertilization the second time, the realities are pretty stark.

In telling his story of finding a new treatment for his infertility and pinning his hopes to it, Steven described how he went about it like a job: finding the right medical practice and having elective surgery to enhance the chances of success. But when it didn't work, he despaired, as the last possibility of having a biological child was removed. He concluded:

When my sperm failed to fertilize any of Anne's eggs, that came as a real shock to us. When the doctor called and said we had no fertilization and that there was clearly a severe male factor, we knew that there was a male factor, but we didn't realize how severe. So, basically, he said, that the chances are zero. Almost absolutely no chance of us having a child together with my sperm. And so, obviously, we were both devastated. Very devastated. It was a very devastating period. After my first shock, my own reaction was, "Well, there's got to be a way." The chances are very slim that we could ever have a child of our own, and that is an important thing for us to begin accepting, and it's very difficult for us to accept. And it brings us to donor insemination.

Steven tries to accept this outcome as final. One medical option remains, that they use a donor to conceive, in which case his wife would be the biological parent and he would be the social parent. Relinquishing the desire to be a biological parent after so much energy has been invested is usually a gradual process. Although some couples turn to donor insemination without much delay, it may take others a year or more.[11]

Typically, men and their partners learn about donor insemination in a roundabout way. With the exception of those who happened to consult a urologist or an infertility specialist who was an advocate for donor insemination, men in this study reported that urologists often did not mention donor insemination in discussing their infertility. Physicians thus are in the position of gatekeepers, with the ability to limit their patients' knowledge of available medical procedures. All physicians have opinions and are more favorably disposed toward some treatments than others. But donor insemination stands out as a procedure about which physicians may be particularly diffident, and their attitudes limit people's access to the procedure. Moreover, starting in the 1980s more constraints have been placed on the use of fresh donor sperm. These have tended to enhance the development of sperm banks as a business and lengthen the treatment process.[12] Although the use of frozen sperm results in an appreciable increase in the cost of treatment, a significant decline in both cycle fecundity and three-month life-table pregnancy rates, and an ethically troubling enhancement of physician income as a direct result of the diminished efficacy of treatment, almost all practitioners follow guidelines set by the American Society of Reproductive Medicine in 1988, which recommend the use of frozen sperm to eliminate the extremely slight risk of HIV contamination. Despite a risk-benefit analysis indicating that the risk of HIV infection using fresh sperm is almost nonexistent given specific screening techniques, this policy has not been altered.[13] Moreover, people who are discouraged by the length of time it takes to conceive may be more likely to drop out of treatment or to move on to more expensive technologies.[14]

Reports from participants in the research describing their experiences with practitioners confirm that some practitioners are ambivalent about donor insemination. This was true both before and after the introduction of new reproductive technologies to treat male infertility.[15] In her study of attitudes about donor insemination and donor egg, Erica Haimes concluded that different criteria are applied to semen and egg donation based on a view of the family that has motherhood as its centerpiece and that is assumed to be heterosexual, patriarchal, and nuclear. While the donation of semen was sexualized by her respondents, the donation of eggs was seen as asexual. She thus demonstrated how practices such as egg and semen donation are gendered and built around

cultural assumptions about male and female roles in reproduction.[16] The
perceived dissimilarities lie in issues of paternity, sexuality, and, ultimately, patriarchy.

Donor insemination is an example—possibly one of the most blatant
examples—of the politicization of reproductive technologies. As donor
insemination has become more complex for the practitioner, other reproductive technologies have become easier to offer and certainly more
lucrative. This emphasis on other reproductive technologies further marginalizes donor insemination as a treatment option. Sean's experience
exemplifies the difficulty many people in this study described in gaining
access to donor insemination:

*I saw a urologist, and he ordered a semen analysis. And it turned out
that I had no sperm. None. Which was a big surprise. The doctor
wasn't all that sympathetic. He said, "Some guys think that they have
to have children to have some kind of eternal life. You don't think
that, do you?" And I said, "No, but I would like to have children."
And he said, "I understand that, but there is nothing else I can tell
you. That is all." And we left it at that. Six months later I called him
back. He said that there could be other analyses done. He recommended a testicular biopsy, so I had that. They found the same thing,
no sperm cells or anything. He didn't ever talk to me about possibilities. He was very clear that medical science knows nothing about it.
He had no analysis as to whether it was an injury or an illness or a
birth defect. I would like to know. We talked to my mother about it.
She was always informed of what we were doing, and she is very interested.*

*So then the summer after that, we saw an advertisement for an in-
fertility seminar and went to that and there was absolutely no talk
about male infertility. Which was disappointing. But we found out
some of the other possibilities. It was put on by a hospital or attached
to a clinic, or something. We found out about it [donor insemination]
through an advertisement. After that, we spent most of our time
thinking about it and talking about it and not really taking much
action.*

Sean's experience is not unusual. Men routinely reported encounters
with urologists and other practitioners in which this treatment for male
infertility was never mentioned.

Men like Jim, who had been searching for treatment possibilities for a long time and belatedly learned about donor insemination, were often prepared to move quickly:

But once we found out that donor insemination was an option, it all happened pretty quick. We did it the next cycle. We found out that I didn't penetrate any hamster eggs on Christmas Eve [suggesting that further efforts to conceive with his sperm would be unsuccessful], and then we did the insemination on January 21. So, less than a month later we had gone through this process, got the donor information, and gotten the sperm.

While Jim moved fast because he and his wife had been in medical treatment for several years and had exhausted other possibilities, Sean and his wife took some months to make this decision:

We finally decided, we talked about using donor sperm. For a while we talked about using my brother, who is a year younger, and I thought that would be nice. We sort of decided on that. We talked to him about it, and he was very supportive.

Then we decided to make an appointment for a consultation to use donor sperm. And that doctor was very supportive, but not about the idea of using live sperm. She said her clinic would not do an insemination with live sperm at all. And she wasn't eager to use a known donor. Which made us think a little bit more. She referred us to a counselor who we didn't ever go see. But we started talking to more people. We talked to Lydia's father, for example. It is interesting that he is from a very traditional society [in Eastern Europe] but he was really, really supportive, and all through this has been. He said that in the future all babies will be born that way, anyway. He is a believer in science, but he also said that it was too complicated a thing for us to involve my brother. So we went ahead: we had several visits with the doctor and lab tests for Lydia. And on the first insemination she became pregnant, and that was just a month and a half ago.

The speed with which Lydia conceived with donor sperm is testament to the relative effectiveness of this practice: the cumulative success rate for donor insemination is usually better than 50 percent. In the past it was estimated that four times as many children were conceived annually through donor insemination as through the combined practices of IVF, GIFT, zygote intrafallopian transfer, and ICSI today.[17]

Gus, who knew about donor insemination before he learned of his own infertility, was not troubled by the use of a donor. He was able to proceed quickly because he saw that decision as separate from dealing with his own infertility. In this story he explains the gains and losses that donor insemination has entailed for him:

There was no hesitation. It was almost like that was the starter gun going off when I failed the test the second time and it was like, "Okay, this sets our course. Now we know what to do—we'll try donor insemination, and if that doesn't work, then we'll do this next thing. . . ."

So I made the decision to do donor insemination immediately, but that was for me a separate issue from dealing with the fact that I was infertile. It was very easy for me to separate those issues. One issue was, "How do we have children?" And it became very clear that donor insemination would allow us to have children and would allow Sharon to become pregnant and give birth to a baby. And that was a totally separate issue from me having to deal with the fact that I was infertile. The hardest part for me to deal with was that I wouldn't be able to give a biological contribution to my son or children. I think that's the thing that I had to come to terms with. I think that was the most difficult thing to have to come to terms with. And it was underscored by being a biology major. For periods of my life the story of evolution was very important to me, and so it was somehow from the school of irony that I had to come to terms with the fact that I couldn't contribute to the biological heritage of my children.

Gus was able to separate his feelings about his infertility from the question of "How do we have children?" This is a first step in moving toward donor insemination. When men are able to separate these issues, they are usually able to consider the prospect of donor insemination in a positive manner. Gus was very clear from the start that donor insemination was a means to an end: his wife would be able to experience pregnancy and childbirth, which were important to her. He was thus able to put aside patriarchal issues about paternity. Nevertheless, he acknowledges the cultural importance of the biological link between father and child, as it signifies what is "natural" for men:

I think one of the reasons I didn't have a great difficulty with the decision to do donor insemination was that I didn't really have a strong sense that my fertility was somehow tied up with my manhood. There was certainly a little of that. I think that it's probably pretty natural to feel that, just as Sharon felt that for her to be pregnant and have a child confirms her womanhood. It wasn't really a strong overpowering feeling that somehow I wasn't a man if I couldn't get my wife pregnant, and that if I couldn't do it, by God, nobody would! I felt a loss, I felt sad and frustrated and upset that I couldn't do it, and as I say, perhaps the hardest thing to get a hold of, to come to terms with, was not being able to give a biological contribution.

Cultural ideals about manhood are intimately bound up with cultural ideals about fertility and related issues, such as sexual prowess. Gus points to a parallel set of cultural assumptions for womanhood that affect his wife. He acknowledges his sense of loss and frustration in being forced to give up the cultural ideal, but he is able to do it. Gus focuses on the child that he will father:

But once you have your child, you enumerate the traits that characterize your child. And you sort of assess them. You just don't do that and think blissfully, "Well, if only . . ." You just look at your child, you love him to death, and that's all there is to it. But, of course, we didn't quite know that, then. While Sharon was pregnant I felt left out. I felt kind of like an outsider. And that was real hard for me to take because Sharon really wanted me to be closely involved with the pregnancy and to listen to the little heartbeat and to the kicking, and I did, but I just didn't feel a connection with it. And so I felt, at times, kind of disappointed that I didn't feel any real closeness to this particular baby. But the moment he was born those feelings just disappeared and were replaced with joy.

Men who opt for donor insemination often have a sense of disconnectedness during their wife's pregnancy: they are working to give up the cultural expectation that men uphold patriarchy through their biological contribution. Gus's response to the birth of his child was the same as that of almost every other man in this study who decided to use a donor: with the birth of the child, feelings of loss were replaced by joy.[18]

CHOOSING A DONOR

One reason men and women may find the selection of a donor appealing is that they can control certain aspects of the process. Matching the donor with the social parent, both physically and educationally, is very reassuring, whether or not the couple plans to acknowledge the use of a donor publicly. Controlling for similar characteristics in donors makes the process much more acceptable. Donor programs therefore work to select donors who will be physically compatible with the prospective parents. Asked how they chose their donor, Jim and Lani responded:

JIM: *Well, one of the things that we chose was what he did for a living . . .*

LANI: *He was still at school.*

JIM: *Right, he was still at school but a lot of the people were really science- and math-oriented and this person was as well, but there was also a lot of artistic stuff.*

LANI: *So, that was really one of the most attractive things, aside from the fact he had dark wavy hair. His eye color matched and his height and weight matched. His ethnic background matched.*

Mara and Keith had similar concerns:

We agreed we wanted the person to be biologically as much like Keith as possible. And in terms of his racial, ethnic, and also nationality background, and all that. And I think that we sort of discovered as we did it [the selection process] that we really had a bias for somebody smart. I don't think we would've said that when we started, but we kept wanting to rule out people with only four years of college education. We kept looking for people with seven or eight years of [college] education, even though we know most of the donors were in school and were doing this to help finance their education.

In their reports of the selection process, couples invariably emphasize finding a donor who is smart and attractive and shares certain attributes of the social parent. From the couple's perspective, such a selection is not only desirable but also gives them a sense of control. Although in the past practitioners usually picked the donor for the couple, relying on their own judgment of who would be physically complementary, current practice almost exclusively utilizes commercial sperm banks that provide details about donors and allow couples to choose. This shift in practice has contributed to the commodification of donor gametes. Very occasionally, couples who want a known donor may find their own donor and a practitioner willing to work with them, but this approach is the exception.

In the United States most donor programs operate under the policy that sperm donors will always remain anonymous; a limited number of programs agree to release identifying information after eighteen years. Government policies on the confidentiality of the donor vary among countries.[19] These confidentiality policies are linked to patriarchal notions of paternity. They are also promulgated because of concern that women will fantasize about the donor—which sometimes happens—and that their partners will be threatened by the donor—which also happens.[20] Semen donors may or may not be willing to be identified, but in the United States most agree to donate on the basis of promised anonymity. Many of these issues and policies are very different for female egg donors.

EGGS AND AGE

When I first began studying infertility over fifteen years ago, women over forty had little hope of conceiving. Although I occasionally heard about a pregnancy in a woman over forty, those cases usually involved women who had conceived other children with no history of problems. The women I initially interviewed were in despair about their potential to conceive as they approached forty. Because adoption agencies favored younger couples and the private adoption movement had not yet become widespread, their chances of parenting through adoption were also slim.

Today, assisted reproductive technologies provide the means for women to conceive and give birth to a child after menopause. When this technological advance was announced, I immediately recognized its implications for a wide range of life issues. These have only recently impressed themselves on the public, with the birth of children to women in their sixties. This newfound potential means that our ideas about aging and the course of life must inevitably change. Indeed, those ideas are already changing, in part because of other technological advances and lifestyle changes. But this particular advance alters women's potential in concrete and essential ways. Even if only a small minority of women elect to use a reproductive option such as donor egg, societal awareness of such options will affect women's roles in later life, extending the period of midlife and deferring what people think of as old age into the eighties and beyond. This technology potentially refashions adulthood and may tear down stereotypes about women and age in the process.

The introduction of donor egg technology also forces us to ask whether we measure age with a different ruler for women and men.[21]

When older men become fathers, they evoke cultural assumptions about ongoing sexual prowess and may also raise questions about an inappropriate display of sexuality. Older women, on the other hand, are clearly not supposed to be sexual; the cultural stereotype of an older woman is asexual and grandmotherly. What is more, when an older man becomes a father, people rarely ask if whether he will live long enough to guide the child into adulthood. The assumption is that since the child's mother is young, she will do the parenting. These views reveal the persistent cultural assumption that women have primary responsibility for child-rearing.

Women who have gone through menopause prematurely, in their twenties or early thirties, may be eager to use the donor egg technology because it represents their only chance for pregnancy and childbirth. Similarly, women in their forties and older may look at donor egg technology as their only option for having children. Women in their late thirties and early forties, however—the majority of candidates for donor egg—find it difficult to give up the idea of a genetic connection to a child. A long period of futile attempts with IVF often precedes the consideration of donor egg. Ruth commented:

I went to the doctor in December and she said perhaps we should consider donor egg, and my response was, "Oh, please." You know, I couldn't consider it. And so in January we had a followup appointment with her, and she felt that donor egg was our only hope. And it was just really hard for me to even think about. I just couldn't let go of one more IVF cycle. I couldn't let go of the biological child. Even though I was processing this. Trying hard to think about it and what to do, and I didn't want to adopt. Then I joined an egg donor support group. They had been going on for a while and they were splitting up, but they had this informational meeting, so we formed our own new group. And a number of people were ready to get started, while I'm still thinking about one more IVF. So we did try one more cycle. I didn't have enough eggs. We had to cancel it. We went on vacation, and my period came on the way home. That was the end of IVF, and it was really clear that this is it. No more IVF. It's egg donor, adoption, or nothing.

Ruth's story of attempting one last IVF cycle is a common one. For many women, this is the definitive moment in deciding to proceed with donor egg, although participating in a group of people who are contemplating this technology may prepare them for this shift. Sometimes, however, there is no single defining moment, a lack that contributes to further delays. Julie, at forty-three, was dealing with the revelation from IVF treatment monitoring that she did not have any eggs:

Not having any eggs that time [during the last IVF cycle]. The doctor had said that your body can be different every month, so he couldn't say whether I was going to respond well or not again. So it's like, "Well, I can produce eggs," and he's still saying I could try IVF again. It's not like something is not working. It's just, again, the age factor. So that is the only decision I'm facing. If it would have been, "Okay, you don't have any eggs," I could have accepted that, too, but it would have been a known fact that for two months in a row, I didn't have eggs and that would have been what I'm accepting: "You can't do it because of this." I like to say that it was in my own control to make that decision, too, about going on rather than saying, "You can't because you don't have eggs." It's sort of ridiculous because it might be that your body says, "You can't do this anymore," rather than, "You have to make the decision." I don't really know what's best. I just know what it feels like, and this is the way it feels best [stopping IVF]. It doesn't feel good, though.

Julie is experiencing the loss not only of the possibility of a biological child but also of her sense of her body as young. She is now considering the losses she associates with donor egg technology: "Now that IVF hasn't worked, I'm being faced with whether to go ahead with egg donor. I find myself thinking, 'I don't want to do that, something foreign inside of me.' I don't know if I can accept another woman's egg. Even though we're considering using my niece's egg, I think about seeing the baby and feeling like it's not mine, it's hers."

Despite her reservations, Julie continued to consider this possibility for a long time, listening to others' experiences and investigating all the ins and outs of this technology. Nearing the end of medical treatment for IVF, she wanted something that would work, and she began to realize that donor egg was not foolproof. She became discouraged:

So we are thinking about doing egg donor, and I was a lot more hopeful about that, but hearing more people's stories about doing egg donor and that they've had several failed cycles at that. Or they've had trouble getting their egg donor with the interview process, or people [donors] backing out, and I'm going, "Oh, no!"

Our egg donor group that I'm in had ten people and now it has thirty, and there's a lot more people I'm talking to. There's barely a place to sit. It's crowded. It's good to hear the stories but it's also kind of depressing because the stories aren't good. We're still thinking about doing it. I'm sort of ready to do it.

The growth of Julie's support group attests to the widespread acceptance of this technology. Julie's experience of learning about donor egg in a group contrasts markedly with the experience of men considering donor insemination: imagine a men's donor insemination group being full! Male infertility and donor insemination are seldom contemplated in a group context because of the reserve and secrecy associated with male infertility. The only donor insemination group that was initiated during this study quickly foundered.

Julie is chagrined to find that using the donor egg technology will not necessarily result in a child. Although "the stories aren't good," she has company; many other women and their partners are attempting egg donor, and they share their experiences in an atmosphere of openness. The social support and group identification that occurs facilitates people's subsequent decision to try this technology.

NORMALIZING A DONATED EGG

Once women's options have dwindled to donor egg, or to other possibilities that do not involve the body, such as adoption, women begin reworking how they will enact gender. Normalizing the use of a donated egg is a central part of that process. By normalizing I mean the process whereby this somewhat exotic technology is made ordinary through its attributes, such as preserving the male genetic line and carrying the pregnancy in one's own body.[22] It is easier for women to normalize the use of a donated egg than it is for men to normalize the use of donor sperm. It is also easier for women to enact gender because women carry the pregnancy and thus establish a biological link with the child.

Eileen explains how she gradually adjusted to the idea of using an egg from a donor:

I was starting to become resigned to the fact of donor egg on some level. I think it started to become obvious that it wasn't going to work with my egg, and so what were we going to do? There was childfree, there's adoption, and there's donor egg, which actually was exciting for me because they thought the success rate was a little higher than regular IVF. So here was something we could do with a better chance, and with my sister, that was pretty good. I mean, to keep it in the family. Somehow, thinking about it that way, the loss wasn't as great.

For Eileen, one of the appealing aspects of donor egg was the possibility of using her sister's egg and thus "keeping it in the family." During the time she was investigating the use of this technology, she did not consider using another donor. But her sister backed out. Eileen, however, had adjusted to the idea of using someone else's egg and went on to use a donor selected through an "egg broker" associated with her physician's office.

I always wanted to be pregnant and go through childbirth. I used to read books on that stuff when I was a teenager. I was really into imagining breast feeding. So that's really important to me. And with adoption you don't get that. It's very difficult to do adoptive nursing unless you have previously had a baby or been pregnant. And if it was either that or childfree, we would pick adoption. But there are things that I would gain if we did donor, and I would provide the environment for the baby. So that's a big thing. It's your body that's doing the nurturing.

Eileen's ultimate decision revolved around her ability to experience biological, if not biogenetic, continuity with her child.

Rebecca, age forty, is mourning the loss of biogenetic continuity in her family that using a donor egg represents:

I feel real sorry that we can't have our own child, and I think with the recent loss of my parents it becomes more acute. This is it [end of the family line]. You know, my parents are gone, and I will not be able to pass their genes on, and my sister is older—she doesn't have children, and my brother has one child, and that will be it for them because his wife is what? Forty-four now.

I have one other brother whose wife has some medical problems, so whether they'll ever have their own is doubtful. It's sad. I would like to perpetuate the family. I'd like to see my child, but I also realize pragmatically that it's not going to happen and that, all right, if I can't have my own child, what's the next best thing? Jordan is pretty opposed to adoption, so this is what I'm left with. And although it's not the best choice, in a lot of ways it's the only choice. The last few days I've been feeling pretty positive about it.

Letting go of the cultural ideology of biological continuity between the generations is the hardest thing for Rebecca to do, but like other women, she has realized that she would be unlikely to conceive with her own eggs. Still in the contemplation stages of this technology, Rebecca differentiates between having her "own" child and a child with a donated egg.

Rebecca's husband, Jordan, thirty-five years old, joined in the discussion. He had his own set of concerns:

It sounded more positive than adoption. It was just the fact that we're late in the [adoption] market. I think maybe the time to enter that market was maybe five years ago, four years ago, and now it's just too saturated.[23] *It's too saturated with people looking for babies and there are not that many babies. I think lawyers are making more money than they should be. That's what I like about the donor egg thing. You know, there's only five hundred of them been done in the world [at the time of the interview]. It's like an over 50 percent hit rate, with couples with our profile, so I don't know.*[24] *It just seemed more positive, and right now it's not a saturated market.*

Jordan's comments indicate that he thinks in terms of markets and supply and demand issues. The relative newness of this technology is one of its appeals, but he sees signs that the market for donor eggs will soon be "saturated," as well:

We can already tell that couples are finding out about it because we went through a book of donors and we wanted one, but this couple had stepped in ahead of us. Then there was another one, and she's thinking about it but she's coming off another pregnancy. It just seems like it's starting . . . it's looking like this is going to get saturated pretty soon, too. So I think we're at the right point now, whereas I think we're a little late for adoption.

Rebecca, asked what she thought, said,

Well, what Jordan is saying is true, but it's also true that he is and always has been opposed to adoption. I dragged him to these adoption meetings hoping that he'd have an open mind, which is the way I felt about adoption at first. I think I was more open to it. But I think the donor proposition works best for us because Jordan feels real comfortable that it will be his child. Whereas I will be the mother, biologically I won't be, and I think Jordan has a real lot of problems with biologically not having your own child.

Jordan responded by laying out the dizzying array of choices that Rebecca had faced: "Yeah, right. And also the whole thing of, you get to be pregnant, and everything like that. I keep asking Rebecca, I said, 'What is it about the baby? Where do you want to start the baby? Do you want the whole process of pregnancy or do you just want a baby and what age a baby?' And she wanted the whole process of being pregnant. Well, this gets closer to that." Rebecca interjected, "And it's true, it does."

Jordan continued, "Yeah. A donor egg is not like buying a baby from a birth mother. It's basically a tissue donation. It's not alive. It's just a tissue donation."

Jordan's statement triggers a small argument. Rebecca takes issue with this biomedical way of thinking about a donated egg: "I feel differently about it."

JORDAN: *Yeah. You feel differently about it. You can't find a donor that looks alike, that's all.*

REBECCA: *No, there's a lot of other things.*

Rebecca is dealing with the emotional aspects of using another woman's egg. An egg has enormous cultural significance, and referring to it as a tissue donation diminishes its cultural and emotional importance. Although Jordan is purposely trying to depersonalize this body part in order to make it more palatable to Rebecca, the use of another woman's egg, for Rebecca and most women, is an intensely intimate undertaking and a huge step in relinquishing the cultural ideology of biological parenthood. Although women seem to come around to this decision more easily than do men contemplating donor sperm, it is still an enormous shift.

Finding someone who matches her own physical description ultimately catapults Rebecca into this decision.

I was feeling less positive when we didn't have a donor in mind and we were just sort of going through an evaluation cycle. We were going to try to find someone. But yesterday we got this phone call about a woman who's twenty-one years old and wants to be a donor, has my hair and eye color and is the same height as me and about the same weight as me. The counselor even said to me that she showed the picture of the woman to someone in the office who had met us, and she said it could be me when I was, you know, twenty years ago . . . she's got the same ethnic background—German on one side and Russian

*on the other side. My family is from Germany and Russia. It's like this
incredible match, and when she said that, I felt maybe this is okay,
because I felt like we were making a lot of compromises with a lot of
the others [potential donors]—people that look like Jordan and I was
afraid that I was going to have a dark-haired, dark-eyed child, and I
would feel even more out of it. Now this doesn't mean that we won't
have a dark-eyed, dark-haired child, anyway. . . .*

*Going into it I feel, at least right now—we may change our minds
several thousand times before we actually do it—but I feel at least a
little more comfortable that at least I can select my physical characteristics, to reflect my genes or biological traits. So it's not the best, but
I don't have that option.*

The idea that Rebecca can select an egg donor who reflects her physical characteristics is compelling, as it is for men and women considering
donor insemination. The donor's physical similarities to the social parent
are important in that they pay lip service to the notion of biological
continuity. Having the child resemble oneself is a way of dealing with
the cultural ideology about biological parenthood. At a practical level,
it reduces the level of "cognitive dissonance" that social parents experience, as it is a cultural expectation that children resemble their parents.
Because use of donor gametes is less widely accepted than adoption,
parents of donor children, regardless of their stance on donor confidentiality, want to maintain a degree of confidentiality about the child's
origins.

When women finally relinquish the hope of conceiving with their own
egg and decide to use a donor egg, they face a range of additional issues.
If women do not use a family member's donated egg, they and their
partners must go through the process of selecting a donor, a system that
differs considerably from that used for donor insemination. Known donors, and donors who are family members, are considered acceptable
for eggs but not for sperm because of existing cultural ideologies: the
same sexualization of sperm and asexualization of eggs that Haimes
found in Britain is present in the United States.

A central part of the process is working with a donor "broker" to
select an egg donor. Egg donation is big business. Whereas sperm donors
are paid $50 to $75 for each sperm sample, egg donors are paid $2,500
to $5,000, and often much more, ostensibly because of the amount of
time involved and the invasiveness of the procedures and medications
that a donor must be willing to endure. It should be noted, however,

that the United States is the only country in the western world that allows egg donors to be paid, and that this practice has resulted in blatant commercialism and marketing of body parts. For example, websites now offer "designer" eggs, and couples seeking egg donors offer incentives such as a "gift" in addition to the fee and expenses.[25] Chris commented on what he and his wife saw happening: "A local egg broker was paying people several thousand dollars, and there's a place in [another city] that pays people extraordinary amounts of money, it's amazing. And we both thought that was unethical, with this feeding into exploitation of women, and particularly people that are disenfranchised who want to make some money. It just opens up an enormous problem." The commodification of donor gametes represents an ethical dilemma for many people because it raises questions of disenfranchisement and exploitation. Although men and women in this study expressed concern about this issue, in all cases they went ahead with their plans. Sid volunteered:

They're generally younger, and they are economically down a couple of notches compared with people already in there [in the clinic, who want to use donor eggs] because you've only got people in there who can afford $10,000 or $15,000 a cycle. So by definition you're going to have a younger person from a lower economic stratum.

Users of the donor egg technology sometimes see themselves as exploiters of lower-income women, a position that makes them uncomfortable but is built into consumer culture.[26] There are middle men to pay as well, as Eileen observes:

Donor costs: you pay the donor, and you pay the egg broker, and you pay the clinic to screen the donor. I wanted to find out the rationale behind charging each time, because we have our donor, but we still had to pay for the screening. And these doctors said that basically the idea is that it costs more than that amount to screen a donor to use her one time, and what they wanted to do was spread out the costs over "the life of a donor." She will donate several times if she is a good donor. And he will screen some people out, so they're spreading the costs out over that, and that's why you're charged this amount each time. It doesn't seem fair.

Despite these concerns, people go ahead. Ruth describes a typical scenario: "A couple of weeks after that we went to see the donor broker. We sat down with the books, and we both looked through all the books.

It was hard. We started out with all these criteria. Not this one, not this one, not this one. But we had a few options by the time we left." Ruth, having known ahead of time how this system works, takes this part of the process in stride. What makes it complicated are the variety of choices. Her husband, Frank, is somewhat overwhelmed: "This was the first time we saw pictures of anybody. With the pictures, you start looking at them as people, and that made it more difficult. I found myself thinking, 'This is a really nice-looking woman.' Then I felt like, 'What do I care? I'm not calling her up for a date!' But it was distracting from the birth data, from the genetic factors."

The use of pictures enables people to visualize—and fantasize—not only about the donor but also about the child that may be born from a donor's egg. Pictures are almost always used in donor egg transactions but almost never in donor insemination transactions. Meanwhile, Ruth wanted to find a donor who shared her own religious background:

I always felt strongly that I wanted a Jewish donor. They are real difficult to find, but we ended up with a Jewish donor. She was one of our first choices. One of the things that attracted me was she had a child. And the picture of her was this xerox of a photo. It was a terrible picture, and it was hard to see what she looked like. She's standing next to the child, who was beautiful. She was this gorgeous child, and I looked at it, and I thought, "Well, I'd take one of them."

The image of a woman and her beautiful child enables the consumer of this technology to become acclimated to, even accepting of, the idea. For Ruth, this was the final step in normalizing such a pregnancy.

We have seen how certain technologies highlight deep-seated assumptions about gender and how those assumptions shape the way a technology is presented to the public and utilized. What is more, we have seen how gender interests are preserved in the policies that are promulgated. The buying and selling of donor sperm and eggs highlight how gender interests are supported through consumer culture and draw attention to class differences, the benefits that accrue, and the ways—both subtle and obvious—that power is wielded to shape the ways in which reproductive technologies are utilized. In particular, we have seen a specific instance of the operation of the moral economy of reproductive technologies. The relatively low-cost technology of donor insemination is marginalized as the new technology of ICSI, which enables men to parent a biological child, takes precedence. Moral judgments are at the root of this shift.

The shift toward greater direct participation by consumers in the selection process has recently led to concerns that a "new eugenics" is being created, in which couples seeking donor gametes select those they consider the best potential donors and reject those who do not measure up to their ideal. Such practices in donor insemination have been upstaged by the excesses introduced into the selection of donor eggs, for example, offering "designer eggs" on the Internet. While it is understandable, at a personal level, that people want to control the use of donor gametes insofar as possible, at a societal level it raises questions about the potential creation of a new elite who have been preselected for looks and intelligence and who are born into the upper classes. The ramifications of such actions for the future of society should be apparent, as, intentional or not, they replay the efforts of earlier eugenics movements that sought to create near-perfect specimens of humanity and, in doing so, may widen the gulf between wealthy and poor members of society.[27] The power of the market greatly facilitates this process.

Although feminists have long complained that women are tenaciously equated with nature, when reproductive technologies such as donor insemination are examined, it becomes clear that cultural ideas about what is natural for men are deeply ingrained as well. There is no way to "naturalize" donor insemination; it profoundly challenges cultural ideas about men and nature. In consequence, it has been eclipsed by technologies such as ICSI that have a slim chance of success but uphold cultural imperatives about what is "natural" for men. Donor insemination, the oldest of these reproductive technologies, is thus displaced by successive technologies that are more effective in normalizing ideologies about gender.

Meanwhile, women carry the burden of representations of what is natural into their interactions with new reproductive technologies, such as donor egg. The attributes of this technology make it attractive to women and possible for them to first normalize, then naturalize, its use through their embodied experience.

CHAPTER 9

Embodied Technology

Leslie and Stan, who told their story of undergoing IVF in an earlier chapter, describe how they envisioned as children the embryos that had just been implanted:

STAN: *Talking about naming the embryos, it was funny, we went on vacation to the mountains for five days, and during the time there we were planning to see if it worked or not, and all we could do was wait and hope. So we'd play games. And one evening laying on the bed, I had my head on her stomach, and I was talking to the embryos, and I said, "If you promise to come out in nine months, I promise that we'll come back here to bring you on vacation every-year."*

LESLIE: *We sent postcards to people that said, "Well, the embryos seem to be enjoying it here, and so do the negotiations for summer vacations."*

I think the other thing it did was about the abortion issue, which we have had different opinions about. To me it had always been a very cut-and-dried issue, that it was simply a woman's right to choose. Period. And I never really thought of it any further than that. And once we did this, I said, "You know, I still think it's a woman's right to

choose," but suddenly I had realized that, for us, in the
room that day, the embryos had personalities. It didn't
change my opinion about abortion but, you know, it
makes you think a little bit more.

STAN: *We thought up names and everything.*

These statements highlight a cultural shift. The new reproductive technologies emphasize transformation, and, in doing so, they naturalize technology.[1] They allow people to view embryos and fetuses as children. As couples become immersed in a complex process, the embryos become children who are part of them.[2]

The specific attributes of new reproductive technologies contribute to the embodiment of embryos. Two key components associated with these technologies are visualization, as in the use of ultrasound and other technologies that reveal what was previously invisible, and ritual. These phenomena imbue the process with cultural meaning, enabling embryos to become embodied by bridging what happens inside and outside the body and making it more accessible, experientially, to women.

Women generally respond positively to visual technologies. As these technologies expand, ways of documenting family life encompass visual images that precede the birth of a child. Visualizing technologies are apparently becoming part of a familiar language of "private" images, such as photo albums, videotape collections, and the like. They also give women a sense of control over the reproductive process and a visible indication that a pregnancy is possible.[3]

For men, too, embryos become embodied, as Stan's comments demonstrate. Men become engaged in and personalize a process that occurs in their partner's body so that they become emotionally connected to the process. For women and men who pin their hopes on technology for years on end, embryos represent the realization of their biological connection to the next generation. So powerful is this process that even before there is a fetus, the much-sought-after child is experienced as alive.

At the same time, from a feminist perspective, the primary danger of transforming the female body into a site for technological intervention is that it may render the body invisible, erasing the woman while foregrounding the fetus.[4] The potential dangers are most apparent when they render women's bodies transparent.

VISUALIZING THE BODY

The ability to visualize aspects of medical procedures has altered the experience of infertility treatment. Microprocesses that normally occur in women's bodies, hidden from view, may now be observed—even conception itself. Because of this ability, moreover, questions that once had no medical answers may now be explained.

Visualizing reproduction actually begins before IVF. For example, surgery, which was first photographed for the benefit of physicians' education and training, can now be viewed later on videotape by patients who undergo it. A laparoscopy is often the last step before IVF. Rebecca describes hers: "We have a video of my laparoscopy, a color video. Just amazing. They go in there with a camera. They speed it up and show you what they did and what they found and how things are." Jordan, intrigued by the technology, interjected: "Yeah, they show them zapping out the stuff with a laser. It's cool!"

Rebecca, ambivalent about the work done on her body, responded, "I probably learned more about my body than I've ever wanted to know."

Through the new technology, the inside of the body, previously mysterious and unknown, becomes accessible to view. Captured on videotape, it can be examined again and again until it becomes familiar. Jordan's comment draws attention to the visual similarity between this technology and a Star Wars–type video game. Rebecca, however, is ambivalent because this videotape represents physicians' efforts to "fix" her body, which they view as faulty. She feels dehumanized by this experience and expresses her aversion. The "virtual reality" of the body becomes enmeshed with challenges to Rebecca's identity. The videotape becomes a concrete symbol of her inability to conceive.

Microprocesses, initially abstractions, make the potential child seem real as treatment proceeds. But the excitement that visualization generates can lead people to forget or overlook issues they formerly thought were important. For example, Colleen, reporting on her experience of IVF, said, "He [physician] said, 'Look at the screen!' He was thrilled that there were all these eggs [embryos] there and was really into the technology of it. Meanwhile, I was focused on these worries about selective reduction. So I looked at the screen and got excited about it and forgot to ask about selective reduction." When women's bodies become a site for technological intervention, the process of medicalization escalates, not only dehumanizing the body but also redirecting both patients' and practitioners' concerns away from humanistic and ethical issues toward the technology itself. Colleen's distraction shows the power of visualization. People become drawn into the process in a series of steps in which their concerns are muted by engagement with the technology. Having made certain choices to begin with, such as the decision to undertake IVF, people often relinquish subsequent choices as the technology takes on its own momentum. Once in gear, the process fast-forwards people through a series of technological steps during which there is little opportunity to pause for reflection or further decision making.

Women and men reported that when they learned what was possible from these technologies, the information often gave them new hope—hope that was often short-lived. Chuck, who had a low sperm count, and had consequently considered using sperm from a donor before deciding to undertake IVF, said, "From that procedure [IVF], we knew that my wife produced four eggs. And two of them were fertilized by my sperm. There was no donor sperm at all. And that was a piece of information we hadn't had before." Marlie, his wife, agreed: "The doctor said, 'Now we know his sperm can fertilize your eggs.' So it was worth it [doing IVF]. Except it gave us, perhaps, false hope."

On the basis of this information, this couple, who had previously decided to use donor insemination if their first IVF attempt failed, attempted another IVF cycle. Once a "high" technology such as IVF was unsuccessful, couples in this study were less likely to try a "low" technology such as donor insemination, even though the latter might have a good success rate. Women and men cannot imagine that something less expensive could be effective when something more expensive has failed. This trend reflects the consumer belief that the greater the cost, the better the product.

The medical information provided by such technologies did sometimes lead to recommendations to use a donor, but almost invariably those recommendations were for using additional "high" technologies. For example, Rebecca said, "From that IVF, we found out that my eggs weren't in good condition; only three fertilized, and none of them planted. So the doctors, after looking at everything, said, 'It looks like you have an egg problem.' " Jordan added,

We have pictures of all our eggs so you can see the form of them. They're fragmented and just not dividing. Like a fertilized egg. A fertilized egg should be at two days, what? Eight [cells] or sixteen, or some-

thing like that. Four or eight, something like that. But, anyway, they
weren't getting up there. They were fragmenting and stuff, which is
okay—some could fertilize, but you know, you want good ones. So
then the doctor suggested, "Don't continue with this."

Pictures personalized the process: to Jordan, Rebecca's eggs became
"our" eggs. But unlike Jordan, who discussed the eggs with some detachment, Rebecca was sensitive about the state of her eggs. Having
them discussed this way added to her feelings of defectiveness. However,
she was trying to be matter-of-fact about this news, so she concurred
with Jordan and described the potential solution their physician offered
them: "After two cycles of IVF, the doctor suggested we not continue
with this. He suggested we should consider a donor egg, instead, because
so many of my eggs fragmented." This suggestion, which they followed,
led to a further cycle of IVF, using donated eggs.

Visualization techniques promote the use of high technology. Not
only does visualization reinforce people's sense of the potential in new
reproductive technologies, these technologies, in their ability to render
visible even an embryo in its earliest stages of growth, turn abstractions
into reality. Actually seeing these stages of the process creates expectations of success, so that the potential for the technologies to fail is difficult to contemplate and may be completely disregarded.

RITUALS OF EMBRYO TRANSFER

New reproductive technologies reshape cultural meanings attached to a
range of basic concepts, such as, "What constitutes human life?" and
"When does life begin?" For couples who have spent years in infertility
treatment, human life begins not in a woman's body but in the lab.

Ritual is one of several elements that contributes to the embodiment
of embryos. The power of ritual to reshape cultural meanings is well
known to anthropologists.[5] Helen describes the process of embryo transfer with donor eggs:

The embryo transfer. Has anyone described to you what an embryo
transfer is like? What happens? I thought it was an awesome moment.
It was really awesome.

Another doctor did the embryo transfer. It was really the most ritu-
alistic piece of anything I've gone through. All the other stuff is so
medical—it's surgical, it's clinical. But this was quite ritualistic. And
it's so incredibly awesome because they're putting these live embryos

*into you! So it's sort of appropriate in some way that it's ritualistic.
But it was quite something.*

*They have a separate room for the embryo transfer. It has dim
lighting. And it's pretty well soundproof, so it's very quiet, and they
have an examining table that does all of these adjustments. I have to
be in a weird position. I was sort of bent over the table with my butt
sort of exposed. Not the usual feet-in-the-stirrups position. I did this
sort of in reverse. Talk about having nothing left [privacy, modesty].*

Helen articulates some of the basic elements of the ritual process.
First, a sense of mystery is established through the use of a special room:
a womb-like, otherworldly environment. Second, the person who is the
focus of the ritual is placed in an out-of-the-ordinary position. Helen is
put in an awkward physical position that maximizes her sense of vulnerability. The ritual principle of removing all worldly crutches from
the novice, so that she is left exposed and vulnerable, is carried out
literally here, as Helen acknowledges.

*So, anyway, there I am with my butt sticking up in the air. They have
a catheter. So first they check to see if the catheter and . . . this was all
happening behind me. I couldn't see it. Then they take it back to the
lab which is right across the hall, which has the embryo. These are
live, growing embryos. It's so amazing. They gave us pictures of the
ones they were going to transfer. Have you ever seen an embryo picture? They gave us pictures of four. They wanted to put them in so
they're high but not so high they go up the tubes. They measure them.
Then they run down the hall and they load the tube. They loaded the
catheter with them. See, I never got to see it. But it's very solemn. A
very solemn event.*

Sid interjects, "Yeah. It was overdone."

Now that the person is in a vulnerable, exposed position, some of the
ritual activity occurs where she cannot see it, heightening the mystery
and sense of suspense. As in a traditional healing ceremony in another
society, in which the healer may go into a trance and then symbolically
cough up the offending problem or needed result, signifying a cure, Helen is given pictures of the embryos. The solemnity of the occasion further marks it as a ritual of the utmost importance. Helen continues:

*And it's very ceremonial. It's very interesting. In fact, I commented on
this to the doctor, that this felt very ceremonial, and he said, "Yes, instead of my scrubbed jeans, I feel like I should have witch doctors*

roaming around." But it is very ceremonial and very quiet and formal,
unlike any other sort of "procedure" that I've had for infertility stuff.
And then they count from five down? What did they do? [asking husband, who shrugs]. But it's very formal, 'Five, four, three, two, one
. . . BLAST OFF!' kind of, not blast off, but whatever.*

Sid irreverently interjects, "Squirt!"

Despite the indignity of Helen's posture and her inability to actually
see what they are doing, the various elements of the ritual have a profound effect on her. Most of all, she finds the transfer of the live, growing
embryos amazing. Having received pictures of the embryos before they
were transferred, she regards them as real: living, embodied parts of her.
For Sid, however, the embryo transfer is not embodied; it is another
clinical procedure that has been overblown.

Helen resumes the story:

*And then they still won't let me move. I'm still sort of in this semi-
bent-over position, and they move my body and straighten out the table and the table is somewhat downhill, had gone downhill. Legs up.
And didn't they whisper? Did they whisper? [to husband] Anyway,
they were very solemn. But I kept forgetting that I was supposed to
whisper, and I would say something in a loud voice, and the nurse
would be whispering to me, "Whisper now." They don't want any
diaphragm exertion in case it might cause an expulsion. I think it's
partly ceremonial. It was really the most ritualistic piece of anything
I've gone through.*

Helen is aware of the ceremonial aspects of the ritual at the same time
that she is impressed by them, thus calling our attention to the most
significant aspect of ceremonial healing: it is an event consciously constructed to set apart the person who is the focus of healing from others.
For the ritual to be effective, the person must at some level be aware of
the ceremony and her special status in it.

Asked whether the ritual associated with this medical procedure dif-
fered from those IVF procedures they had done without a donor egg,
Sid, still unimpressed, responded, "We went through the basic GIFT
procedure, we didn't go through IVF, so I don't know. But in the basic
GIFT procedure, she's out [unconscious], so it's irrelevant. They take the
eggs and they immediately mix them with the sperm and blast them
back up. There is no ritual." As an afterthought, he added, "It would
be interesting to do a study across clinics to see whether the ritual does

any good." This comment suggests that perhaps Sid was not entirely immune to the ritual.

The ritual of embryo transfer also calls attention to the way in which women's bodies are manipulated. Helen is put into an ignominious position, immobilized and helpless. Her body is treated as a receptacle for embryos. Her enforced passivity is underscored by most of the action taking place behind her back. She is chided for her irreverent loud remarks. Although she complains, all the negative aspects of this experience are erased by the thrill of having live embryos placed inside her. Through this action she begins a transformative process. The decision to undertake conception with a donated egg was an enactment of gender that is now being realized.

Women see such procedures as enacting gender even when they are simply physically there—because they see their actions leading up to this event and following it as the critical parts of the process. The procedure itself, whether purposely staged as a transformative ritual or not, signifies their mastery over a process that is outside their control only in the immediate sense. This moment is a bodily expression of their actions.

Another aspect of ritual activity surrounding embryos is the use of the word *family* in referring to embryos, humanizing them even before they are inserted into a woman's body. Dennis reported on meeting the embryologist:

She had participated in this ritual of fusing people's gametes in an IVF lab, but she had been an invisible participant in this process. We made this good connection [with her], so she allowed us to go in and look into the microscope, and it was like, "There is your family." It is a very profound thing to do. I will die with that image on the back of my eyelids. Looking down and seeing one two-cell embryo and two four-cell embryos and one six-cell embryo, and the knowledge of what they were.

Describing the transfer of the embryos, Dennis continued:

We decided to transfer four of the embryos. The doctor was walking down the hall with this catheter with four embryos, and he said something like, "Here's your future family." And he put them in, and then they looked under a microscope to make sure they had all come out of the catheter. One of them was stuck. So there was this quick decision, whether to fill it up again with fluid and do a second injection of this fourth embryo or not. He said to us, "One thing you risk by doing it

is that you can wash them all away by adding more fluid into the
uterine cavity." So we said, "No, we'll just have to go with three."
It was like being crushed on some level. Because you get focused on
four, and all of a sudden you've lost one. You're already down 25
percent!

Dennis's sense that this is his family is reinforced by the physician's
words. In describing the loss of one embryo, Dennis expresses his attachment to these embryos. To him the embryos have already taken on
life and become children. The fact that these activities are being conducted in a lab does not diminish his sense of connection either to the
embryos themselves or to the process. By the time couples have reached
this step, they have integrated technology into their expectations about
the creation of life and their active role in it.

Even when such efforts do not succeed, women and men think of
their embryos as alive. Polly reports how she talked to her embryo:

A few days ago they retrieved a healthy egg and it fertilized. It divided
into four cells, then by the time they implanted it, it was up to eight
cells. I had to lay completely still in the OR [operating room] for an
hour and a half, then another two and a half hours in the recovery
room. I went home and spent the next couple of days off my feet.
I talked to the little thing, telling it what life would be like, why it
should stick around. In the end it didn't. But I was a mother for a
minute.

As a step in the embodiment of embryos, embryo transfer carries
cultural meanings about the creation of life. Even when chances are slim
that an embryo will turn into a fetus, men and women become attached
to their embryos and regard them as living, investing them with cultural
meaning as potential children. Steven described what happened when a
delayed fertilization occurred after using his sperm in IVF:

I called the doctor's office, as I was supposed to do, and the reception-
ist said, "Oh, we're so glad you called. One of the eggs fertilized. We
need you to come in." After expecting nothing, there had been what
they called delayed fertilization of one of the micromanipulated eggs.
They had manipulated six of the twelve eggs by drilling a hole to facil-
itate fertilization. And seventy-two hours later, after they were put to-
gether, there was a delayed fertilization. We had one two-cell embryo.
*   I tracked down Anne, and she rushed over there, and they did an*
embryo transfer, and, on top of that, they give you the picture of the

embryo. Which we bonded to immediately, predictably, and in a pretty unnatural way. We got very attached to that embryo. And statistically we knew that the combination of delayed fertilization and a micromanipulated egg meant that the chances of successful implantation and pregnancy would be very low. Probably 5 percent at most. But, you know, that was better than zero percent.

So we went over there and did the embryo transfer. And you know, it was amazing what a leap that was in where we were at. Because when nothing had fertilized, I cried and cried. These roller coasters.

It was just a whole different stage than we had ever expected to go to. Even if we didn't succeed, it was much farther than we had ever experienced before, and it was pretty high. But realistically, I think we knew it wasn't going to take. We also didn't know quite what to tell people, because those people that we had told, we had already told them there was no fertilization.

And then it did not implant. And we were back to depression again.

The roller coaster metaphor, pervasive in people's reports of infertility treatment, succinctly describes how people are affected by the unpredictability of the process.[6] Steven's reference to going "farther" shows how people may become enmeshed, and then entrapped, in the process. Even though this attempt was unsuccessful, their appetite was whetted. Having had seen pictures of *their* embryo, they had experienced new hope, and they decided to try again.

VISUALIZING THE FETUS

Ultrasound represents another step in the process of bodily incorporation of embryos. The use of ultrasound to mark the progress of fetal development reinforces the view of the fetus as a child. Chuck said, "When we heard the news, I thought, 'I'm going to be a father!' That was really exciting. I was giddy with it. They did an ultrasound." Marlie interjected in excitement, "You could see the little guy!" Chuck continued, "Yes, not only the little sac, but you could see the heart tone in the fetus." She interrupted, "And he had a name!"

Chuck continued: "We named this child. We were really into it. A couple of weeks later, when we went back to have a test, the sac was really diffused. There was nothing in the sac that could be visualized. We both knew something was wrong."

Marlie amplified on this: "The doctor came in and said, 'I'm sorry.' It felt like this black cloud had been drawn down around both of us. I fell apart. Totally grieved. This time I had trusted it would be real."

When a miscarriage occurred, having seen the fetus on the ultrasound screen reinforced the couple's sense of loss. Another woman, who conceived after four years of effort, was reluctant to believe she was pregnant until she saw the fetus on an ultrasound screen. Anxious that something would go wrong, she underwent another ultrasound despite her physician's reassurances. That time, "Where the baby had been, there was nothing but a black hole." The miscarriage after seeing a fetus triggered an extended period of mourning.

But for others, reassured by their good news, the ultrasound signaled the actual start of life. They were excited: "We have pictures!"; "That's Waldo, that's what we call him for now"; "We call him the Creature"; "We think it's a little girl." One woman concluded, "The whole thing feels so fragile. But then you get to see the fetus on ultrasound, and you get to see the heartbeat."[7]

Marlie, after recovering from her previous pregnancy loss, underwent another cycle of IVF. Ultrasound was used with this pregnancy as well. Several years later she reported,

I still have the ultrasound photo tucked away in my appointment book that I carry around with me. I had gone to have an ultrasound taken and the doctor said, "Don't get your hopes up about this kid," and I said, "Why?" And she wouldn't tell me. So I looked at that little thing. Up in the corner the picture says, "No FHT." What's that mean? So I asked the infertility specialist, and he said, "No fetal heart tone." So he scheduled another ultrasound for us a couple weeks after that. It was fine.[8]

Although there can be inaccuracies with ultrasound, for couples who have been yearning for a child, the ultrasound picture signals that life has begun.

TRANSFORMATION OF THE BODY

The idea of making a biological contribution to one's child is rewritten when women use a donor egg. When integrating a donor egg into their bodily experience, women place a heavy emphasis on the naturalization of the donated egg. When the bodily incorporation of embryos culminates with a successful pregnancy, women experience a resurgence of bodily knowledge. Both women and men use metaphors to characterize bodily phenomena that reflect their shifting understandings of the pregnant body. Visibly pregnant, Sandra, thirty years old, was sitting on her sofa with her feet up. She had been married a year. A college graduate, Sandra worked in business administration, but her work was completely eclipsed when she developed a chronic illness that triggered reproductive problems. "I was diagnosed with premature ovarian failure soon after I met Ken. We were about to become engaged. After a few tests, it seemed conclusive that I had already gone through menopause. I have a blood disorder which is an autoimmune problem. A simple way of describing it is that I'm allergic to my own red blood cells."

Sandra was determined to have children, however, and the time immediately preceding her marriage and subsequent to it had been dominated by efforts to conceive. The egg that had made the pregnancy possible had been donated by her sister. She talked about her efforts to create order in her life out of the disruption caused by her illness:

A few months ago I was going through a hard time and questioning the baby we're having. One of the things Ken said to try to pull me out of that sadness was, "This baby is going to be more you than it is your sister. Your life force and your blood is going to be the central thing. Your body is nurturing that baby for months. And the only thing that helps from your sister is the fact that she was a DNA model. The rest is going to be you." So I have sort of stolen that from Ken and adopted that philosophy and have said it to other people, like an affirmation to myself, to try and convince myself that I believe that. And it's part of my healing process.

This series of disruptions—the onset of a chronic illness, premature menopause, and the decision to use another woman's egg to conceive a pregnancy—affects Sandra's bodily knowledge of herself. Bodily knowledge represents a lifetime of self-understanding, which encompasses women's expectations about their bodies in pregnancy. Part of what Sandra describes as her "healing process" is the identity work she is doing to experience her body as essential to the pregnancy. It enables her to repair her bodily knowledge of herself as a woman and a mother.

Sandra's comments illustrate how biomedical models of heredity are being incorporated into belief systems to inform people's sense of self and are also being used as metaphors. In characterizing her sister as "a DNA model" and Sandra as a "life force," Sandra's husband metaphorically demotes the sister's role in the pregnancy to a mechanistic part of the biological process and highlights Sandra's role in carrying the pregnancy to term. Still not convinced that the baby she carries is *her* baby, however, Sandra remarks:

I try and repeat those thoughts and I say that to other people when they ask me how I feel. I'm partially trying to convince myself that it's true. And I think that the more I do it, I do believe it. Intellectually, I do believe it. But in order to feel it in my heart, I need to say it repeatedly. Especially when people say, "How does it feel to carry your sister's baby?"

Here the baby is embodied metaphorically as a part of her "heart," an affirmation that the baby is part of her both physically and emotionally, body as well as soul. When others ask how it feels to carry her sister's baby, Sandra experiences cognitive dissonance, a disjuncture between her bodily knowledge and an alien representation of her situation. Convincing herself that the baby she is carrying is her own is critical to efforts to reestablish her bodily knowledge. Moreover, doing so facilitates her ability to link her bodily knowledge to her gender identity. In grappling with her feeling of being disembodied, Sandra reaches for a metaphor that reconnects her to her body:

When I deliver this baby, I want to look at that baby and think, "I really did make that baby." And I know, intellectually, that without my womb, it would have never gone anywhere. And I really am making the baby. Even though what it took to start that fire didn't come from me. But the fire doesn't burn on its own. It needs fuel. And I guess I really provided that.

The fuel and fire metaphor, representing the nurturance that is associated with being a woman, enables Sandra to gain a sense of coherence. The equation of her body with fuel, and its ability to keep the fire of conception alive through nurturance, reestablishes Sandra's bodily knowledge. The baby becomes tangible proof of her living, nurturing body, in contrast to her recent experience of her body as unable to sustain another life.

This story illustrates how women must rework the cultural ideology of their bodies as "natural" when they use new reproductive technologies to conceive a child. Sandra's embodied knowledge has been reconfigured by the technology. The construction of the female body as natural is embodied from the time of a woman's own birth through a cultural process that is entwined with her own physical and social development. Sandra's story illustrates how deeply embedded this assumption is in bodily knowledge and how profoundly disruptive women find it when their bodies do not function as expected. Women who persist in their efforts to become pregnant through new reproductive technologies must rework cultural meanings of nature and nurturance so that they can bring their bodies into a semblance of accord with this cultural ideology. They rework their bodily knowledge to create synchrony between their gender identity and the cultural ideology of womanhood.

Sandra's story brings a new dimension to bodily experience. Something that was formerly impossible has been made possible through technology: another woman's egg has been planted in her body, and a conception has taken place. The integration of new science models into existing cultural interpretations of reproduction are mediated at the level of the body through metaphor.[9] In this process the infertile, menopausal body is transformed into the body of a mother, and the technology is naturalized by the body: the transformation to motherhood takes place *within* the body. Sandra reframes the donated egg as the starter, thus naturalizing the technology and placing it in a subsidiary position to her own, embodied contribution, the "fuel." She further draws the technology into her body and appropriates it when she says, "The fire doesn't burn on its own." The technology, now humanized, becomes part of the process of transformation.

This example graphically depicts the process by which technology alters bodily processes that were formerly viewed as natural. The technology is humanized and made natural through a process of replacement. Embodied knowledge, of the body as it should be, is reshaped through the use of new technology as an adjunct to bodily processes. Thus, not only does technology alter bodily processes, but the role of technology is altered by its engagement with the body: technology is subsumed by the body and becomes part of it, naturalized and embedded in a woman's life.

Sandra's story illustrates how bodily experience reflects the cultural foundations of metaphor as well as the moral force of cultural ideologies. All of these phenomena interact. Sandra is about to give birth to a child. The pregnancy is embodied; the child is hers. She draws on bodily metaphors. But, at the same time, Sandra needs to establish the baby as hers in the eyes of those who regard it as her sister's baby. In representing it as hers through her choice of bodily metaphors, she asserts control over the situation. She is simultaneously responding to and resisting those cultural ideologies that stand for normalcy.

New reproductive technologies undergo a process of naturalization in which women and men, as well as practitioners, take part.[10] These technologies transform the experience of conception and pregnancy, and at the same time are transformed by those who use them, in ways that are explicitly cultural. Two aspects of transformation, visualization and ritual, facilitate the naturalization process, which culminates in the reworking of bodily knowledge and the redefinition of the meaning of natural.

The various technologies have the capacity to turn women's bodies into objects, thus dehumanizing them, and, all too frequently, to divert people's focus to the technology itself at the expense of addressing moral questions. But there is another, often overlooked, side to the use of these technologies: the actions that people take as they put them to use. People see themselves not as passive recipients of these technologies but as active masters of the process. They see the technologies as instruments of their own gender performance. We will see in the next chapter, however, that when conception does not occur, people's sense of engagement with these technologies evaporates, and efforts to naturalize them cease.

Technologies utilizing donor gametes can be seen as transformative of nature and culture. But they also reflect the ways in which ideologies about nature and culture are reproduced. Men as well as women are absorbed by this naturalization process. On the one hand, this is cause for some concern. As many feminists attest, reproductive technologies facilitate male control over women's bodies, first because the majority of scientists and physicians developing and using these technologies are men, and second because new reproductive technologies can be seen as reinforcing a patriarchal agenda.[11] Under some circumstances men remain distanced from their partners' bodies and may be more detached and coolly analytical. On the other hand, they are also engaged in a collective process with their partners in which embryos, pregnancies, and fetuses become "ours." The ways in which men express their engagement with the technology indicate that they too experience these technologies at the bodily level. These technologies are an expression for men, as well as for women, of the performance of gender.

CHAPTER 10

Shifting Gears

Although couples were quick to embrace technology when success seemed likely, the embodied aspects of these technologies quickly faded when conception did not occur. Whether the process took months or years, those who did not conceive gradually ceased to be receptive to the allure of these technologies and instead became resistant to them. Once disillusionment set in, it rapidly affected women's and men's attitudes toward further medical procedures. Polly, a veteran of four IVF attempts, reached her limit suddenly:

I sat in that last group meeting listening to these women; it was a well-attended group. I think probably fifteen people were there. And I was just about the last one [to speak]. I was second to last. By the time they got to me, I just . . . I couldn't . . . I don't know if this is terrible to say, but I couldn't stand the sight of them. I felt like saying, "You know, you are losers. What's wrong with you? What are you all doing all this to yourself for? Don't you know you're going to just end up exactly where I am? Only you're just at the beginning. You pathetic little creatures. You're at the beginning and you're yacky-yacking and feeling all positive and hopeful, and you're not looking at where you're going to be."

'Cause all this stuff has such a minuscule success rate, and they just keep going on and on and on. It just makes me sick. I don't want to hear it. We women are becoming fertility experts. We know more

*about our bodies, and all these procedures—it's like another language.
It's like we're a subcult of some sort, you know, the infertile, and here
we go around yacky-yacking to each other, and we know the latest
high-tech this, and the latest way to do that, and let's see, "Why don't
you talk to your doctor about doing a combination this and this and
doing a that and that and then three months later repeating it with
a . . ." And I'm going, "Oh, my God. I can't stand this anymore."*

*So when my turn came, I just said, "I am so sick of this. I don't
know what's going on with me, except I just want it to be over and I
want my own life again. We have one more time, and that's it." I just
cried, and I said, "I need some time with my husband. I need some
time that's stress-free. I just . . . I need to not be thinking about the
next step." I'm looking at these women, and they've got years of next
steps. I just want it to be over. Absolutely over.*

Although many people reach a stopping point more gradually, Polly's
sudden loss of faith in the technology is not unusual. Once people have
tried everything, they express increasing impatience with medical treatment. As Polly so eloquently asserts, they need to go on with their lives.

As women and men near the end of treatment, they subject their
previous actions to intense scrutiny. They examine cultural ideologies
more critically, as when Polly analyzes herself and the other group members as a "subcult of the infertile." Her notion of women as fertility
experts who speak a special language indicates that she is feeling increasingly removed from this process.

Polly's insights signal a dramatic change in how she thinks about
unwanted childlessness. She is reworking the meaning of normalcy.
Whereas she once saw the intensive pursuit of infertility treatment as
both normal and legitimate, now she views it as abnormal and "pathetic." Her portrait of women as "losers," among whom she includes
herself, signals the depth of her disillusionment. Her view of herself is
changing; by differentiating herself from other women experiencing infertility, she is beginning to rework her gender identity.

Efforts to reorder the world and restore a sense of order begin with
the body. An essential step in reordering the world after life has been
disrupted by infertility is withdrawal from medical treatment. Polly
notes that women know about their bodies in the context of these technologies, but she now finds this knowledge uncomfortable, even unpleasant. Women's bodies are rendered unpredictable by infertility treatment, and renewing their sense of bodily predictability restores stability

and enables women to begin reworking their gender identity and moving on with their lives.[1]

The hope with which people imbue new reproductive technologies gives way to a sense of despair and futility about the ability to achieve the desired ends. It amounts to a loss of faith, and people respond in ways that are similar to loss of faith in religion.

THE CUMULATIVE EFFECTS OF MEDICAL TREATMENT

When time wore on without a pregnancy, women and men in the study began to note the cumulative effect of infertility treatment on their lives. The pursuit of treatment initially ameliorated women's sense of failure and made them feel they were taking responsible action. After they had been in treatment for some time, however, women began to feel engulfed by infertility treatment and frightened by their dependency on medical technology. They felt out of control and observed changes in themselves that they viewed as negative. For example, Justine, thirty-seven, said, "I started to feel like I am insane, I need help, I need something. It scared me that I was becoming dysfunctional. That's what I felt like." Later she observed, "There is that terrible period of time when you're waiting to see if you're pregnant or not. Some of those months were just horrible. I thought I might have to check into a mental institution a few times because things got so intense."

Despite their emotional exhaustion, women were slow to relinquish medical treatment because treatment symbolized hope for a pregnancy. Giving up this goal meant that women and men had to rethink their entire lives. Julie described the dilemma she faced when she contemplated stopping treatment:

I think the whole thing is about when you put your biological child to rest. I hadn't been ready to do that with the other cycles, so I think that it was helpful that way. I could have done it without that last cycle, but it would have been more difficult. It wasn't like I had to do it, it was like I had to figure out, "Well, when and how am I going to do that?" So doing that cycle was my limit. It's like saying, "Do one more," and when it wasn't complete, I had a hard time saying that, and so doing one more for me was still going to be the marker. So I think it was helpful for me, but I don't think it was necessary. I don't know how to say this, but I think everybody has these different things

*they get set on, like, "How is this going to end?" and "How am I go-
ing to accept it?"*

*I'm sure [husband] will do it [donor egg] if I say, "It's time to do
it, we should do it." But he's always been the optimist, and he's depressed now, and he's not optimistic. He is an optimistic guy. This is
a guy who believes in the goodness in life that will always carry him
along. I think we'll do it at least once, and we might do it twice, and
my feeling is that he really wants to do it too, even though he drags
his feet. I mean, he might let it go. If he was the leader in this [fertility
quest], he would let it go. But I think that's what we'll do. I have no
idea after that. He's talking more and more about not having kids
and being childfree.[2] He's really talking like this is how he sees the
future.*

*It's probably taking its toll on my body and on my emotions, but
it feels like the decisions are coming. Getting used to the disappoint-
ments. It's like anything you get with a debilitating disease or getting
into a car accident, and things totally change and you have to live
with doctors, or whatever. With a changing physical condition, after a
while you cope and accept it. But it's still living with it. It's harder to
think about it, not having kids.*

When Julie begins to talk about letting go of medical treatment, she
is contemplating how to reframe her life. In trying to conceive for a
number of years, she has imagined herself as a woman with a child.
Because her husband is unwilling to adopt, she must seriously consider
the possibility that she will be childless. Having subscribed fully to cultural ideologies about motherhood, parenthood, and family, she must
now begin to fit herself into a different picture.

Julie observes that making decisions about treatment is a process of
adjusting to disappointment. At this stage, Julie is having difficulty imagining life without children: it is difficult to find other things that are
meaningful. Her husband, however, has begun to alter his vision of the
future to being childless. This difference between them strains their relationship and adds to the strain Julie feels on her body and her emotions. Giving voice to her sense of loss is essential to her ability to come
to terms with her situation and reestablish a sense of synchrony with
her partner.

In this phase of medical treatment, women and men are confronted
with questions about whether their relationship will endure. Women and
men both work very hard at maintaining their partnership because of

the latent threat of ending up both childless and without a partner. The potential for this combination of losses makes contemplating the future even more difficult and provokes a crisis of meaning as women and men seek to find some vestige of order and predictability in their lives. Lani describes how the entwined issues of fertility and the relationship affected her and Jerry at a late stage of medical treatment:

That was the beginning of the time when Jerry was working out of town a lot. And then we really got crazy because I was doing all this treatment, and then he got sent to Hawaii and was going to be there, so I flew over to Hawaii when I was ovulating so we could make love. And then he went and stored some sperm in a sperm bank because he was going to be gone. And it didn't store very well. Even though I did pay to retrieve it and use it the following month. But it only had a 17 percent survival rate after the freezing, which is not very good. And we now know that is a good indicator of the viability of the sperm, that there could be some kind of sperm problem.

So then he was gone for a few months. It was almost like a time of separation in our relationship, and I just wanted to get my body back to some kind of normal. What would it feel like not to be on drugs and doing all this stuff? It felt great, actually.

Faced with a period of separation, Lani's first expressed concern is with her body and returning to some kind of bodily normality. After a long period on fertility drugs, she is relieved to have a respite. This respite led to a decision to try further treatment, however, because although she had been in treatment for a long time, she had not yet been to a specialist:

And then we started getting scared about how much older we were getting, and we decided we needed to do something soon. Either, not to be doing this or looking into other alternatives such as adoption, or whatever, that we need to get a lot more aggressive. And the nurse practitioner said we should be trying intrauterine inseminations. From all my reading I thought this should be my next step. So I decided to go to a specialist.

During the couple of months before that, I really felt that I had gotten into a spiritual crisis with the infertility. That it was really affecting my faith in God or the higher power. And I was really starting to lose hope and lose faith about that. And so I sought out a spiritual community to give me some support and to seek some answers for

*myself, and which I did find and which was very helpful to me. . . .
And the day before I got the name of this specialist, I was talking to a
practitioner in the church in a healing group, and I was saying that I
really wanted some healing around this, and he said that I was going
to be led to the right specialist. And the next day I heard about her.
And she did take a much more aggressive approach.*

Lani's story illustrates that medical treatment does not happen in a
vacuum. It is part of a much bigger picture that, in this case, involves
Lani's bodily concerns, her relationship with Jerry, their fertility, and
her spirituality. Through finding a new church she is able to restore her
sense of spirituality and hope for the future.

The removal of the last hope of treatment often created a crisis for
women in the study. Justine, who had been denied IVF by her health
maintenance organization, expressed the desperation typical of women
when their medical options dwindled: "I told my doctor, 'There has to
be something else.' I feel like I'm not that old. There have to be more
options. I didn't break down and start sobbing in front of her and beg
her to give me the authorization to get in vitro, but that would have
been more honest. My doctor responded, 'Have you thought about
adoption?' I said, 'I'm not ready for that!' "

Six months later, however, when Justine had run out of medical options
and thought about how medical treatment was affecting her, she began
to consider adoption seriously. A year later she and her husband adopted
a child.

LETTING GO OF IVF

When women and men use reproductive technologies to ameliorate infertility, it is common for them to put life "on hold." The combination
of repeated failures to conceive and the need to go on with their lives
often catapults them into a crisis. Peter, a thirty-seven-year-old man,
and Jennifer, thirty-five, suddenly nearing the end of their treatment
options after three years of infertility, expressed anger and sorrow. A
year and a half after I first interviewed them, their hopes had been destroyed, and they had become cynical about the effort to have a child.

Peter sat at his kitchen table, reflecting on several years of infertility
treatment: "I think by the time we will have finished with all this stuff
I will be so sick and tired of everything having to do with a family that

I will want to play tennis for a few years and just have some fun."
Jennifer joined in:

Yes, I think with the IVF that things hit me that I wasn't really expecting. For instance, like the idea of not having children. One more or maybe two more of these things [IVF cycles], and they are done. And if they are negative, or if they don't work, it is like the option has gone. I mean, except for adoption being out there somewhere.

And I guess I started looking at bigger things. Like if I don't have kids. It is a whole different way of looking at my life. Do I want to live my life as I am right now? This is not what I want to be doing thirty years from now, and not just going through all this stress, but going to work. . . . My daily routine is not how I want to be living my life.

So your goal is to have a family and you have to . . . we have to rethink this whole thing. I don't think it is just the disappointment of the cycle not working. You start looking globally at your whole life, and your expectations, and you ask, "What was my life going to be like, and how it is going to be now?"

Women and men often earmark a specific procedure as their last attempt ahead of time. Then, in the midst of IVF, they begin to ask, "What if IVF doesn't work and life becomes completely different from what we anticipated?" Sometimes people experience a sense of disruption belatedly. When this happens, they dread the end of IVF and sometimes delay final treatments while they try to adjust to a view of life without biological children. Until this point it was unthinkable to Jennifer that their efforts might end without a child. The idea that IVF might fail forced her to examine her life and question her expectations. She continued,

So those are the bigger issues that hit me this time which weren't out there before. Because before it was like, "Yes, IVF, that will work, we will get pregnant." That, and then sort of trying to get geared up for another cycle. I think I don't want to do it [next IVF cycle] because I feel it gets me closer to not having children. It is like I still have one out there, and maybe it will work. It is hope. There is hope out there. Whereas, if it is done, it is gone.

Jennifer and Peter had begun infertility treatment optimistically, expecting that medical intervention would soon bring results. As time passed and one kind of treatment gave way to another, there was nothing left to try but IVF. Now, with the end of medical treatment in sight,

Jennifer and Peter were trying to face the painful possibility that all their
energy and effort might be for nought. Jennifer's response was to put
off the unbearable end of this chapter in their lives by deferring the last
IVF cycle.

Peter and Jennifer were facing a very different life from the one they
had anticipated for so long. They were trying on the prospect of life
without children. Reflecting on the IVF cycle they had just finished, Peter
said, "Three [cycles] is my limit. Not hers, but mine. And two may be
mine, too, I don't know. I will have to wait until we get two. I know
that I won't do any more than three. I am sick and tired of putting my
life—our life—on hold. But it is just an easier thing for me to come to
than for Jennifer."

Agreeing, Jennifer said,

*So I know that they [physicians] prepare you when they say, "Okay,
here is how the cycle goes, blah, blah, blah," and you get to this point
and the results are, "Well, it could not work." It is like, "How do you
mean, it could not work?" So I think having it not work has brought
up a lot of stuff with me, thinking if the other one or two [cycles]
don't work, are we going to be childfree? Because right now adoption
is not appealing to either of us. We haven't put much energy into it.*

Peter responds,

*I think that the reasons why you would perhaps not go for adoption
are different from mine, and I could be wrong. I am not so much worried about getting somebody's used car kind of syndrome, as it is even
more my experience from watching our friends—that it is even more
disruptive than the medical intervention. It is a nightmare. At least
with this stuff [medical treatment] you go through the protocol and
you are going to be taking a pregnancy test on this day, and it might
not be what you want, but that one is done.*

Jennifer agrees with this: "Yeah, you deal with it and get over it."

It becomes apparent they have had similar discussions with each other
many times. Peter's and Jennifer's comments on IVF are closely linked
to a deeper issue—the disruption to life posed by their infertility, and
their efforts to resolve their childlessness and carry on with their lives.
Their comments about adoption reveal their continuing attachment to
the cultural ideology of biological parenthood and their rejection of alternatives. Even though they think IVF is almost hopeless and have negative feelings about adoption, Peter and Jennifer are fearful of childless-

ness. It represents endless pain and mourning, and, perhaps, lifelong disruption. Facing the end of medical treatment, Jennifer calls attention to her profound sense of disruption:

This last break that we had in the fall was really helpful. I felt happy, I was playing tennis. I was doing a lot of stuff and feeling good, but you [to Peter] and also my therapist did point out to me that I should take a break before going for the next one and try to feel healthy again. When you are doing these cycles and you stop exercising, you just feel horrible. Do I try to get myself back to how I felt good, to start into another one? Or just go for it and get it done, and get it over with?

Meanwhile, the need to get on with their lives is creating pressure to bring this period of medical treatment to a close:

Peter has been trying to do a job search but it's like, "No, limit your-self to the local area. You can't go anywhere else." We talk about, "Can we do this?" or "Can we do that?" and we can't make plans. So we plow ahead and just do the next cycle and get it over with. Can we resolve it? Because I look at how I feel, which is, "If this were it [end of treatment] and if we were done, could I be accepting?" Right now I am so teary about it. I think, "Oh, I might never have kids." Could I accept it if it was a final statement? And people promise that you do resolve these things, but I look at it and ask, "How will I resolve it?" I feel cheated. It is unfair. The chance that I had has gone. It is not how I wanted things to be. So how do you accept that? It is not like you just said, "I don't want to have kids," or, "We tried, so it is okay, we did everything." I don't see how it feels good. When you are so enmeshed in it, it is like, "How am I going to get over it?"

Peter responds, "It is not supposed to feel good."

Jennifer counters, "How do you resolve it?" to which Peter responds, "The way that you do with other things."

Jennifer, aghast, says, "Just with time? Or do you just accept it?"

Peter responds, "I think so. Because I, for one, am not going to let us do what we have seen other people do, which is they seem to go to any extreme on the face of the earth to have a frigging family. That is just too far for me."

Hope is inextricably linked to notions of progress, which are embed-ded in U.S. values of activity, achievement, and focus on the future.[3] Giving up hope represents loss of meaning.[4] As they face the loss of their hopes, Jennifer and Peter are engaged in a struggle to find meaning in their lives. They need to regroup and find another focus for their energies. Peter struggles with how to set limits on an experience that he feels is out of his control, while Jennifer, having just begun to face the end of treatment, cannot yet imagine another route through life. For women who have always imagined themselves as mothers, finding alternative ways of envisioning their lives may take years.

LIVING WITH MULTIPLE DISRUPTIONS

Not only did women and men in this study consider infertility itself to be a disruption, they were also subject to other disruptions, such the illness or death of parents, the onset of other illnesses, and job losses. The cumulative effects of these disruptions took a heavy toll and heightened the sense of loss caused by infertility. Looking back over several years, Jane, thirty-eight years old, and Ted, forty, describe the chaos they lived through. Successive infertility treatments have been only one disruption in their lives.

JANE: *We knew we wanted children when we got married. But there were some things we wanted to do first. So once we started trying, we tried for two and a half years. So we kept trying. We did about six cycles of IUI [intrauterine insemination]. Or seven maybe. But somewhere in there, every time they did an IUI they examined the sperm under a microscope. One time the doctor told us it looked pretty low, and then one time another doctor told me she didn't see any of it at all. So we went to see a urologist who she [physician] recommended. And he came up with a million sperm count [20 million or more is considered normal]. He recommended . . . he told us that the only thing that he could imagine working was IVF. So we went to see this other doctor. We heard that she was a good person, so we sought her out, and she wanted another sperm count. Now, did we do one? Yeah, we did one and it looked really . . . oh, I know what it was. She did a sperm count and it looked low, but then she wanted another sperm count where she would do some regulation to look at it. Oh, she was going to try to freeze it.*

TED: *She would freeze it and see what would be there after the freezing process to see if they could save a number of speci-mens.*[5]

JANE: *They concentrate them. Oh, and at the same time we were looking into adoption. And so that same week we had an appointment, the first adoption appointment with an attorney. And Ted had the appointment to bring the sperm in for freezing, and the Sunday before that our house burned down.*

But there's something actually before that, which is at the end of August or beginning of September I got diagnosed with Graves' disease, which is a hyperthyroid. And okay, so then our house burned down. And in between that we kept on trying [to conceive]. But then the house burned down and I was struck with Graves' disease, and so we stopped trying. Probably the house burning down was the main thing, but also I got referred to a specialist, and he said not to try to get pregnant until they could fix my thyroid. But we wouldn't have been able to try, anyway, by then. We were just dealing with our basic needs.

This litany of disasters not surprisingly affected how Jane and Ted viewed their fertility problems. Jane looked back on these losses and their consequences:

It's been a really wild couple of years for us. And in terms of our relationship, it's been probably, if anything, positive. You know, we really have stuck together, and it's been fine for us, and I know that for a lot of people whose houses have burned down, it could go either way. Either strengthened their relationship or the things that are already . . . the pebble that's already in the shoe starts to really rub. So we really stayed very busy working on dealing with getting our lives back in order, and we're pretty proud of ourselves that we came out of that. We decided not to rebuild, and six months after the fire we moved in here, so we feel like it has worked out as well as it could. There are a few things that we lost that we are still sad about. But I'm not sad about that much. I'm actually pretty happy we're here. So then we started to talk again about starting to try [to conceive]. That was March, maybe, when we were still over in the other rental house. And I think that was right before we moved here. The week we bought the house.

And Ted went and got another sperm count. That doctor's theory is that it's related to the fact that Ted had Hodgkin's disease when he was in his early twenties and had radiation.

A lot of people we talked to said they weren't able to emotionally pursue adoption and biological stuff at the same time. And I know before the fire I didn't feel that way. I felt like I had so much sort of frantic energy about it that I could juggle twelve balls. Probably I was feeling that more than you [Ted] were and you were saying, "Okay, go ahead, whatever you want to do." And after we started the donor insemination, I mean, some of it was that maybe we were reenergized. That there was maybe now a new chance. But I think it was that I didn't feel anymore like I could . . . like I had the emotional stamina to be doing both at the same time.

In concluding that their relationship has been made stronger as they have dealt with all these troubles, Jane emphasizes triumph over adversity, a core aspect of the ideology of individualism in the United States.[6] Weathering disruption is not new to them. Although she emphasizes the strengthening of their relationship, Jane also acknowledges that the "frantic energy" she was previously able to invest in the effort to have a child has been consumed by the disruptions in their lives. Dealing with other life problems has diverted their attention away from infertility and put it into another, more all-encompassing, perspective.

Disruption to life serves as a catalyst for rethinking common assumptions about life. Disruptions often reveal deep-seated cultural expectations and cast new light on everyday practices. The pursuit of continuity itself can be seen as a cultural ideology that is built on a constellation of factors embedded in American life.[7]

LETTING GO OF BIOLOGICAL PARENTHOOD

Giving up medical treatment means giving up on biological parenthood. After several years of infertility, it has finally been discovered that it is Judith's husband, and not Judith herself, who is infertile. Resisting all Judith's efforts to persuade him to have tests, her husband finally agreed to be tested when their physician declined to proceed with IVF unless he did so:

I was disappointed and sad for him because we had—he had finally come around to it that it was him. And that was tough for him in the beginning. And now all of a sudden he can't say, "I'm sorry" enough. What have I really put him through? And then again, we still don't know. We can sit here and say, "I don't think that I would have a doctor tell me today that it is the egg." I mean, they just say it could be. But logically—I am a real logical person—logic says here is the only thing. I just felt bad for him because we had put all our hopes on it. And all of a sudden you come crashing down.

In trying to come to terms with her husband's infertility, Judith relies on logic, a core element of the American ideology of individualism, to find an explanation she can live with.[8] Part of her concern is about the relationship and how it will be affected by this belated identification of the problem.

I think it's women's intuition. You are just not surprised that something is wrong, whereas he had always been surprised that something was wrong. I wasn't, for some reason, some gut feeling, and I had no way of knowing. But I don't think I have blamed him. If anything, the only time I would become frustrated was earlier on when he didn't want to accept what the doctors were saying. Never did I ever blame him. I was just saying, "Let us keep moving on."

The different responses that women and men have to the identification of a cause for infertility reflect different cultural dialogues about manhood and womanhood and the role fertility plays in these dialogues. The cultural ideology about manhood assumes potency. Motherhood has other meanings, and in her anger about infertility Judith belittles men's role and highlights women's role:

So we know that there is no way his sperm are going to penetrate my egg. Number one, they can't get through the cervical mucus, and number two, they don't have the enzyme, they are missing the enzyme. They get through the cumulus. So we know there is no way. We were both disappointed. I think that it probably hit me the hardest, and I was mean. I am not normally a mean person, but I didn't handle it well from that standpoint. I was just mad that I was never going to be a mother. I think that there are things that people say that from a father's standpoint, they are a father, no matter what you call a dad, but you don't go through something really prior to that to make you that father other than your sperm swims around.

But in motherhood, motherhood really starts at the time that you become pregnant. And I realized that I was never going to have those things. That I was never going to see the birth of a baby. Never going to have all those sensations that everybody else has talked about. It is still a fairly emotional decision because they were the cards that were dealt to me.

In differentiating motherhood and fatherhood, Judith ascribes much greater importance to motherhood, and, in enumerating what is being lost, she demonstrates that she has begun to mourn the loss of biological motherhood:

One day you sit there and say, "Okay, we have got money, we will survive it." The house that we have been putting off buying until we knew how many kids we were going to have and everything was going to be perfect. We were going to do that, buy the new car and do all the exciting things and be just a couple, right? That was going to be our family, but that lasted about twenty-four hours with the two of us.

Reporting how briefly she considered being childless, Judith then returned for a final consultation with her physicians: "We had a talk with the doctors. They said, 'You could do one of the new procedures, which is where they inject it [ICSI]. So I explored that. And I was bored to tears. I just didn't want to hear about it. I just honestly didn't believe in it anymore, that $15,000 later I would have a baby." Having finally closed the door on these technologies, Judith was able to consider adoption: "So we started the adoption process and I got all encouraged, and I thought, 'This is it; it is going to happen.' We are not a beautiful couple, but we are not real bad—somebody will pick us. And the doctors also said try donor insemination, and Roy has been real anxious for me to try that, but I just wasn't interested anymore. Adoption is going to work."

Most, but not all, couples are unable to contemplate adoption seriously until they have finally abandoned medical treatment; they may express negative views about adoption up to the point of stopping treatment. Once adoption becomes the only remaining option, however, like Judith, people may experience a shift that constitutes the beginning of alternative ways of viewing parenthood. Although contemplating adoption means giving up biological parenthood, it enables people to rework their ideas about parenthood around a culturally acceptable alternative.

At the same time, Judith is coming to terms with the extent of her grief at missing out on pregnancy:

I don't think I had really realized that the next step that I had to face, which is not being pregnant. I didn't think that was going to be a big deal for me. I didn't think I cared anything about getting fat and all those things. I don't think I realized that I was going to miss mother-hood. But that is okay. The bottom line is that I want a baby.

So I want to adopt. I was watching Phil Donahue, and the woman he was interviewing, they have been trying to adopt for ten years. I was sitting there going, "I can't wait. I don't have ten years." When I get depressed I go and buy something, so we have gone and bought strollers. We have two strollers sitting in there. I feel like I have to have hope. I have to believe that someday I am going to have a baby.

Sometimes couples plan for adoption if medical treatment fails. Openness to adoption *during* medical treatment makes treatment seem less of an all-or-nothing issue. According to Susan, it reduced the stress of medical treatment:

My reactions to the fourth IVF made me see that I didn't want to do it [IVF] again. When the doctor told me in January that I had to re-peat some test, I said, "Come on! I've done this three times. How could it change?" I didn't say that to her, but that was the way I felt. I thought, "This is telling me it's just too much of a hassle, and I need something that will produce a baby at the end, and adoption will." It's just a matter of time. If one of us had said the most important thing is biological, that would have put so much pressure on the IVF. I might have had a different stress level during the whole thing. But because I always knew I could just quit and do adoption at any point, and we'd both be happy, then it really took a lot of pressure off it.

When people are able to let go of the cultural ideology of biological parenthood before undergoing final medical options, they experience those medical treatments much differently from people who feel they have no other recourse. Everyone who goes through infertility must grapple with cultural ideologies they cannot live up to, but the point at which people seriously begin to resist those ideologies varies greatly and affects how they will weather this disruption. Larry, who learned about his infertility several years ago and has already come to terms with cul-tural ideologies about manhood and biological parenthood, looks at the questions he and his partner face as they prepare to discontinue medical treatment:

My mind is clear as far as the fertility problems. But I wish something would either happen, or, what it's gonna feel like when we decide to make that decision to stop. We're gonna have to be able to handle that. Our decision is something that's gonna be hard to handle, maybe. Like, "What is our next step?" Or, "Is there a next step?" Or "Let's just go on with our own life." Of course, we'd say, "Adoption next!" But I think we need to let some time go by and maybe give us a chance to settle. Give ourselves a chance to . . . I don't know if it's to grieve or to just pass some time. Pass a little water under the bridge until you are ready to take on a new challenge.

Larry's comments call attention to two ways that men and women reconcile failure to conceive with reproductive technologies. First, implicit in his statement, "My mind is clear" is the cultural notion that since he has done his best, it is okay to stop treatment. Second, his comments illustrate the process by which hope is reframed by identifying a new challenge. These ideas are deeply embedded in American cultural ideals, enabling people to find culturally acceptable ways of reconciling unfulfilled desires.

CHAPTER 11

Redefining Normalcy

When infertility goes on for years, the goal of parenthood becomes an abstraction whose realization may seem increasingly unlikely. If biological parenthood finally occurs, women and men meet it not with complacency but with surprise and sometimes ambivalence. Marjorie, a forty-year-old woman who has had three miscarriages and experienced preterm labor prior to the birth of her child, sat on her couch talking about how it felt to become a parent after so many years of infertility.

It is hard to explain. We got the Jeep — we have a Jeep now — and we have a golden retriever. We are like the all-American family. We leave the hospital [after birth of their baby], and with the baby in the Jeep we would have been a great commercial because we had all the flowers and the gifts, and it looked like we had been there eons. We are coming home, and we have a car seat, and she is in the car seat with Daddy in the front seat, and I am in the back, and we are only two or three miles away from the hospital, and we said, "Oh, my gosh, there is no turning back." It is very scary, all of a sudden it hits you. You wait these nine months, and then you are responsible for this life. But it has been wonderful.

In the early chapters of this book, women talked about their feelings that not having children is un-American. Now Marjorie talks about being the all-American family. She draws the analogy to a commercial, and indeed her family portrait sounds picture-perfect. Living out the cultural ideology of biological parenthood is normalcy, American style. Marjorie is uncomfortable, even ambivalent, about it: "There is no turning back." During years of medical treatment she became accustomed to a life scenario that is distinctly abnormal: multiple miscarriages, difficult pregnancies, and constant grief and pain. The new picture superimposed on the old one makes the whole experience seem somewhat surreal, except for one thing: there is a new life for whom she is responsible. After all the years of focusing on herself and her relationship with her husband, she has someone else to think about.

Restoring normalcy means reconstructing the life story, and leaving space for new possibilities to emerge is part of this process. For Marjorie, the shape of the future has changed. She concludes, "A baby changes your whole perspective of things. My tomorrows are all associated with her and what's to come. My future has changed."

Marjorie is not only reexamining the past in relation to the present; she is also rethinking the future. It is not surprising that she sounds tentative. Neither is it surprising that Marjorie responds to her baby by looking at her own future. When a child finally arrives, both the future and the past must be reconfigured.[1] After anticipating childlessness as a likely outcome for so long, the birth of a child forces parents to rethink gender identity once again. Now that Marjorie has finally given birth to a child, she must rethink the ideologies of motherhood and continuity in relation to her own altered life.

Even for parents who eventually have a biological child, the experience of infertility shatters any sense of complacency about the predictability of life. Such parents often express persistent worries that something will happen to the child. The anguish they have experienced during the period of infertility makes an indelible mark. Normalcy itself thus becomes suspect: hence Marjorie's expression of disbelief that she and her family now epitomize the all-American family. Yet despite people's discomfort when they belatedly find themselves fulfilling the cultural norm of parenthood, the desire to fit in is a strong one. Under such circumstances, what constitutes normalcy must be redefined.

THE LONGING FOR NORMALCY

Biomedicine reinforces moral dialogues about normalcy, most specifically the cultural ideology of biological parenthood. Redefining normalcy is a gradual process in which women and men rework what "normal" means at the same time that they rethink their relationship with each other. Alison and Scott illustrate this process as they reach a turning point in their efforts to have a child. Asked how infertility had affected their relationship, they responded:

SCOTT: *We have our ups and downs.*

ALISON: *I think it has brought us closer.*

SCOTT: *Yes, I think that it has brought us closer overall. I think, part of the reason, I am now moving more willingly towards adoption because I want to move on from this. I don't want to be defined as a couple who is infertile and doesn't have a child. I want to start enjoying other parts of life with Alison. And so I guess for me there is a little more of a sense of urgency because I want to enjoy other parts of life. I have a sense of being stuck.*

Alison, too, longs for normalcy in life and describes what she now considers would be a normal life.

ALISON: *I have heard people in our discussion group talk about how it is an issue for your whole life, and the grief and the pain, and I guess I just can't buy that. I sort of think that there is a regret, but I don't know, I am just not the person to hang on to that sort of thing. Like if we never had children, I see that at least for me it would really be debilitating. But were we to adopt children and become an adoptive family I don't really see . . . unless, you know, if we are not able to integrate as an adoptive family and somehow that becomes a lifelong failure and we are screwed-up parents with screwed-up kids. I could imagine hanging your hat on that and say, "What if we had our own?" But if it is sort of a normal life, I can't see obsessing about it. It just doesn't make a lot of sense to me. But who knows what will happen?*

SCOTT: *I think it will pass. I don't think I am going to forget it. But I don't think it is something we will ruminate over a lot. I think that we are going to have a child, maybe more than one.*

ALISON: *I don't know. I think that your life fills up with love and relationships. Like when I think back to my most miserable lonely times when I was single or broken up with some love affair, that pain was so intense, but I can barely*

*remember it now because my life has now been filled up
with a real constant, you know, healthy love. So I sort of
imagine it being the same thing. That if the adoption thing
works out and is fairly normal, and we integrate as a family, and I think that is going to be its own challenge. But
I see that as a lifelong challenge—being adoptive parents
with an adopted family. But I guess I don't see that loss
sort of looming in everyday life. I think that it will fade.*

After years of attempting to conceive without success, normalcy to
Alison now means having an adoptive family. Underlying this shift is
her definition of family. It means "integrating" as a family and having
healthy family relationships. She hopes for "a normal life," in which
everyone gets along, but she fears being part of a dysfunctional family.
She therefore sees creating a healthy adoptive family as a lifelong challenge.[2]

Scott, however, has not let go of the idea of having a biological child.
He does not see adopting a child as a foregone conclusion:

SCOTT: *I think this interview would have been different three
          months ago. Or even a month ago. We have gone through
          so many phases, and three months from now it is going to
          be very different. I just feel like we are entering a very
          critical phase where some major decisions need to be
          made about in vitro, and adoption, they are going to be
          made in a very short period of time. And you have caught
          us just before those decisions are going to be made.*

ALISON: *Before the disasters happen in our life. So it is a good
          moment.*

SCOTT: *So you can see our temperaments.*

In this interchange, Alison is more definite than Scott, now that she
has redefined normalcy, about what a normal life would entail. She is
more fearful of things turning out badly, however. Their interwoven
uncertainties create tension as both of them slowly let go of the cultural
ideology of biological parenthood.

COMBATING THE MORAL FORCE OF NORMALCY

When people are working to reclaim their lives after ending medical
treatment, one of their biggest challenges may be sharing their decision

with their families. Their parents, in particular, may subscribe to cultural ideologies about parenthood and about biological reproduction that women, especially, feel poorly equipped to manage. The attitudes of others can hinder the redefinition of normalcy. Susan and Stacy describe how differently their two sets of parents responded to the news that they were going to adopt a child. Susan observes, "So when we told his parents we were adopting, they said, 'Oh, that's wonderful.' They were perfectly fine with that. They don't want to interfere. So they are helping us find a kid."

The situation with her own parents was much different, however:

SUSAN: *I would have preferred not to tell my parents until much later, but the day I had a miscarriage with my last IVF, my parents had come to visit. One day we had this argument when they were visiting because my mom just kept saying, "You have to keep trying." I said, "We're going to adopt."*

STACY: *She was very negative about that.*

SUSAN: *She said, "Don't give up. You shouldn't give up." I said, "I'm not giving up." We had this whole discussion—not discussion because we were screaming at each other—of it's not her business, it's my business and Stacy's business, and we've done enough medical things and I'm tired of it, and we're going to adopt, and she just didn't want to hear that. Finally, I said something to her like, "Mom, it's either adoption or no children, and it's my choice to have children, so you can either choose to be a grandparent or choose not to. But I'm choosing to be a parent." So she did kind of shut up a little bit after that.*

Megan's mother was more adamantly opposed to her decision to end medical treatment, and her opposition lasted several years, making it much more difficult for Megan to move on:

I know that if we announced that same kind of choice [living without children], it would not be joyfully received by at least one section of the family. Although most would probably be really cool about it. There is just one person that would be a problem with it. My mother. And that's hard, it's hard for me. When it's hard for me, it makes it hard for him [husband]. There is just so much emotion surrounding that, and I don't feel at all free to express myself to her because she just tears herself apart over it whenever I even mention this. So there's this big thing between us that can't be talked about. It's the elephant in the room that nobody is talking about. Everybody knows it's there but no one's talking about it. Everybody is trying to tiptoe around it. We just can't do it.

When I try and bring it up, she just gets defensive and angry, and all of the things that she wanted when I did not get pregnant. I feel so pressured by that. Oh boy, that is really hard. Sometimes she says things I can't believe: "It would be okay if your brother didn't have children, but not your children." It's like I'm the perfect child. I just want to say, I don't ever want to be a mother like that. I don't want children if I'm going to do that, and that's unfair to her. But it has made it very hard and almost impossible for me to settle into it with her. Because if I ever say to her, "That's it. We've decided not to have them," what do you think she'd do? My mother is very confrontational in many ways. She's very emotional, she's very forthcoming, she doesn't hide anything, and she's not prone to sitting down and logically discussing things. Which I think we are. She'd burst into tears and not talk to me for weeks. Building a wall. She makes this issue very difficult to get around because I can't resolve it with her, even if I can resolve it between us [self and partner].

So one day when Mom and I had been talking and we were really in this good place, and I thought that we were pretty comfortable, so I brought this up. I said, "Sometime when you're in the mood—it doesn't have to be now—we need to talk about some of the things around this infertility and how you feel about it." And there was this instantaneous change. She was cooking, and she just stopped, got stiff like a ramrod, and said, "Well, you know exactly how I feel about that." Not, "I can't even imagine how you feel." But just this huge tirade that rolled out like a giant wave, and I was going, "Whoa!" And she ended it with "Is that clear enough for you?" "Oh, yeah. No problem. Is dinner ready?"

My mother, who only ever expected to raise kids, is as deprived as we are in some ways because she feels that it's something that she is entitled to. That was her entitlement in her old age—my kids, and to live close to us and have her grandchildren around her, and she didn't get it. So the fact that she can't cope with that is something I'm going to have to cope with. Sometimes I feel a lot older than she is.

Megan's story of her mother's response is a reminder that powerful cultural ideologies impinge on the process of letting go of biological parenthood *through other people*. Megan's mother expected to have grandchildren and, indeed, feels entitled to have them. Megan's only sibling has no children and shows no sign of having any in the future. The fact that Megan is unable to provide her mother with grandchildren suggests that, in her mother's view, Megan is somehow at fault, because if she were willing to try hard enough, she would have them. In Megan's story, the cultural ideology of generational continuity joins together with the cultural ideologies of biological parenthood and individualism, in which perseverance looms large.[3] This combination of normalizing ideologies almost overwhelms Megan and stymies her efforts to bring this phase of her life to a close. The conflict in which Megan and her mother find themselves is intense because it engages multiple, interacting cultural ideologies. The moral force of the ideology of the family interacts with both the ideology of biological parenthood and the ideology of continuity.

In the United States, where the nuclear family is the dominant model, cultural dialogues about the family give little overt attention to the rights and responsibilities of the extended family. Yet the extended family continues to be very important, and perhaps never more so than when questions of attenuating generational continuity are raised, thus engaging the cultural ideology of continuity. When other ideologies simultaneously come into play, the moral force of those ideologies may swamp the culturally agreed-upon rights of the individual.

This dilemma raises questions: Who is entitled to children? Does entitlement extend beyond the nuclear family to extended family members? It also raises questions about responsibilities within the family: What are a family's rights and obligations? Does a daughter have special obligations? What extenuating circumstances are sufficient to release a person from her obligations? Megan has been forced to address such questions repeatedly because of her mother's stance on Megan's responsibilities as a daughter. These questions are implicit whenever infertility is diagnosed. They were a consideration for everyone in this study in one way or another, and they played a role in lengthening medical treatment.

MOVING PAST GRIEF

Grieving for unborn children is a catalyst for redefining normalcy. There are no rituals or other public markers to help people define or manage their grief when they have experienced infertility.[4] Such grief may be liberally laced with anger. Indeed, anger may be, and often is, the dominant motif immediately after women and men relinquish efforts to conceive through reproductive technologies. The intangible nature of infertility—most often there is no dead child to mourn—makes coming to terms with this loss all the more difficult. Such experiences lead women and men to question their assumptions about normalcy.

The grieving process often makes it possible for people to reconsider cultural ideologies to which they previously subscribed, such as the cultural ideology of biological parenthood, and to resist those ideologies in favor of alternative solutions. Alicia looks back on her experience after four miscarriages, adopting a child who was reclaimed, and other tragedies in her life:

My mother died, and my sister died. And I had four miscarriages, and I had one of the most immense professional projects that I've ever had. And this was all in a six-year period. So you're in a position with infertility that pretty much normal people, without some sort of superhuman effort or tremendous support from somebody or another, a lot of people would just not make it. If anything else in your life goes wrong, there's no room.

It's a process of continual loss and grief. I feel like I have four dead children and one kidnapped child. And I'm a pro-choice person. I've never had an abortion. When I was pregnant . . . the first part of the child is the dream of the child, and I felt very much like these were children for me. The other thing about the continual losses is, you feel like you are a damaged vessel. It's one thing not to be able to conceive, but it's another thing not to be able to protect your child. So you feel maternal and unable to protect your child. Even though it was thirty days [the length of each pregnancy]. It was the same day, almost, with every pregnancy.

Alicia, in recounting this long series of tragedies that led to profound bodily distress, refers to herself as a "damaged vessel" who cannot protect her children, either in the womb or outside it. She captures the embodied nature of these pregnancies when she talks about the "dream of the child," which is what turns them into real children, even in the first thirty days of pregnancy. She describes her helplessness in feeling maternal about them but not being able to protect them.

The other thing I have great difficulty with, I think there's a real strong issue among women. I have lots of problems with my closest friends who are busily having babies. I think when you have your own child, you're totally absorbed by that. Especially if you're a late-in-life mother. And that's your life. And all of a sudden, I was losing babies and losing my friends. And then I also think there is a competition. I think that historically, maybe forever, women have competed [with each other] by the men they are attached to and the babies they can produce. And however enlightened you may be, you'll feel that surging through your body.

Alicia's suggestion of competition between women to have children is startling but plausible. It is borne out in the reports of women undergoing infertility who report women friends with babies being insensitive to their feelings of loss and emptiness. Women who conceive with ease not only may be absorbed in the pregnancy, they may also be responding to cultural ideologies that promote the ideas that pregnancy and childbirth are primary roles for women. Of course, women who are trying to conceive are also often hypersensitive in their relationships with friends who have become mothers.[5]

Because Alicia is now thinking about trying to adopt another child, she recently turned down a big promotion at work. She is mulling over what she has gone through and trying to put it into perspective so that she can come to terms with her losses.

I may never have a child. I have to accept the fact. No one cares about that. Everyone says, "Of course you will." There hasn't been a person I've talked to that doesn't say, "You will have your baby. This wasn't meant to be." I think that's bullshit. I may never have a child. That is the truth. I may never have a child biologically, and I may never have an adopted child. It just may not happen with me. Then, if you're going to spend your life without a child, then the other things in life that are extremely valuable and rich become the focus for you. Your ability to be a childless person. And have all the enriching things, that a childless person can do, that everyone else envies. And you celebrate those things! It might not have been your choice, but you play the hand you're dealt with. And if you're going to survive and be healthy and happy and you don't suffer the entire loss of your whole family and not figure out ways to be, then you're not going to sit around being miserable about something that you can't do anything about. You do the best you can and then you go on. And try and have what you have and enjoy it.

So I had to make a decision about taking that job or waiting for this

*other thing [adoption] that may never come — they were on a collision
course. And I feel it is yet another price that I have to pay. I may get
another crack at it [job she turned down]. People that are pregnant or
people who are trying to be pregnant or people who are trying to adopt
make very different life decisions. And if you're trying to do this for six
years, seven, eight, ten years, then you are forgoing other things in your
life. We never did. I mean, we did it all! We had deaths in the family, infertility, breakdowns, we were full throttle. But now we're worn out.
You can only do one thing at a time. You wear out. Just your endur-
ance. And then you start having to make those tough choices.*

Alicia is simultaneously trying to address her sense of grief and loss,
make sense out of it, and redefine what is normal. As she faces the
unknown future, she is trying on the possibility that she will be childless
at the same time that she is again trying to adopt. At this first interview
Alicia had already relinquished the social imperative of a biological
child, which she mourned along with her miscarriages. With the "kidnapped," or reclaimed child, she mourned the possibility of having *any*
child. But, shortly after this interview, she phoned to invite me over to
see the adopted baby she had suddenly received twenty-four hours earlier. She was anxious that this child, too, would be reclaimed, but, one
year later, when the child was starting to walk, she and her husband
looked back on this time and concluded that, although their ten years
in limbo were over, their sense of normalcy had changed. The chaos
they had lived through had receded. Their primary focus was on their
family life. Women and men undergoing medical treatment for infertility
tend to lose sight of two things: first, that it is possible to live out the
cultural ideology of the family with a child who is not biologically related, and second, that the cultural ideology of the family holds greater
power than the cultural ideology of the biological child.[6]

Redefining normalcy is a process that occurs only under extreme du-
ress, when it becomes apparent that living out cultural ideologies is unlikely to happen as originally planned. But even if it is eventually possible
to embody those ideologies through the birth of a biological child, the
ideology has been weakened, undermined by people's own experiences
and by other forces. For example, voices from within Resolve may incessantly question the need for a child to be a biological child, leading
people eventually to believe that where the child comes from is unimportant. Charlie and Ellen describe how their view of adopted children
changed:

CHARLIE: *When you adopt a child, you realize that child is so
            much your own, it just blurs the distinction entirely
            [between biological and nonbiological children].*

ELLEN: *At least it did for us. But initially we didn't know any-
            thing about it. Of course we were hesitant because we
            . . . well, we didn't know anything about it. We decided
            that doing it privately was the way we wanted to go, and
            my initial feeling was that I didn't want to feel like a ba-
            bysitter. I wanted a child and then wanted to dump the
            birth mother on the other side of the earth. As I educated
            myself [through Resolve], I came to realize that all my
            fears, all my insecurities, really weren't feeling good.
            There was always the struggle, "Could you love someone
            who's not biologically related to you?" I think everyone
            goes through that struggle. I knew someone who had
            done a private adoption. I knew the child and I realized
            this was a great kid, and his parents really felt like his
            parents. It became clear to me that it was something that
            I could do. And when I realized that I could, when we
            realized that . . . When the doctor said to us, "This is
            your child," that was it.*

CHARLIE: *Oh, yeah, the first time I laid eyes on him, that was it.
            That just eliminated the issue right then and there. It
            took half a second. Ellen was sitting in the waiting room.
            I was standing there—they had a little viewing area.
            I was looking through the big glass window, and they
            brought out this hairy little thing. I thought, "This is our
            little monkey."*

The key to this story of redefining normalcy through adoption lies in education. As Ellen and Charlie explored adoption, primarily through resources provided by Resolve, it began to seem less scary. After beginning the actual process, they were connected with the birth mother early in her pregnancy, and by the time their child was born they had no hesitation in accepting this child as their own.

ENACTING GENDER THROUGH THE FAMILY

At the same time that women and men are redefining normalcy, they are engaged in reworking their gender identity. In doing so, they re-

peatedly question not only the importance of a biological child but also
how they live out other parts of their lives, and how and whether those
other parts of life fit with parenthood. The family becomes the focus of
this work whether or not women and men eventually have children.

Linda, who gave birth to twins after going through IVF, felt a need
to reclaim her body. Although this is a common lament among new
mothers who have not gone through infertility, it is unusual for women
who have gone through infertility to call attention to this need. They
may feel that having put so much energy into conception, they cannot
complain about the outcome. For Linda, however, bodily consciousness
and an inner sense of harmony were necessary for restoring a sense of
normalcy, which she had lost with infertility and the subsequent birth
of twins. When they reached the toddler stage, she felt her life was out
of control. In order to recapture her life, she began several types of
therapy:

*I went back to therapy. I had to stop when I was on bed rest [during
pregnancy]. But when I was too overwhelmed with the babies, I went
back to therapy. And that has helped me with all of my stressors. I
also go to a body worker. She does this thing that's sort of like a mas-
sage except it's more like working with your breathing patterns and
then you are also doing talk therapy. I've been doing that for the last
three or four months. It's been nice for me because one of the things
that I definitely felt for a long time was I kept going through this
thing of feeling like I wanted to have my body back. I felt like I
hadn't had my own body for a really long time. And I really had a
need to be in touch with my body or have it be my own body. I'm
sure that was part of weaning the babies. I still haven't gotten to the
point of having any time at all to get any exercise. That's one of the
things that I think will have to be next stage for me, finding some way
to get out and swim or walk or do something where I can get some
regular exercise.*

*But this body therapy thing was very nice to help me to start feel-
ing like I had my body back, and I was sort of getting back to being
my own person a little bit. It's been just an incredible transition. And
I'm sure it has been exacerbated by going through all the infertility
workup and tests and all the stuff you have to go through with the
IVF. I never thought about it like this before, but in actuality I'm sure
that this also contributed to my feeling of not having my own body.*

And then the physical problems I had during my pregnancy certainly was part of all that.

Linda has experienced this life transition primarily through her body. After infertility treatment and her serious illness during pregnancy, she is trying to regain her bodily knowledge, which she feels grounds her in reality. She needs to feel in charge of her body in order to deal with twins. In addition, her relationship has been under great stress since the birth of the twins. She and Josh have no time for themselves as a couple, and not much time individually, either. Reclaiming her body is the first step in redefining normalcy. A second step is negotiating with Josh over rights and responsibilities, an important aspect of enacting gender in the United States to which both of them have given priority in their years together. The arrival of twins, however, has intervened:

So trying to find time for ourselves individually has been hard. When I started going to therapy every Saturday morning, Josh was complaining about it and then he sort of put his foot down and was able to say that he definitely felt like I shouldn't get every Saturday morning, that he wanted some of them. So then we started doing it back and forth. So it feels more equal now. I think Josh is doing better at saying what he needs more rather than just being kind of unhappy about it and grumpy. You're definitely seeing us at a good moment. We don't have lots of them.

We've been working on being parents to twins for almost a year now. We know a little bit more, and there are good days and bad days, and you [interviewer] are definitely getting a good day. The children have actually been very good all day long, and that really helps. When they are both fussy simultaneously, they can completely wear out two adults in ten minutes. Absolutely knock you down and exhaust you.

Linda introduces a new idea, that parenting twins entails a learning process all its own. She and Josh have to learn how to get along all over again. She places the arrival of twins within a larger perspective:

I guess I see this as part of a long process for Josh and I of learning how to live together and learning how to cope with stresses. I think the whole infertility process was a huge process of learning how to make decisions together and cope with hard things. We did have what I thought was a pretty terrible big fight about a month ago. It was

pretty upsetting to have that happen. I think that's part of the reason
why Josh has decided to go into therapy, and I'm really happy about
that. I think both of us really need to have some place to go outside of
the house and outside of our relationship and outside of the kids.
Have a place to get some help with all the stresses that we go through.

Linda's story demonstrates that parenthood is only one aspect of gender performance. The bigger issue, for her, is one of "learning how to
live together and cope with hard things." Both Linda and Josh feel
shaken by threats to their partnership. Their gender negotiations emphasize the cultural ideology of individualism and autonomy: both partners negotiate for time for themselves, away from the children, to follow
individual pursuits. Children are only part of the equation in living out
the cultural ideology of the family, and for some people they are not
necessarily the most important part.

Enacting gendered expectations is a complex process for men who
have gone through infertility with their wives, regardless of their own
fertility. As Mitchell, thirty-seven years old, suggests, much more is at
stake than simply becoming a father. Questioning the meaning of manhood is a comprehensive project, fraught with anxieties and ambivalent
feelings. When he lost his job shortly after he and his wife conceived, he
was forced to rework his gender identity:

It was real interesting for me to come to grips with who I really was,
with my identity. I felt real solid about my identity of being a father
and now having a family, but I was kind of shaky in the identity as
far as any productivity in the society or something like that, as far as
career or job, that got shaky, so it was like going back and forth be-
tween the two. Coming to grips with who I thought I really was. I
was offered some jobs and part of me was desperate to take them, not
financially, but in an emotional sense, in an intellectual sense, but I
didn't take them, which I thought turned out to be really smart, and
even some jobs that I was kind of interested in because they were in
the industry that I came from, so I knew that I could do it.

Asked if he thinks U.S. society fails to prepare men to think of themselves in parenting roles, he responded,

I think so, because in my experience, and certainly speaking about
myself and from what I can understand from other guys that I have
known, that guys don't really talk about it or read about it or watch

*TV shows that might speak to these kinds of issues. I don't think that
really exists. Because men probably don't really want to talk about it
much, but you really don't prepare, you really don't think about it,
somehow. I get the impression that it just happens, and then it is an
evolving process, and either it evolves well or evolves badly and people get divorced or somehow it works. But I don't see a lot of preparation, and certainly not in my case, and not in the cases of most men
I know. You get married and then you deal with that, and then you
have children and you deal with that, it is not like there is a lot of
forethought about it, and what would a marriage mean to you, or
what a family would mean to everybody concerned.*

This portrayal of how little men think about and prepare for family
life distinctly contrasts with women's reports of intense preparation for
marriage and children. As Mitchell portrays it, men perform gender primarily through their careers:[7]

*And I think to my detriment, I place an undue amount of weight on
career and career planning as opposed to any other kind. I think that
even though certain things have changed a lot in society, I think that
it is weighted toward career. It is simpler for men, in a sense. They are
expected to go out and achieve, and then you deal with other stuff.*

*I think that is wrong, and I found out that is wrong. There needs
to be much more of a balance, and certainly in my mind, my family is
more important now than the job, but things get skewed out of whack
when you are so wrapped up in a career path. I think men are
brought up that way and geared more that way, who you are and
what you have achieved, and then based on that, you get married and
have a family, but that seems ancillary. But I think it has changed. It
used to be much bigger, this kind of ratio, but now it is coming more
this way, and also you have to throw in the economic factors because
when you don't have a job you don't have a whole lot of choice about
what quality of life you have. You just try and get a job and put that
out there again. I think that it has been much harder for women to
break the mold of having to be the one who stays at home and raises
a family and then to go out and create quality in the job force and yet
still having the burden of not only physically having the baby but the
burden of care being on the woman while trying to juggle some kind
of career identity. That is much harder, and there is not a lot of help
from society.*

Mitchell took the step of entering into fatherhood without a job so that he could spend as much quality time with his son as possible. Despite the urge to take almost any job in order to affirm his identity as a man, he stayed at home with his son until the baby was six months old. Discussing this period, he concludes: "We did it together. I wouldn't say that it was equal. But we were both there and we shared all the things that we needed to do all the time for the baby, which was great. It really made us a family unit, a true family unit." To become "a true family unit" epitomizes the cultural ideology of the family. Mitchell and his wife finally became biological parents after many years of effort and began to draw this era of life to a close.

REDESIGNING THE LIFE PLAN

Redefining normalcy for oneself means rethinking specific aspects of gender identity in relation to changing life experiences. Enacting gender entails a process of personal change that is informed by social mores and cultural dialogues. After years of experiencing a sense of difference because of infertility, women and men no longer accept cultural ideologies without question—if they ever did—but they do continue to wrestle with those ideologies within a culturally circumscribed arena, bounded by the known and familiar. People are unable to imagine possibilities outside their cultural worlds, and thus when personal change occurs, it does so within the boundaries of that cultural world. Perry, forty-five years old, describes how he is altering his life plans following the birth of his child:

I thought my future would change more. He is so insidious. He is so overwhelming. Always there, always in your face. I thought I'd be more accommodating. I just worry about getting through the day. I am definitely not futurizing as much about him as I thought I would. But I guess my vision of the future hasn't changed radically. I'm even talking about retiring before he's out of high school. You know, quote retiring. Just quitting work and enjoying something that I like to do instead of driving this long commute. I'm still focused on those same kinds of things I was focused on before he ever came into the world.

Despite his assertion that his plans haven't changed, Perry acknowledges that the presence of a child does affect his future:

My blueprint of life. There's rice cereal and formula spilled all over the here-and-now, okay? But the vision of the future, again, it's back to my blueprint. I do want to quit work by a certain time. You hear a lot of, "We can't do this until the baby gets out of high school." Or that kind of thing. And maybe that will come as he gains friends and stuff but right now it's not. So no, I don't think the blueprint of my life beyond tomorrow has changed dramatically.

Perry's plans illustrate the increasing fluidity of life phases, in which retirement and new parenthood are not mutually exclusive. The birth of their child also leads him to think further about what parenthood and fatherhood mean:

I keep beating on this "aha" I had in my life, that the whole idea of parenting versus creating life was just an incredible "aha," and I know it's going to definitely affect the way I raise him. Just from a standpoint of "I'm not perfect." We're muddling through this thing together. I think the idea of parenting further reinforces my feeling of, "Look, you didn't come with an instruction book. On the day of your birth we toasted you and said, Good, we've completed the birth process. Now we have to figure out how to be parents. There wasn't any class that we could sign up for. So here we are, Johnny, we are muddling through this together."

One of Perry's insights is that parenthood is separate from creating life. He feels ill-equipped actually to be a father and raise a child:

The whole idea of parenting is something that is not biological. It isn't something that you come fully equipped to do. It's something that you just grope your way through and try your best. When I grew up, it was kind of like, "Parents are up there. They got their stripes. I am the parent." You know, have you ever heard that? "We are going to do it this way because I'm the parent." I think that mindset that kids have looking up to their parents, like somehow they have this qualification. Now it's gonna be a lot of difference for him because I'm going to run out with him and say, "I'm a little more qualified than you are to do this." They don't give classes, you don't have to get a license, in fact, you have to do even more to get a driver's license than you do to be a parent.

I would say the infertility work is clearly a transition into a new paradigm. We are here and this is our life. The blueprint of life just got recast.

Perry's insight that parenting is not biological is one that people usually have belatedly, whether they eventually parent a biological child or not. The strength of the cultural ideology of biological parenthood makes it difficult for most people to see this in the early stages of infertility. For those who do view parenthood as a social phenomenon early on, the actual experience underscores it. Perry's observation that the "infertility work is a transition into a new paradigm" affirms this view.

CHAPTER 12

Women Rethinking Parenthood

Redefining normalcy is the prelude to redesigning one's life. When women do not conceive, they begin to turn their lives in new directions. Reworking their gender identity continues while they are rethinking the cultural ideologies to which they previously subscribed. Megan described what had been happening since the preceding year, when her IVF cycle went awry. The effects of the drugs were so distressing that she decided she could not endure any more IVF cycles. She has been rethinking her life:

Boy, these last few months have really been a challenge. I'm not a mother, and I don't have a job forever, so that was a good time to examine all these issues. I know I'm going to feel a twinge if I get to the end of December and Christmas is here, and all the kids in the family are doing kid-type things. . . . I know that by December 31, that it's going to be "Ouch!" Just from what it isn't going to be. But it isn't going to be that knife-in-your-gut thing that it was for a long time. I guess we could probably say we're resolved at this point.

Although Megan acknowledges that being childless is still painful and her career switch somewhat uncertain, she is regaining the self-assurance that was undermined by infertility treatment. Her relationship with her husband—always good—is taking new directions, as each of them explores what they want to do next.

We have gotten really productive. We have traveled. I met a group of women that I really enjoy. We meet and talk about art. We just have lots of things going on that I know we would not otherwise have. I have come into a little more confidence about myself that I don't have to have a child to be patient or tolerant. That I have a lot of other avenues to do in dealing with people.

I'm at an age now where I'm comfortable not having children, and it's amazing to see these people say, "I'm fifty-two and I just had a kid!" If we were to get pregnant naturally, I think both of us would be thunderstruck.

At thirty-seven, Megan is becoming comfortable with her childlessness. She has managed to free herself from cultural ideals that say women must have children to be complete, and from cultural ideologies that say parenthood—especially biological parenthood—is essential to life. Having been thoroughly indoctrinated in cultural priorities, she is now resisting them.

STARTING A NEW LIFE

Although infertility treatment may go on for years, sooner or later people start to rethink the overall direction of their lives. During this process, which may also last for years, people may face questions about gender identity, age, and relationships with a partner and the extended family. The process may be more profound for women than for men because of cultural ideals that equate womanhood with motherhood. But no woman, even one who has succeeded in having children, is exempt from this life transition. Infertility is a life-changing experience because it challenges so many cultural assumptions about how life should be. Women's experience with medical technology is part of the catalyst for this subsequent reworking of life.

Polly, after multiple cycles of IVF, is asking herself what happens next. She describes how the process snowballs:

I have one foot in the world of fertility and one foot in the world of childfree. I have tried my foot in those waters [childlessness], and they don't feel so bad. When I knew that this [medical procedure] was going to be the last time, I had to think about what would happen if it didn't work. Because I'm a planner. I like to be in control of my life, so I started thinking. I remember doing a series of group sessions. We talked about childfree one night and the group leader said, "Well,

*how would you feel? Each of you, how would you feel? What would
you do if you didn't have a child, if you were childfree?" I remember
saying that I think I could accept that as long as I could make some
changes in my life.*

*So I started thinking about what would I want to change in life? I
started thinking, "Yeah, I'll get out of that job, and I'd get rid of this
and I'd get rid of that." You start out thinking, "It's just a job. All I
want to do is get rid of the job." Then you think, "Maybe it's not the
job that's so bad, maybe it's a career. Well, maybe it's not that I want
any career that I could now, maybe it's time to go back to school and
do the things that I didn't do before." You just start throwing stones
in the pond and the rings go out and out and you're going, "No, no,
no, don't go any farther," but you can't stop. It just keeps going and
going and going. I just thought about everything. It took on its own
force and spread out my whole life. You know, do I want to live in
this house? Do I want to be married to Colin? Do I want to live in
this part of the country? I mean, everything.*

*Everything. Every little thing. And that was really frightening. Be-
cause, you know, I build these security blankets. I cover myself with a
certain lifestyle. You're not sure of how that is false. How much of
that is really what you want? How much have you grabbed onto because it was the closest thing or the easiest thing? If I could choose all
over again, would I really choose this? That was kind of scary.*

Having experienced a long period of liminality when she was an infertility patient, Polly is now both intrigued and frightened to find herself
questioning her entire life.

When people are able to let go of adherence to cultural ideologies,
they begin to explore alternative dialogues into which they may fit themselves. As those competing dialogues take hold, specific cultural ideologies may begin to lose their power. During medical treatment women
and men are aware of exerting agency on the situations they have entered, but they usually see their own actions as limited, such as negotiating the details of a particular medical procedure or making decisions
about the next step in medical treatment. When all of that effort becomes
irrelevant, they often nevertheless realize how much power lies in their
own actions and become newly aware of their effectiveness.

Polly and Colin, her husband, approach this phase of the process very
differently. Colin was much less involved in medical treatment than
Polly was. Although he has tried to be supportive, he has been somewhat

detached. Their communication styles are also very different. He is typically quiet and low-key, whereas she is talkative and outspoken. Colin introduces his growing ease with remaining childless:

I got through very little medical stuff when it happened, and um, right now, I'm pretty okay about it. I mean, I'm dealing with not having children. I seem to be okay about it. There was times when I was really bummed about it. I still get bummed about it when, you know, sometimes when I'm around a lot of my family . . . because all my relatives live around here. When I get together with my brother and all the children, my brother's children, my sister's children, sometimes that's hard. Although it gets easier every day.

I look toward the future. I don't think about having children. We have this one more thing [medical procedure] that we're going to do. I just don't know. I really have my doubts this will work 'cause it's never worked before. We've been in this group [Resolve support group] with all these other people, and it never worked for any of them. I don't know anybody it has ever worked for, so.

I just go on with my life. I spend more money now. I guess I'd like to be closer to my brother's and sister's kids, and maybe that would compensate for not having children. If you have a missing leg, you have to go on with your life and make the best you can. If you don't have children, you just go on with your life. You don't sit there and be depressed about it.

Clearly, children continue to be important to Colin, and he is thinking about ways to have children in his life, as most people do who remain childless after infertility treatment. While he talks about making the best of his life, the missing leg metaphor makes it clear that he feels incomplete without children.

Polly takes issue with his comments:

Well, see, I don't want to go on with my life. I want to begin a new life. I want to do things I've never done before. I want to do traveling. I mean, I really have a lot of things I want to do. Like I said, I'm really . . . I'm there. My body is in fertility work, but my mind has gone way beyond it. It's like, "Yeah, okay, okay, let's get it over with." I've really thought about not doing it [medical procedure], but I don't ever want to look back later on in my life and think maybe if I had just tried that one more time, I wonder what it would have been

*like. To me, having a child is a real adventure. It's not something I
want to do because I feel like I have to, it's just a real adventure.*

Several things are being negotiated in this interchange between Polly
and Colin. One of them is the perennial issue about having a child. Polly
is considering adoption as one of her potential directions after she undergoes her final treatment. A second issue is their relationship: will it
continue, and if so, will it be rewritten? How will it change? This relates
to a third issue: what life will be like. Polly asserts she wants to start a
new life. She is unhappy with her job, which she has previously referred
to as "a glorified secretary," and bored with her daily life routine. She
has plans, and whether or not they include a child and a husband, they
definitely include adventure. Colin, however, is quite content in his work
in hotel management. His job requires him to be there, dependably, on
a daily basis. Lengthy travel is not possible for him.

When people undergo such significant personal change, they may
question assumptions they previously subscribed to. Having started to
explore changing her life, Polly looks critically at herself and at her past
life. She examines the last transition she went through—*before* she decided to try to have children—with respect to cultural norms, or
"shoulds," as she calls them:

*That time I decided I needed to be a completely different kind of per-
son. The kind of person I thought I should be, it was all the shoulds:
you should clean the house, you should go to work every day, you
should do this and you should do that, and you should have a relationship with a guy who your mother should just adore, and you
should have a house, and should . . . you know. So I just created it.
I just forged my life into this whole life of shoulds. Recently, when I
went through this big thing about "What do I really want to do with
my life?" I realized that I hate my life. I hate my life. Because all I'm
doing is a bunch of shoulds.*

In saying she hates her life, Polly is, intentionally or not, including
her life with Colin. Rethinking the relationship is common when the
effort to conceive a child together fails. When adherence to cultural
ideologies is suspended in this in-between, liminal phase, cultural dialogues about marriage are also challenged. Not having children poses a
challenge to marriage because it questions the whole basis for marriage
for many people. If they want to stay together, Polly and Colin must
find new reasons to do so.

Although the relationship is vulnerable at this point, Polly is feeling still more fragile. Having rethought everything she thought she believed in, Polly recognizes her own vulnerability and her profound sense of loss:

I am in a really delicate period now. I was just drowning in my own sadness over this. This lack of life is a nonlife. It's like nothing belongs to me. And here I am, a really free individual who could do so many things and all I'm doing is all the things that I decided I should be doing. So I had to wipe out every routine for emotional survival. I had to approach every free moment as what would I like to be doing. If I decided too quickly, "Well, I'd like to just go home and rest," maybe I should rethink that. Maybe what I'd really like to do is go take a hot tub. I would just force myself to try all these new patterns and just mix my life up. Get out of my schedule. And now I'm really into that. It worked really well for me, really well.

Polly's approach to dealing with this inner conflict is novel: experiencing a sense of chaos, she undoes her daily practices so that nothing stays the same. A more typical approach is to cling to the routine, predictable, part of life. This approach once worked for Polly, but now she is questioning her previous decisions, such as the decision to have a child:

Now I'm thinking "I don't know if I really want to get into this whole schedule with a child." I mean, that's kind of putting back what I just removed. . . . I would still like to have a child if I can. I'm still willing to have that adventure. I'm still willing to list that as one of my adventures that I'd like to do, but it is no longer the be-all and end-all for me. It doesn't break my heart anymore.

I think there's two stages of big disappointment. The first big disappointment was knowing that it wasn't going to be my biological child, and the second one will be knowing that there will never be any child.

Letting go of her hopes for a child, which propelled her through multiple medical procedures, including five cycles of IVF, and acknowledging the depth of her loss, puts meaning itself into limbo. For years her life revolved around the desire for a child. Now that she is letting go of this goal, much seems meaningless. Questions about what in life is worthwhile dominate her anguished statements.

Polly's emotional rampage, in which she attacks everything stable in her life, is part of the tearing-down process many people undergo to find new meaning in life. This process is a necessary precursor to efforts to find meaning in other, alternative cultural dialogues.

Like Polly, Pauline, thirty-five years old, is reevaluating everything in her life, including her career. The pivotal issue for her, however, is age. Stopping medical treatment and remaining childless makes her feel old:

I'm reevaluating life in major ways. At the foundation of my being. I have no fears of living the rest of life with Bruce. I really enjoy him and I really enjoy our relationship together. But still, it's different than what I expected it to be. That's one of the things that you sort of look at when you're forty. I think I told you this before but I've taken on Bruce's age a lot in my mind. When he turned thirty-nine, I went through a crisis because next year is forty, and forty means old. Forty means the end of the childbearing era. Even though I'm five years younger, I really went through this crisis with his age.

Who did I find out was pregnant recently? I had a good cry over that one. I can't think of who. But sometimes it takes me a long time. But overall, I do feel like I'm doing better and I do feel like there's a little light at the end of the tunnel. And that's real encouraging. I feel like it's so important for me to get a goal long-term, like if I could take a certain job and kind of go with that, so I can really have some purpose to get me through the next five years.

I just feel like I'm aging, like I'm getting on. I feel very old. And the body is just boring. I have lots of things like arthritis on my knees and my back and my neck is real stiff, and just all this stuff. So I feel like I need something to keep me going for the next five years, and I will reevaluate at that point. I know I'm only thirty-five but in my mind, I think of myself as about fifty. It's so weird. I think it's just part of the state I'm in. I've gained a lot of weight in the last couple of years, and I'm just slower and my body creaks, and I just feel like an old person. If I start lifting weights and increase my exercise again, maybe I'll feel younger.

I've been evaluating life from the standpoint of, "Is my life almost over?" And it's like, "Why?" I think it's just feeling tired. I can't figure out why. I don't feel like I'm losing hope, and I certainly don't have any kind of suicidal ideas or anything like that. It's just this sense of oldness. Maybe that will change as I have more time and more energy.

Pauline's response to childlessness—to start feeling like an older woman—is not unusual among women who do not conceive or adopt.

Gender identity and age are linked, and women readily make this connection. Indeed, throughout medical treatment and afterward, women wonder if they are too old to take on the duties of motherhood. And, if they are not to be mothers, does that outcome somehow age them? The cultural dialogue on age and womanhood has been given recent impetus by the donor egg technology that makes it possible for women to become mothers after menopause.

Six months later, when interviewed for the last time, Pauline has become more reconciled to the idea of being childless. She says:

I am realizing that it's the proverbial turning a ship around. Like an oil tanker—they say that it takes miles in the ocean to turn it around. And to get going in another direction—it takes so much energy and so much working through all this stuff. If all of a sudden out of the blue I got pregnant, I would be very angry and annoyed. Because I would have to take this oil tanker and turn it around yet again.

That women may become resistant to the idea of having children when they have pursued parenthood for so long is not surprising. In part, it is a pragmatic response to an untenable situation. But, equally important, it attests to the multiple expressions of gender identity to which women gain access once they move away from viewing themselves in the framework of motherhood and biological children.

LETTING GO OF BIOLOGICAL CONTINUITY

Megan, whose story introduced this chapter, was making considerable headway in resolving her infertility and remaining childless. But one of the things she continued to wrestle with was her sense of obligation to persist with infertility treatment. Even though she responded poorly to the drugs used in IVF and had become sick from attempting such medical procedures, she continued to feel that she had failed to live up to cultural expectations of motherhood and biological continuity. This sense was underscored by the imminent deaths of older family members.

I don't even know how we finally arrived at this decision, but it is very hard for me to say, "We're not going to have kids, and we're not going to carry on [the family line]." I'm sort of in the process of losing a couple of people in my family right now, and to think about how the family will not continue is a hard thing, but yet, it took me a long time to be able to say, "I don't want to have medical treatment."

I always felt that the responsibility was on me and that if we didn't have children, it would be my fault and it was nothing he ever did. He [husband] never made me feel that way. He always said that it would be okay if we didn't. He didn't want me to go through procedures, and I was struggling a lot with myself. And I felt that it was wrong for me to be the one to say, "I'm afraid to do this, I don't respond to drugs well, I don't want it." I felt like I should be able to say, as my mother has said, "I'd do anything, anything, to have kids," and I'm sure she would. Of course, she got them.

The notion of maintaining generational continuity through biological linkages is at the root of the cultural ideology of continuity.[1] It is the driving force behind many people's lengthy efforts to bring about a conception. To relinquish the effort to live out this ideology is considered a radical departure from normal behavior.

Megan, in struggling with this dilemma, has captured one of the most significant aspects of cultural ideologies: although they are abstractions in themselves, they have symbols attached to them, in this case the image of the child.

I don't remember, anymore, what my vision of our child was like. I lost it. But I did go through some very serious soul-searching between the time that I left the job recently, going through this crisis and saying, "Okay, I'm not working. I'm in school getting a degree, I'm not getting younger. As a matter of fact, I think I'm a little too old for this. If we're going to do this, this is the time." And I kept checking it out. Every time I said, "I'm going to make an appointment, I can do Lupron." I can't handle that stuff. It's not healthy. I can't even get through an IVF cycle because I get sick from the drugs.

Now that Megan has lost her vision of a child, she has also lost her drive to persist with medical treatment. The child is a cultural image that people personalize. It is what keeps people in treatment. But the very fact of having had to go to such lengths in the first place runs counter to what the vision represents. The vision of the child becomes blurred and begins to fade as people undergoing treatment gradually come to recognize that it has already eluded them. Profound distress follows, as Megan attests:

It ruined our life for a fair amount of time. I was never comfortable, certainly emotionally, and it took me a long time to recover. And I thought and thought about it, and decided that we have a great life.

We're very active and interested in a lot of things. Why go through that again when there's a very high probability that it won't work?

One thing that surprised me was our doctor. When I went to see him about this [stopping treatment], I expected him to say, "Oh, you have plenty of options left, and you're still young enough, and yes, you should go for it." I expected him to say all that. I expected that would be the sales pitch. I said, "I'm not really panicking about this. I'm not desperate to do this treatment. Is that indicative?" And he said, "Absolutely! You ought to think hard about that." And I told him I feel guilty because I haven't gone through nine IVFs like a lot of my friends have. And he looked at my chart, and I could hardly wait for what he said. He says, "What do you mean? You've done IUIs, you've taken the drugs. What do you mean you haven't done this? That's ridiculous!" So finally, when almost everybody around me started being able to say, "This is okay. If this is what's right for you, this is okay," I began to feel less guilty about saying, "No, I don't want children."

Megan's sense of responsibility for bearing a child was so great that she felt she needed permission from others, including her physician, to discontinue medical treatment. Surprised by his supportive response, she felt somewhat released from her sense of responsibility. In fact, Megan's physician was voicing another part of the ideology of personal responsibility: that once a person has given a major effort to an enterprise without success, it is okay to stop trying. Megan was also able to remind herself of something that she—and many others going through medical treatment—had forgotten: she has "a great life." The burden of trying to live up to the cultural ideology of continuity often blinds people to the pleasure they once took in life, pleasure that is still available if only they begin to look at their lives differently. Being able to recognize this pleasure is an indication that a sense of normalcy is returning. But, more than this, looking at one's life anew, as Megan is doing, is an indication that a person is reconstructing the life story to emphasize other aspects of life that are meaningful.

I think that's been the last final step in working past that and saying, "Oh, I don't want to admit that I'm at all comfortable with this, because if I do then it will mean that we won't try again." So in a funny way, I think we've been through a lot of the issues, we understand them. We're not fighting with them anymore, but I have been having trouble being able to say, certainly to myself, but definitely to any-

body else outside, "I am resolved. We are not going to have children."
In fact, we saw something in the Resolve newsletter that I thought
was fabulous. The Good News section, the last one, said, "So-and-so
have decided to cease medical treatment and not to have a child, and
to celebrate their decision, they are looking forward to a trip to Swit-
zerland. They plan to live a happy, childfree life." And I just wanted
to call them and say, "Do you want to have dinner?" I have never
seen that in any of the newsletters ever before. Ever.

Megan found this newsletter announcement to be enormously affirming of the decision she and her husband had made. The support and
agreement of peers is a critical factor in resisting the moral force of
cultural ideologies because peer support gives credence to another ver-
sion of normalcy. To resist these moral forces in the absence of such
support, people must begin by asserting their sense of normalcy based
on their bodily knowledge and forge alternative dialogues by engaging
with others whose interests are different. Megan began new friendships
with people whose focus was not on having children, and she spent
much less time with her friends in Resolve, whose lives continued to
revolve around how to become parents.

It's very sad, it really is, but as we get further and further away from
it [becoming parents], you find that there are just so many things to
do in life. It doesn't make it okay, but I think we've found some kind
of a balance for ourselves. And the hardest thing is just to say, "I
quit." I admit that I quit, and I admit that I feel badly about doing it,
and feeling like it's okay to quit, which sounds so contradictory I can't
even believe it. But for a long time I was saying, "It's not okay to feel
all right about not having kids." And that was very self-destructive, so
I stopped saying it, and now I feel like it's going to be okay again, and
it will if the two of us can work it out together. I think we can and
that we are.

Megan resolves these issues by reasserting the primacy of the marital
relationship. In the context of the extended family she redefines her role,
shifting from being a mother to being an aunt:

So we will be the perfect aunt and uncle. I think that everybody needs
an aunt and uncle that they can go to when they get really upset with
their parents, and they want to go and hang out some place and have
a member of the family that they can go to and talk to. I suspect we'll
be that. We're making more time to do it now.

I think it has strengthened our marriage immeasurably [working through these issues]. We had to be pretty honest about some things. It's either going to break you up and make you feel like crying, depending on how effectively you can or cannot communicate. We don't do beautifully every time we talk about it [life after infertility], but I think that we can talk about the way we feel, and that makes a big difference. Basically it's okay. But it's going to be better.

By placing herself and her husband in relation to each other (having a strong marriage) and in relation to their nieces and nephews (on her husband's side of the family), Megan finds an acceptable means of connecting herself to the extended family. Having resisted the moral force of multiple cultural ideologies, she is initiating an alternative cultural dialogue—on marriage without children and on the role of childless people in extended families.

By focusing on women in this chapter, it has not been my intent to suggest that only women made this decision. Sometimes men took the lead, and often the decision not to have children was a joint one. But when women had primary responsibility for the decision, the issues they wrestled with were especially complex, because they had to forge a new self-definition that was independent of societal views about normalcy for women.

Deciding not to have children is perhaps the most difficult decision for women who have gone through infertility: much commitment has gone into this effort to conceive, and this option is the least socially acceptable. Not having children has been characterized by women earlier in this book as un-American and unwomanly. Indeed, there is a renewed emphasis on family in the United States, and even those once associated with childlessness, such as gay couples, are now parenting in considerable numbers. Deciding not to parent is therefore a dramatic departure from the renewed trend toward parenting in American society.

Turning one's back on motherhood is apparently much more difficult to do later in the infertility treatment process than it is initially. There are indications that for women who do not pursue medical treatment in depth, as the women in this book have done, shaping one's life around other aspects of identity is easier. Mardi Ireland has found that women contemplating motherhood, who did not pursue it to the same lengths as women in this book, were able to realize their identity through other aspects of life without undue distress.[2] Conversely, the more women persevere with medical treatment, and the more unattainable the goal becomes, the more committed women become to realizing it, necessitating at last a difficult about-face. For women to reject this cultural ideology, self-definition has to change.

CHAPTER 13

Rewriting the Family

People start out on the fertility journey wanting to be a normal family and wanting others to see them that way. Years later, those who are faced with giving up the idea of a biological child are still concerned with being a normal family; indeed, they become more concerned with this issue than they were before. The question of how to proceed so that people see them as a normal family and the child as a normal child becomes the centerpiece of their efforts to become parents. Jordan, talking about using a donor's egg to conceive a pregnancy, was worrying about how others might view their actions: "You know, they might think, 'These weirdos went through this weird experiment and did something weird.' I'd just like the kid to be normal. You know, just be a kid. It's not going to be a martian. But it's going to be a martian if we call it a martian." The desire for normalcy, for the kid to be "just a kid," is paramount for the sake of both the child and the parents.

The cultural ideology of the biological child is a major stumbling block for women and men who want to have a family. Few of the people we interviewed worked through this issue quickly. Only a handful of people chose to adopt within the first two years of trying to conceive.[1]

When people are able to consider nonbiological alternatives, it is because they have ceased to equate gender identity with biological functions. Those people have stopped being preoccupied with the assault on their gender identity, and the cultural relevance of biology for their identity has diminished. When people are able to do this kind of identity work, they shift their focus away from themselves to the potential child. It is at this point that they begin to ask, as Jordan does, What is in the best interests of a child?

In choosing an alternative route to parenthood, women and men must address three intertwined issues. The first of these is, of course, coming to terms with having a nonbiological or nonbiogenetic child. The second is how to imbue the child, and the family, with a sense of normalcy; in other words, how to manage the fact that the family will not embody the cultural ideology of biological parenthood. What approach will give the child and the parents the greatest comfort and ease? What policies do the parents wish to adopt to make this experience as "natural" as possible? In considering the best interests of the child, parents in this situation confront a third issue: the degree of privacy, confidentiality, or openness they wish to maintain, and the possible role of a third party (such as a birth mother) in their daily lives. The stories that follow address the new issues that arise when issues about biology recede.

PARENTING WITHOUT BIOLOGY

When people opt to parent without biology, they are forced to rethink the purpose of parenthood. Eddie, mulling over the issues of third-party parenting, made these observations:

I went to a Resolve workshop where a guy discussed his reaction to adoption. He just starts out, "I was certain that I would take my perfect genetic material and my wife's perfect genetic material and produce a perfect baby that would never throw up," and he talked like a guy talking to guys. And you go, "Yeah, this is what this is all about." I mean, we're trying so hard because we both had such incredibly perfect genetic material, you know? That we want to see what we can produce. He says, "The whole thing really does get down to, we're talking about families, we're not talking about biological processes here," even though you do. But you're constantly thinking about biological processes, right? And so then you get into something like this symposium. I mean, you hear about people who are having [nonbiological] families, you know?

You could get involved in this third-party parenting and get so analytical about it. But guess what? You weren't that analytic in getting married. I didn't look at you and say, "Well, now, what would our kids be like? And maybe I should pick somebody a little shorter or a little . . ." You don't do that. So why not pick somebody who you think is going to produce a healthy baby, then you have the privilege of raising it?

Eddie is describing a basic paradigm shift from a focus on biological processes to a focus on the creation of a family. He is also drawing attention to the assumptions with which people begin relationships. People's assumptions, the ideas others have referred to as "the dream of the child," are rudely destroyed when they confront infertility, and often give way to highly particular desires about the "perfect" child. With his newfound insights, Eddie proposes an alternative.

Eddie and Phyllis had heard a woman speak about her philosophy, developed as a surrogate mother, that the child does not "belong" to anyone except itself and that the role of a parent is not genetic. These comments had a powerful effect on them. Phyllis said: "It was so touching to both of us, the philosophy of this surrogate mom, that the child is really not yours. I mean, just to get into thinking that way, that a child is really not yours. You are there to help them learn and grow up, and they never really belong to you, anyway. And it was like a very profound thought."

Eddie continues:

That was how she was able to answer this question of "How can you give up this child?" It was one of those things where you didn't question the honesty of her response, because she just kind of wore it as a mantle of serenity. I thought, "Wow! This is centered! This lady knows where she's coming from." Just talking so quietly, and she just said, "My son asked me, 'Are we going to have to give up this baby?' " And she said, "I told him it's not ours. I have the pleasure of giving it life, and somebody else is going to have the pleasure of bringing it up."

I was like, "Wow!" That works on my brain. It says, "All right. So this whole thing that men typically get into of, 'This child is a reflection of me,' isn't the program here. The program is showing somebody small how to become big one day." You know? That really helped my brain deal with parenting in general. And specifically, the third-party parenting thing, I realize, is all of the questions you can ask, and all of the hand-wringing that you can get into, and the distress, and the "What if . . . ?" The bottom line is it really, really doesn't matter.

Separating the task of parenthood from the preoccupation with maintaining genetic continuity enables Eddie and Phyllis to consider third-party parenting seriously. Their old assumptions, emanating from the cultural ideology of biological parenthood, have been replaced by a new vision of parenthood. This alternative vision frees them to attach new meanings to parenthood and examine the picture from another angle. Most people who turn to third-party parenting do so after deciding that parenthood is much more important to them than biology. Their reasons are practical: they want to parent a child, and this way gives them a reasonable chance of becoming a parent.

Sean, together with his wife, had decided on donor insemination to conceive a child. Asked whether he felt any sense of loss, such as about not passing on his family line, he responded:

Not so much my family line. Maybe it is egotism or something, but I do feel a loss that some of my . . . I don't know where my personality came from, or my talents or feelings came from, but I do feel a sense of loss to know that if any of that came from my genes, it won't be passed on. I don't know where everything comes from. But I know that I am different enough from my genetic father. It is not the most important thing, but it is something that is always present. But just talking about that is funny, also, because the goal isn't to make an ideal person, it is to have some kind of a family, and the way that family turns out is certainly our business, and it is in every family. And ours is maybe a little different than other families, but it is still our family.

Although Sean and his wife, Lydia, have conceived through donor insemination and the baby will be born soon, he has not finished reworking his ideas about parenthood. Indeed, when a donor is used, the nine months of pregnancy are a time of intensive emotional work for both men and women. The parent who has had a donor substitute must rework previous ideas about gender identity and about what constitutes the performance of gender.

In response to a question from the interviewer about how they came to consider donor insemination rather than adoption, Lydia said:

Sean was thinking about adoption. It was his first idea, but I decided I wanted to bear children, to give birth to someone, and I was offended by him a little bit—not because I don't think adoption is such a good

thing, but I think that at our age [late twenties] and in our financial
position, we can't do it now [because of the expense]. And especially
this moral position. I think that when people are a bit older, and they
understand things a little bit better, they can do it. I think that I was
not ready. And I think I was offended by his egotism, that he can't do
it and so I am not supposed to do it [create a biological child].

Lydia speaks directly to the issue of women being deprived of pregnancy and childbirth for the sake of a man's ego. Her refusal to consider
adoption has been driven by her unwillingness to go along with this
patriarchal approach as well as by financial concerns.

Asked by the interviewer if he thought Lydia's observation was correct, Sean responded: "Probably, probably. Not anything that I would
ever admit to, at least to myself. Now I am [admitting it]. But there is
probably a little bit of jealousy that if we are going to cope with this
problem, that it has turned out to be both of our problems."

INTERVIEWER: *You mean, do it on equal ground, or something?*

SEAN: *That is really silly. Maybe there was some feeling*
                 like that. I like the idea of adoption, anyway. I like
                 the idea of a large—not a large family—but more
                 than one child, and certainly I don't like the idea of
                 being childless. And I also have some idealism that
                 says there are children who need a good home, and
                 I think we will provide a good home. So now we
                 think we will have another child by donor insemina-
                 tion.

LYDIA: *It is hard to say. I am going to do it once, and then*
                 decide what I want to do about the next one.

Bill and Carla, after many years of childlessness, also realized that
what mattered most to them was parenthood. Years of infertility treatment had led to nothing but pain and heartache. Bill had been ready to
adopt before Carla was. He said, "We were missing something in our
lives. We were missing a child, and I was ready to adopt, but my wife
wasn't ready." Carla describes the catalyst for this decision:

One of my friends in Resolve phoned me and told me, "We just
adopted a little girl yesterday!" I said, "You're kidding!" She said,
"No, we just brought her home." She was born the day before. And
she [friend] is Jewish, but they adopted a little Mexican girl. A few

weeks later, I went over to see her. I just fell over her! When I left after seeing her the first time, I just felt so . . . lifeless, because I knew that's what I needed. I went home that night, and told Bill, "I'm ready."

Once they decided to proceed with adoption, they were enthusiastic, especially when an adoption counselor told them that their chances of finding a Latino baby were good because Carla was Latina. She observed: "So once we decided, I was really excited and enthused. And started working on the letter right away. I was taking my time. I wanted it to be just right. Then, since we're targeting for a Latino baby, we had to make the letter in English and Spanish. So I needed my mom to translate the letter for me. So now it's out there, and we're waiting." A little over a year later, they adopted a baby. At the next interview, Carla said:

Our lives revolve around him. I feel like I will be able to talk to Randy [baby] about anything. The only thing I'm uncertain about is how I'm going to handle it when he has some questions about his biological father. I'm not going to be able to give him answers, and he's gonna be left wondering. So the only thing I can turn to is other people with other kids that he can talk to who are in the same situation. They give each other support. I'm hoping that he won't really think that it's any big deal.

Adoptive parents in private adoptions must decide whether to have any contact, especially in the long term, with the birth mother. The possibility of long-term contact raises the question of who is the "real" mother, and related questions about the birth mother's role. The commonest worry women and men express is that ongoing contact with the birth mother will lead her to reclaim the child. Most adoptive parents in this study expressed a desire for no further contact once the child was handed over.[2] Carla and Bill, however, have maintained sporadic contact with the birth mother, who has another child and lives in another part of the state:

We went sixteen weeks ago or something like that, just a really quick visit because we had to do it on a weekend. We got a nice room in a motel and we had them spend the night. Randy and Johnny played together. We'll probably only see them occasionally. I'd like to talk with her. I tried to call her the night before Mother's Day but I couldn't get hold of her. She's not living at the women's shelter any-

more, and when I call she's usually busy cleaning somebody's house or doing somebody's yard work. We'll probably see them twice a year.

That Carla is comfortable in maintaining contact with the birth mother may derive, in part, from the vastly different economic situation of the birth mother, as well as from the fact that the birth mother has another small child. For these reasons she is not worried that the birth mother will try to reclaim the child. But Carla's sense of security also derives from her strong feelings that she is the true mother of this child:

Some people go through grieving periods with a child that they never gave birth to, and maybe I felt like that at one time, but I don't feel like that now. Sometimes it just comes out where I'll be explaining to someone, and I'll say, "We tried to have one of our own but we couldn't, so we adopted." And after I say that, I ask myself, "Why did I say that?" Because that's not how I feel. Randy is our own. I should say that we tried to get pregnant but we couldn't, so we adopted. So that's how I feel. Randy is our own. So if he's our own, how can I grieve?

Carla and Bill have reworked their vision of the child so that the adopted child becomes "our own." They have thus abandoned the cultural ideology of biological parenthood in favor of a social and emotional definition of parenthood. The connection Carla experiences with Randy has assuaged her desire for a biological child. She is Randy's mother.

REDEFINING FAMILY MEMBERSHIP

What to do about the third party is also a question for those who choose to use donor egg technology. (Because donor insemination continues to be primarily anonymous, the issue seldom arises for those who have used this method to create a family.) This is uncharted ground. Some people using this technology may decide that the donor has no place in the family. Indeed, the donor's very existence may seem threatening to people using donor gametes. Yet because the question of confidentiality versus openness is an important one in the use of donor gametes, the additional question of the donor as a potential family member must be taken seriously.

Eileen and John talk about how much to involve the egg donor, with whom they have developed a personal relationship, in their family life. The question they raise is where to draw the line.

We were talking, and Shana [the egg donor] was talking about the big question, "What do I say to my daughter who is eight now? If you don't get pregnant or if you do, I don't want her to feel a sense of loss," that is, in the sense of our children and Shana's children would be half-siblings. Because they share half their genetic material. And our feeling is that we have to come up with a definition of family. She agreed.

John interjects: "A *different* definition of family."

EILEEN: *To draw the line. Because you have to draw the line some-
             where. What we decided on and articulated was that
             whether you adopt or you have stepkids or whether you
             have a donor gamete child, the family is the emotional
             thing.*

JOHN: *It's an emotional unit.*

EILEEN: *And a social unit: this is your family. And it doesn't have
             to be people who are blood-related, but it's defined as that.*

Eileen and John, reexamining and questioning all of the cultural rules about who is kin, decide they have to come up with their own definition of family. In doing so, they are rejecting the cultural ideology of the biological family, and, moreover, they are saying that their definition of family will be their own, not a standard definition.

Once they have embarked on this process, they discover that the issues are complex. Eileen continues:

And that's okay with Shana because she has half-sisters, and family she calls sisters, which are no blood relation through marriages and families. And so in some ways, they have a working definition of family in that sense. And something else she was telling her daughter was, "When a woman has a period every month, it means that the egg that was getting ready to make a baby to be fertilized, dies. Every month I have a period. Every month these eggs die. I never use them to make children. I'm giving these eggs that would get flushed down the toilet, to people like [Eileen and John] to help them make babies because they

can't do it because Eileen doesn't make eggs." And her
daughter's just about old enough to get it. She understands
how babies are made and that was the explanation, and it
seemed to be fine, and it's fine with us. We don't have an
issue about the kids meeting. She asks, "What am I sup-
posed to call your children?" And I said, "How about Ei-
leen and John's baby?" We don't have a word for someone
like her child and our child, our future child. We share ge-
netic material, but it's like animal breeding or using some
term. But we don't, and you have to be really careful be-
cause they're not half-siblings — that implies a family rela-
tionship. And we also decided when the kids are older, if
they decide to recognize each other as siblings, that's fine.

JOHN: *But that's going to be their choice.*

EILEEN: *That's their choice, and there will always be some kind of*
bond between our families. If this whole thing works, she's
giving us something incredible that we can never repay,
and it becomes this bond with them, and that's fine. But
again, we felt that for everybody's sake, we had to draw
the line over the family issue.

Although Eileen and John are leaving some things open to chance
and future generations, they are also defining degrees of family. The
donor and her children are being thought of as distant, rather than close,
family. Indeed, it seems at times that they are indicating there is *no*
family relationship, as when Eileen asserts that their child and the donor's child will not be half-siblings. With this comment she also indicates
how cautiously they are proceeding. They acknowledge the gift of the
egg as one they "can never repay," which creates a bond with the donor
and her family. (This acknowledgment is despite the fact that this donor
was paid.) However, in Eileen's eyes, the question of indebtedness has
the potential to raise another threatening question: Whose baby is it?
Eileen is very clear about the answer: the child will be known as "Eileen
and John's baby."

Given that biological kin are socially and legally privileged over nonbiological kin in the United States, the use of donors in reproductive
technologies presents a significant social challenge. The trend toward
increased openness appears likely to persist; if it does, traditional cultural assumptions about how the family is constituted are likely to expand.

Although the definition of family has already been reworked to some extent to accommodate families created through adoption, donor insemination, and step-parenting, the donor egg situation is somewhat different. While its use may undercut the cultural ideology of the biological parent, at the same time it may give new weight to a biological connection that may be devoid of the social and emotional parameters that are an expected byproduct of kinship.

Viewing the donated egg as a gift that cannot be repaid adds an additional complication, as reciprocity is very much a part of United States ideas about fairness and equality. What can the donor be offered if, as Eileen implies, money is not enough?[3] For Eileen and John, the only way to reciprocate is with a gift of equal magnitude: family membership.

KINSHIP RITUALS

The cultural ideology of the biological child does not lose all its power once a child is born. It is perpetuated in myriad microcosmic ways, and parents of a nonbiological child must negotiate their way around it. The following story shows how the assumption of biological kinship is played out in a ritualized set of commonplace interactions.

Helen, forty-five years old, and Sid, fifty years old, conceived with a donor egg. Although they chose to be open about the use of a donor, they told only close friends and family. Helen has black hair and brown eyes, unlike her daughter, who is blond. She comments:

One area that continues to prick at me is when I'm out in the world and traveling around with her. I encounter people on a fairly regular basis who don't know about our daughter, and one of the first things people always ask me with the baby is, "Who does she look like?" Nobody says she looks like me. Some people have said, rightfully so, that she looks like Sid, because we have some baby pictures of him, and there's a very marked resemblance as infants between them. So I had lunch with this friend, and I never told her about using a donor, so she's looking at the baby's hair and commented on how her hair is coming in lighter and it's blond and where does the blond hair come from, and on and on, and I'm about ready to . . . I mean, the choices are all uncomfortable. There's no such thing as a comfortable choice to answer the question. I mean, I can make a comfortable decision but it's either mak-

ing up a cover story of some sort, deflecting from a truthful answer in some fashion or telling her the whole story, and I wasn't up to telling her the whole story that day.

It's the "who does the baby look like?" part that comes up all the time.

Helen has stumbled onto the widespread belief that kinship is "natural," that is, biological, and that family members should therefore resemble each other. Asking which parent the baby resembles reinforces the primacy of biological kin over other types of kinship. The scientific field of genetics and popular American ideas about kinship apparently share a normative framework, that a child's biogenetic makeup comes 50 percent from the father and 50 percent from the mother.[4] Helen's black hair and her daughter's blond hair immediately raise questions about their biological relationship to each other. If Helen's baby were a boy, her explanations would probably be more readily accepted because of popular ideas that physical mirroring is less likely across genders. The cultural ideology of the family is replete with ideas about physical similarities in families and by gender, which tell us not only that kinship as a system is gendered[5] but also that assumptions about gender within kinship are patterned in specific ways.

Sid examines the social dimension of Helen's uncomfortable lunch:

It's a standard comment. It's more a ritual between people like, "How are you?" No one gives a shit. You're supposed to say, "I'm fine." But the answer to this is that we are acknowledging our meeting in a sort of respectful manner. It's a symbolic event so you know people are supposed to show respect for a mother with a newborn where they inquire about their newborn. Their life is not turning on the content of the explanation. We are discussing a baby.

Identifying whom the baby resembles is one enactment of the cultural ideology of the family that occurs almost incessantly in the early phases of a child's life. (This activity rests on a particular kind of circular reasoning: the claim to see a resemblance is based on the assumption of a genetic link between parent and child. If the observer did not know or believe the link existed, he or she might not claim to see any resemblance at all.) Parents whose children are not biologically theirs experience themselves as outside the norm when such interchanges occur. Helen and Sid both need to analyze this behavior because it poses so much discomfort for them.

HELEN: *What is the meaning behind the ritual? I agree it has an absolutely ritualistic quality. It's as if people ask the question. They get an answer, and it's like everything is placed now. It's the blond hair from so-and-so. My father had blond hair and blue eyes. "Oh, okay." Everything is in its place now and we can move on. So it's true. I've not thought about it as a ritual, but it really is a ritual and it's somehow a ritual that, like all rituals, everything is in it's place and in order now. Why it takes that particular form sort of mystifies me. It's as if to say, "We have to do this ritual to establish that this baby is yours or this baby is you now."*

SID: *You're in a culture in which lineage is important.*

HELEN: *And legitimacy, I suppose.*

SID: *It's an issue of preserving the lineage.*

Turning to me, Helen says, "Finding out what the rules are that govern the interactions and then disrupting them—that's Sid."

In identifying the underlying reason for people's need to "place the baby" in a lineage and thereby legitimize it, Helen and Sid come to the heart of the cultural ideology of the family: this is the perpetuation of Americans' origin myth in action, and it therefore fulfills an important function in the maintenance of kinship traditions. Gender is an important part of this process. Sylvia Yanagisako and Carol Delaney observe that issues of gender and procreation are at the center of contemporary debates about new reproductive technologies because new beliefs and practices challenge the entire cosmological order, of which gender and procreation are an intrinsic part.[6]

Sid places the dilemma in the context of society as a whole: "Continuity is decreasing in this society, so it's more important. We're struggling for some sense of continuity. It also provides a ritual bridging the gap between individuals. Particularly in a society which is so separated from their neighbors. Somehow it's an opening line which is acceptable." Helen agrees:

That explains why it is such a powerful ritual. I find myself doing it, thinking who a child looks like. Even when I realize the children are adopted. I don't know how to describe it. It's about how much family they are. How much the glue is there, and the adopted child fits. I also think there are continuity and immortality in some sense of the word

that you probably get more intense in this society than others. Some-
how you wake up and ask the question, "Why am I doing all of
this?"

The meaning of the word family *I don't know. In this society it*
gets even more complicated.

Cultural meanings of continuity are tied to biological reproduction
and, consequently, to definitions of family. The cultural ideology of continuity is deeply embedded in life in the United States.[7] This ideology
operates at various levels, from bodily understanding to views of how
society works, but particular views about order in the United States
permeate all of them. The family is seen as a primary conduit of order
and continuity. Thus the simple question, Who does the baby look like?
taps into multiple, overlapping cultural ideologies. When the answer to
this question is "nobody" or "not applicable," these ideologies are undermined, and what is commonly viewed as the natural order of things
is challenged.[8]

SOCIAL PARENTHOOD

We have seen how deep the ideology of biological determinism runs in
U.S. society and how difficult it is for people to let go of it.[9] Women and
men dealing with infertility go through many phases in letting go of
biology; it is a process that takes years and may never be completed.
Many of the issues are dealt with when a child finally arrives, as the
parents' focus shifts from their own concerns to their concerns for their
child.

When Terry and Kelsie were interviewed for the first time, they had
not yet had a medical interview for donor insemination but had given
the procedure a great deal of thought. They had an appointment at a
sperm bank for the following week, but they were still ambivalent about
using a donor:

KELSIE: *We have thought about our one option, remaining child-*
            free. That one was not one that we wanted to consider.
            Donor insemination came first. But the thought of it was
            completely repugnant to me.
TERRY: *I'm a little bit threatened by the procedure.*
KELSIE: *The thought of somebody else's sperm—a third party—*
            being involved in this whole thing, which is usually a very

private thing. We wouldn't be talking about it with you or anybody else. So bringing this third party in feels like we were sort of being violated or something. It was like our little circle of marital privacy had been breached. I mean, it had really been breached, and it was through no fault of our own. I was very, very angry about the choices we had available. It was like either a really crummy choice or a really crummy choice. So for a while there we didn't even consider it. We felt personally singled out.

Terry reiterates the private nature of conception and the difficulty of finding others who shared their problem: "It was very isolating because no one else had this problem, and if there was anybody else, we wouldn't normally find out about it. So we got into Resolve." He has a nagging concern, however:

That [donor insemination] was the next closest thing [to a biological child]. That's one way of looking at it. And at least this way, we'll get to go through being pregnant, and I think you start bonding with the fetus before it's born. And at least Kelsie's genes will be carried along. So in the end, that seemed better to us than adopting, which is, I think, more difficult in some ways. Although adoption may be more socially accepted. . . . Adoption is now almost universally accepted. But donor insemination is not. You never hear about DI children.

Being able to have a child that was partly biologically theirs, going through the pregnancy and birth process, and having the opportunity to bond with the fetus were the factors in their decision to proceed with donor insemination. Terry's observation that donor insemination children are never heard of—that they are essentially invisible—is a concern because it calls into question the social acceptability of this method of conception.

Asked how they planned to handle issues arising from using a donor, they responded:

TERRY: *That's not going to be just between the two of us. I mean, I think it's always going to be a private matter. But our family already knows and other very close friends know. The appropriate people know, definitely. We don't want to do something that we feel uncomfortable with to the point where we don't want to tell anybody about it. And I think we're at the point where we're feeling more comfortable.*

So we've made the decision that those that are closest to us will know so that we can be close to them and talk about it.

KELSIE: *Right, rather than pretending that it didn't happen.*

TERRY: *Right, and we don't want to do something that we have to spend the rest of our lives trying to forget. That doesn't seem right to us at all.*

KELSIE: *Yeah, but yet this whole issue of privacy versus secrecy, you know, has these shaded areas. It's like a person who might make a comment about "Oh, your child looks like your husband," or something. I wouldn't necessarily . . . I hope I'm not going to feel obligated to set them straight, like, "Well, he can't possibly look like him. He's not the biological father." I don't think we want to get into that sort of a pattern where we're having to set everybody straight all the time. I think the more open we are with it, the more comfortable our friends and family will be, too. And we're hoping we'll be comfortable with the child as well, even though they're going to have some difficulties just as adopted children do. You know, when they're doing the family tree in school and people try and ask you in biology exercises where they're matching up eye color and stuff. I mean, they're going to have difficulty with that because not many people know about DI and are comfortable talking about it. But we hope that we'll be able to deal with those issues as they come up in as open and honest a way as we can. It will be a challenge.*

TERRY: *Yeah, you can't predict everything a child will ask except that they will ask everything!*

Terry and Kelsie feel forced to attend to what other people may think:

TERRY: *I don't want my actions to be affected by what other people think. On the other hand . . .*

KELSIE: *You don't want your child to be the experiment.*

TERRY: *Right. But inevitably we are affected by what other people think. So there is that conflict that goes on.*

KELSIE: *Well, part of it was sort of an advocacy issue too. We thought, "Somebody's got to start talking about this." People are never going to find out that this is a viable op-*

*tion for couples where male factor infertility is a problem—
unless people talk about it. So you don't want to be the
one to subject your child to ridicule because you want to
be an advocate for it. A procedure which is unusual, but
yet if you truly believe it's a mistake to pretend, and you
truly believe that it's an option that you're comfortable
with and think that it is right to do, you just have to live
with the consequences.*

One year later, Terry and Kelsie were parents. I returned for another
interview. Asked how he felt about having used donor insemination,
Terry said,

*Well, it was clearly the right thing to do. We are very, very happy
about him. It has just been wonderful. I think, especially, initially after he was born, I would say the first two or three weeks, it brought
back a lot of feelings about the sperm condition. It was really an expression . . . he was an expression of my inability to provide the genetic material, so that was difficult. That was difficult because it was on
my mind quite a bit, especially during the first few weeks, but at the
same time it is so wonderful to have him here that it didn't really matter, but it did bring back a lot of that, definitely. And I would say that
has improved, and has gone away quite a bit. So as time goes by, I am
becoming more and more comfortable with the fact that we used it.
That he is not, he doesn't have my genetic material. You still have
people saying, "Oh, he looks just like you," and you find yourself saying, "Isn't that amazing?" But he is just so much fun, it doesn't matter. I don't think about it nearly as much as I did the first few weeks.
But initially, it was, I guess, not a feeling of regret of having done it at
all, but a feeling of regret of not having been able to do it in the normal way.*

Terry expresses conflicting emotions: the baby is a source of emotional pain at the same time that he is "wonderful." He is still having
to confront the cultural ideology of biological parenthood whenever
some unknowing person exclaims how alike father and son look.

Terry is determined to make the most of fatherhood:

*I feel so lucky, just that he is so alert and he is basically happy most
of the time, and really into things. He is not disconnected at all, like
some babies that kind of lie there. Who knows? The next one could
turn out that way, but he is so into everything, that is wonderful and*

that makes a difference. Once he smiles at you a couple of times, you forget about everything.

I was initially worried about having enough time to go through this bonding process, which is why I made plans to have three weeks off [work]. So I am with him a lot, as much as I can.

It is Terry's emotional connection with the child that he regards as the crux of parenting. In choosing donor insemination he and Kelsie have rejected the cultural ideology that says biological parenthood is the only acceptable form of parenthood. Terry is subscribing to an alternative dialogue that accepts social parenthood. This dialogue has grown stronger in the United States in recent years.

Interviewed separately, Kelsie commented:

This baby feels just like Terry's, he doesn't feel like some strange baby that came from nowhere, although with the pregnancy I felt a little more like that. It was not concrete until he actually came out and we saw that he was okay and knowing that he didn't have a big D on him for donor. No scarlet D.

So, the major problem that I have now dealing with the whole thing is who to tell and when to tell and what to say in front of people because now he [baby] can't understand me, so I can say things like, "Yes, we went and got the donor." I can explain to people how we actually did it because most friends are curious, and I am happy to tell them and demystify this whole thing, you know. It is not like it is a big secret, but yet when he is able to understand, I don't want to be talking about it in front of him but I don't want to be not talking about it on purpose. I don't want to be walking around the issue, but I don't want to be talking about his conception like he is not there.

So that is something that we are going to have to continue to struggle with, I think. There is just not an easy way. We try to come up with criteria of who do we tell, what do we say, we just decided that we needed to have a clear understanding about why we did what we did and what our feelings were about, but other than that, there couldn't be any real rules. It didn't really work for us to have rules about who to tell and what to say.

Attitude is everything, rather than rules and all of that stuff. But we wanted to tell him and show him with our actions how much he is loved, how we are not at all ashamed of having used this donor, but we do respect that it is private, ultimately, so that is why we may not always bring it up in front of people when they say, "You look like

your daddy." We won't always say, "Well, he can't possibly, we used
a donor." And that is why we don't do it. It is not that we are
ashamed of it, but it is just that he has things that he may want to
tell people, and we don't always have to tell people that.

Over time, Terry and Kelsie have shifted their focus from themselves
to their child. They have compromised over biology: the child is partly
their biological offspring and partly not. However, in deciding to tell
the important people in their lives about their child's conception, they
are emphasizing the nonbiological aspect of parenting. They retain lin-
gering concerns about how society will view their son.

Terry and Kelsie are also concerned about advocacy, however, and
about making this an easier world for children like their son to live in.
Alone, they may have little effect. Collectively, however, such parents
will influence cultural practices, and in the long run they are likely to
alter cultural attitudes. As Anthony Giddens has observed, "Social practice has effects that sometimes remake the world."[10]

CHAPTER 14

Performing Gender

In this book I have focused on one aspect of reproductive technologies: how women and men consume them. Consumption is a window through which we can examine technology as a cultural phenomenon. Technology is not independent of the social and cultural contexts in which it occurs; indeed, it can best be understood through the cultural meanings people ascribe to it.[1] We have seen the complex meanings with which people imbue new reproductive technologies and the consequent changes in ideas and practices linked to the use of these technologies, in particular notions about gender and its performance.[2]

Because new reproductive technologies reflect cultural meanings and become a conduit for changing cultural practices, they signify both a challenge to and a reinforcement of the moral order. They have become a focus of moral dialogues in the United States and other countries because their use has transgressed social boundaries. Earlier cultural notions of nature have been displaced, assumptions about bodily integrity (especially of women's bodies) have been altered, and cultural ideologies about biological parenthood have become a locus of debate. In many instances the body itself has been bypassed in favor of the laboratory, raising issues about personhood, the distinction between human and nonhuman, and the transformative nature of these technologies.[3] But, as I have tried to show, what is occurring is not completely new. Many old ideas have had new life breathed into them by the emergence of the new reproductive technologies. Although some old ideas have been displaced, others have simply been reframed. We are in the midst of major social changes that are the more complex because they are occurring globally. The historical vehicle for all of these changes has been processes of industrialization and consumption, which have shifted over time from mass production to flexible accumulation. The uses of new reproductive technologies are a prime example of this shift.[4]

Although I have emphasized how the experience of women and men who engage with these technologies becomes increasingly politicized, I have also tried to show the broad social, cultural, and economic framework into which these technologies fit. The moral economy of new reproductive technologies, built on a cultural ideology of productivity, maintains the status quo. Angela Davis observes that anchoring these technologies to the profit schemes of their producers and distributors results in a commodification of motherhood, a process that complicates and deepens power relations based on class and race.[5] This study, by focusing primarily on white, middle-class, heterosexual couples, has illustrated how the current system of delivering new reproductive technologies to these consumers works in their favor despite their personal experiences of frustration and despair, and how other, less favored groups are rendered invisible. The moral economy impedes efforts to initiate needed social change.

The ways in which these consumers negotiate power have been a particular focus of this book. In particular, I have tried to illustrate the interactive nature of ideology, institutional forces, and people's actions by juxtaposing gendered bodily experience and enactment with cultural notions about normalcy and the use of new reproductive technologies. What emerges is a clear view of technology as culture, with technology as the template on which issues such as gender, nature, and the body are being rewritten and continuously altered.

GENDER ENACTMENT, NORMALCY, AND RESISTANCE

Women and men who struggle with infertility confront cultural ideologies surrounding gender norms. They are seeking a fit between their life situations and the cultural ideologies to which they subscribe. Stymied by the implausibility of this task, they have been forced to work intensively with cultural dialogues in order to reconcile their experiences with cultural expectations. In doing so, they have been performing gender. Initially, as women and men in this study tried to bring about a conception, their performances attempted to adhere to gender norms.[6] These intensive efforts continued over long periods, reflecting their importance as the enactment of gender identity.[7] But as time passed and their efforts to enact gender along normative lines were thwarted, women and men sought to enact different ways of bringing their divergent experiences into some kind of congruence with cultural dialogues about gender.

In enacting gender and redefining normalcy, women and men face a series of challenges. First, they are forced to rethink cultural ideals of womanhood and manhood. Seeing themselves as not fitting those ideals, they question the ideals, often for the first time. Inevitably, they find the ideals wanting. Not only do they find that cultural ideals are often narrowly and rigidly defined, but they also observe that those ideals often have little connection to their lives. The rethinking of these ideals is a catalyst for the reworking of gender identity, on which their actions hinge.

Questioning the cultural ideology of biological parenthood is a further step in tearing down an edifice of culturally defined normalcy and replacing it with alternatives. Rethinking biological parenthood becomes a process by which women and men examine how they feel and what they think of a plethora of related issues, such as the primacy of biology and the definition of family.

Women and men both subscribe to and resist cultural ideologies embedded in reproductive technologies. My emphasis on people's negotiations around cultural ideologies emerges from their own statements about how those ideologies affect their lives. Cultural ideologies not only shape actions; they also become a locus around which people marshal their resistance.

Women and men try to act in accord with the social order, but when those attempts fail, they give way to efforts to reshape definitions of gender, family, and parenthood, efforts that are bolstered and reinforced by the collective context in which they occur.[8] Women and men pursue their goals with intensity. They take matters into their own hands, seeking or rejecting medical care, joining self-help groups, negotiating with physicians, and critiquing reproductive health care.

These actions can be seen as political performances because they are involved in negotiating with the status quo through both accommodation and resistance. Making choices is a political activity, although it is important to recognize the constraints on choice.[9] As we have observed people making choices, we have seen how they come to identify themselves as consumers in a market economy and go on to identify risks and constraints. We have also observed how resistance grows over time, as women and men examine the system in which they have become immersed and find it wanting. Their actions lead to collective resistance that exerts influence on the reproductive technologies industry. Women, and sometimes men, experience the huge creative potential of this movement both personally and collectively as the performance of gender.[10]

In these efforts at resistance, women are paradoxically helping to maintain and reinforce the status quo.[11] Their efforts to resist these powerful forces are aimed not at destroying the reproductive technology industry but at improving its ability to meet their needs. In making demands on the industry, they are supporting it. The conjunction of these forces with cultural ideologies of parenthood can be seen when women who want to stop treatment are urged by others to keep trying and not give up.

These new reproductive technologies are embodied, even when bodily processes usually thought to occur inside the body take place outside it. The process whereby the body encompasses such activities can be seen as one of naturalization, in which women and men use the cultural tools at their disposal, such as metaphor, ritual, and visualization, to take ownership of the process of creating new life.

The forces behind the new reproductive technologies have a hand in this naturalization, but it is the women and men using these technologies who integrate the technologies with their lives. Although there is conflict between women's understanding of their bodies and their use of these technologies, when the technologies work men and women absorb the experience into their bodily knowledge. They are remaking nature, as they understand it. In doing so, they are creating a cultural shift in how people think about what is natural.

While consumers of these technologies have many reservations about their use, naturalization serves to neutralize negative moral dialogues about them. As we have seen, the naturalization process comprises many different cultural phenomena, and those phenomena not only make sense of the technologies' different components but humanize them as well. The technologies embody cultural ideologies, such as the ideology of continuity, that tend to reinforce their use.

After pursuing conception for several years, women and men construe their efforts to live out womanhood and manhood much more broadly. Although efforts to conceive continue to be central to their search for meaning, their primary efforts shift over time to emphasize rethinking what is meaningful in their lives. This broader agenda is initiated when their previous sources of meaning in life are challenged by infertility. In their efforts to rediscover what is meaningful, they live out gender in every action they take, engaging bodily knowledge in endless new ways. The performance of gender after it has been unexpectedly assaulted is a self-conscious process. That is, women and men continually analyze themselves and the cultural phenomena that affect them as they strive to regain their sense of equanimity.

For most people who participated in this study, the outcome has not been what they originally expected or hoped for. But they have done more than make the best of it: they have engaged with the possibilities, and in doing so they have made a series of political choices with specific consequences. These decisions were not made blindly or casually, but neither were they necessarily made rationally or autonomously. They were, however, made with the cultural resources that people had available. They involved much care and reflection, often with great attention to broader political and philosophical issues.

New reproductive technologies signal a specific cultural ideology, the ideology of the biological child. In electing to use these technologies, consumer-patients are subscribing to culturally specific forms of consumption that demonstrate their membership in the middle class.[12] Status and identity are enacted and negotiated through consumption, and, indeed, the use of new reproductive technologies can be seen as a form of identity politics.[13] New reproductive technologies, as an expression of how people attempt to live out gender expectations, reflect efforts to reestablish a sense of normalcy. That is, new reproductive technologies affirm gender identity, and when they work and a child is conceived, they symbolize the return of normalcy.

At the same time, although new reproductive technologies are being integrated into people's lives, they are a long way from being seen as essential or taken for granted. Rethinking one's life—for this is what happens in the aftermath of the discovery of infertility—goes on and on. It doesn't end even for those who get what they wanted from the start—a biological child—because for people who go through this process, life can never go back to the way it was before. People have rearranged their lives and the way they think about things. They question cultural phenomena they once took for granted. They may find themselves fitting the picture of normalcy but finding little comfort in it because their experience has varied so greatly from what they consider to be normal. When people are able to reestablish a sense of normalcy in their lives, it is precarious at best.

But in embodying the U.S. ideology of individualism, new reproductive technologies further reassert a sense of normalcy, whether they work or not, because they mirror what middle-class U.S. society stands for. By using them people have demonstrated their commitment to "progress."[14] Having persevered to this extent frees them to move to other endeavors, for there is an alternative cultural dialogue that says, "Do your best, but when you have made every effort in your attempt to meet cultural expectations and it is apparently hopeless, it is okay to relinquish this effort." We have seen the cultural theme of "do your best" voiced and lived out in this book, and we have also seen that people ultimately do come to terms with their situation if all their efforts fail.

It is at this point that women and men reconsider cultural ideologies and engage in alternative cultural dialogues. They are reworking the cultural assumptions they started with, sometimes rejecting them and sometimes resculpting them. These alternative dialogues fit the familiar cultural ideal of what constitutes family membership. Thus, we see women and men dropping the effort to have a biological child and concentrating on efforts to parent without biology. A woman who decides to remain childless may reaffirm her role as a marital partner or redefine herself as an aunt. In all cases people find a cultural category into which they can fit themselves, though it is neither their first choice nor as socially desirable as being the parent of a biological child.

GENDER AND NEW REPRODUCTIVE TECHNOLOGIES

Are cultural notions about gender reshaped through new reproductive technologies? These technologies perpetuate some assumptions about gender and undermine others, ultimately unsettling gendered categories and opening the door to change. The transformative nature of these technologies lends itself to ongoing negotiations around gender.

New reproductive technologies uphold the emphasis on biology, which underscores traditional images of women as conceivers and bearers of children.[15] This cultural trend has made it more difficult for women and men contemplating parenthood to entertain nonbiological possibilities, and it has also made it more difficult for people who have used other means to parent a child to normalize the experience. Moreover, it has reasserted the cultural notion that women's bodies are the medium through which parenthood is invariably attained. Anne Balsamo notes that the female body is persistently coded as "the cultural sign of 'the natural,' 'the sexual,' and 'the reproductive.' "[16] Women thus carry the burden of these ideas into their interactions with new reproductive technologies. Their bodies have become a laboratory. But, more than this, women's bodies have been rendered transparent by these technologies. This turn of events has implications for the perpetuation of associations of "the natural" with women's bodies. It also raises questions about how women maintain their rights over their bodies as the fetus takes priority over the woman. It remains to be seen whether concepts of what is natural will be reworked or whether they will fall into disuse as it becomes clearer to all concerned that there is nothing natural about gender.

The transformative process of questioning and resisting cultural ideologies does not occur without a struggle. Mary Douglas has observed that women's bodies have often been a site for the transgression of social boundaries.[17] Women are aware that this process is being worked out on and in their bodies, and they experience a significant conflict about it. Women often sacrifice their own health and well-being to conceive and bear a child. But a woman may also put herself first, set limits on what she can tolerate, and question why she, or any other woman, should go to such lengths. Women are simultaneously addressing multiple, often competing, imperatives: their desire to parent, the moral force of cultural ideologies, the promise of the technologies themselves, their sense of responsibility to become parents, and their sense of responsibility as consumers. The forces propelling these technologies along constitute another pressure.

Women experience their bodies as naturally ordered, but in undergoing medical treatment they observe that this sense of natural order is being undermined and reconstructed.[18] When a child is born, the birth compensates to some extent for this disjunction in bodily knowledge because it restores some sense of normalcy. But when these technologies fail, women reject them in favor of other means of finding normalcy in life. We have seen women engaged in both accommodation and resistance to efforts to place their bodies second to a potential biological child. The contradictions inherent in their actions indicate the enormous conflict in which women find themselves over questions of conception and childbearing.

Identity undergoes significant changes as women find their bodies being put at risk and move to protect themselves. They shift from the role of patient to the more assertive role of consumer. They make choices about these technologies, usually after lengthy self-education. Marilyn

Strathern comments that "choice" is a consumer idiom.[19] In the United States choice stands for autonomy, independence, and freedom of will, signifying women's sense of themselves as having an influence on the process in which they are engaged.

The way choices are formulated and presented by physicians can have major effects on consumers' decisions, however.[20] Treatment may be taken to extremes when a physician's sense of responsibility to offer patients all available technology is teamed with a woman's persistence in the quest for a pregnancy. Physicians may also ignore the financial cost of care. They have a long-standing preference for resolving ambiguity through intervention. Although they point to pressure from patients to act (and in the case of infertility that pressure can be considerable), physicians play a considerable role in fostering patients' expectations.[21] Biomedical perspectives thus provide legitimation for actions and reinforce women's views about the dangers of inaction.

As we have seen, women never simply surrender themselves to these technologies. The entire experience of medical treatment is enacted in an atmosphere of heightened surveillance and vigilance.[22] In this case, the surveillance is not simply by institutions of power, such as biomedicine; it is undertaken by women, as the objects of the technology. Women's vigilance as they reluctantly take steps to use new reproductive technologies may contribute to the exhaustion that so many experience during treatment. They are the watchdogs of the system, questioning and taking issue with virtually every aspect of the technologies as they encounter them, and raising those issues, gently or stridently, with their practitioners. Sherry Ortner observes that acts of resistance, whether individual or collective, are often conflicted.[23] We have seen throughout this book that this is so, especially in women's actions.

It is readily apparent that patriarchal gender interests are perpetuated in the policies and practices of reproductive technology, especially those involving donor gametes. Power is wielded in biomedicine to promote very different approaches to certain technologies. Whereas an atmosphere of openness and "naturalness" surrounds the donation of eggs, sperm donation continues to be treated as illicit and is being superseded by new reproductive technologies that reinforce the importance of paternity. Egg donation is normalized in ways that sperm donation is not. Institutionalized patriarchal interests thus make it difficult to bring about social change.

Although specific constraints on donor use tend to preserve the status quo, the use of donors represents one of the transformative effects of these technologies. Women and men are using these technologies to undermine the cultural ideology of biological parenthood and to transform the meaning of family. They are introducing new social practices such as increased openness about the biogenetic contribution of donors. Such practices promise to erode the cultural ideology of the biological child and remake cultural views of parenthood.

New reproductive technologies have also fostered the potential to look at women's lives differently and to uncover age stereotypes associated with women. Until recently, most women over forty had little hope of becoming pregnant and giving birth. And, prior to the emergence of new reproductive technologies, no woman could expect to conceive after she went through menopause. Now donor egg technology makes conception and motherhood possible for older women. It contributes to a broader societal process of reimaging women by making former biological markers such as menopause irrelevant and thereby making age itself irrelevant.

In consequence of such changes, women need to rethink what womanhood means. Does it mean having a child no matter what the emotional stakes and financial costs? Does it mean enduring medical treatment that dissects a woman into body parts? Does it mean mourning unlived lives—the miscarriages and ectopic pregnancies that occur in significant numbers among older women? Does it mean becoming a mother at any age? Does it mean, in the words of one woman, "I am nothing without a child"? Or does it mean that a woman can shape her own life as she sees fit, to have children or not, and at any age she wants? The traditional script for how women are supposed to live their lives has been thrown out, and in its place are a stack of blank scripts, waiting to be filled in. Women, especially older women, have more choices than ever before. There are almost no limits: women have to set their own.

CONSUMERS IN A BURGEONING INDUSTRY

Although I saw the burgeoning of reproductive technologies as a cultural phenomenon when I first began this work, at the outset I did not fully grasp the importance of issues of power and control. It was as if the stage on which I had been observing a small cast of characters enact their concerns became crowded overnight with a Greek chorus, as people representing myriad interests and perspectives tried to elbow their way in. Such concerns as basic infertility care for low-income people were crowded out as preoccupation with the new reproductive technol-

ogies and their markets took over. Meanwhile, other interests, such as
the insurance industry, tried to exert control over technology indirectly,
through withdrawing from the arena. My own focus—on individuals'
experience of infertility and treatment—was inevitably affected by this
transition. I could no longer focus simply on basic cultural phenomena
such as reshaped meanings of kinship or the effects on women's lives of
extending the childbearing years.

The moral economy of the United States shapes the use of new reproductive technologies. Productivity is a moral priority emanating from
cultural values such as individualism, autonomy, and the work ethic.[24]
Financial success is the reward of hard work, and in examining the use
of new reproductive technologies we can see how the moral economy
justifies monetary rewards for physicians and others who provide these
technologies, as well as for consumers who can afford them.

The long list of competing interests that I detailed in chapter 1 not
only reflects the range of forces in this industry but also demonstrates
that what is at stake is power. My task in this book has been to examine
how people's experiences of infertility and their efforts to empower
themselves are entwined with cultural ideologies and with broad institutional forces that reflect those ideologies, particularly those that provide new reproductive technologies and represent powerful industrial
interests. The negotiations of consumer-patients over new reproductive
technologies demonstrate how they simultaneously use, accommodate,
and resist these technologies. The cultural ideologies to which people
subscribe are reflected in the social institutions in which the technologies
are grounded and through which commodification occurs: business and
biomedicine.[25]

It can easily be seen how these forces converge in the case of donor
gametes, for example. The policy set by the American Society for Reproductive Medicine in 1988 to use only frozen sperm has led to a proliferation of commercial sperm banks. Meanwhile, the development of
donor egg technology has become big business, and the cost of donor
eggs continues to rise. Because consumers can now select donors directly
and persistently choose donors for intelligence and appearance, not only
are donor gametes now highly commodified, but the manner in which
they are being used suggests that a new form of eugenics is emerging.

Despite their participation in processes of commodification, consumers are ambivalent about the amalgamation of such institutional forces.
Although other medical specialties are also increasingly converging with
business interests, the coalescence of business and medicine is nowhere

so obvious to consumers as in reproductive medicine. When medical concerns take a back seat to business interests and patients become aware of that shift, they act as consumers and apply their own repertoire of business skills, thus participating in the redefining of medical treatment.

The ambivalence people in this study express about the technologies and their cost reflects underlying dissatisfaction with the moral economy. In trying to live out the ideology of the biological child, these consumers express anger and cynicism that they should have to go to such lengths to become parents. When consumers continually question an economic system that puts some people into debt in order to have children and leaves others out completely, they are expressing opposition to the dominant moral economy, which distinguishes between those who are viewed as deserving and those who are not.[26] The implicit stance of these women and men is that these technologies should be available to them without the added burden of demonstrating that they are deserving by having to find the money to use them. This stance suggests that the dominant moral economy is not, in fact, as widely accepted as it would seem, and that resistance to the status quo is widespread. Self-help groups for infertility have lobbied the federal government to introduce insurance that would cover the cost of these technologies, so far to no avail. While the moral economy of the United States is grounded in a utilitarian approach that, in emphasizing the importance of wealth, ignores distributive justice and commodifies human life, consumers in this study apparently subscribe to an alternative approach, one that would give priority to meeting human needs.[27] This disparity reflects a deep conflict within American society about which values matter most.

Other industries interact with this emerging industry in complex ways. For example, the adoption industry both affects and is affected by new reproductive technologies in several respects, including the cost of private adoption, the availability of children for adoption, and the regulations—or lack thereof—that govern this industry. Women and men in this book frequently compared adoption with the new reproductive technologies, thus testifying to the complex linkages that exist.

Adoption, once viewed as the logical option for infertile couples, is now beyond the means of many families who have used up their financial resources on infertility treatment. But, more important, with the growth of the independent adoption industry has come an increase in the cost of adoption. The demand for children and the resulting cost have escalated greatly during the fifteen years of this research. Couples are thus likely to view adoption as unaffordable and instead devote their resources to infertility treatment.

These effects of new reproductive technologies raise questions about whether limits should be placed on their use. Respect for individual autonomy is apparently a major factor in contributing to technological interventions. Because American ideals favor minimal intervention by government, regulation has been left primarily to the industry itself. Physicians have not attempted to impose limits on the medical use of new reproductive technologies. This tendency suggests that physicians' respect for individual autonomy impedes the modest efforts that have been made to institute controls. The U.S. government has limited its intervention to consumer protection efforts, such as truth in advertising, accurate reporting of success rates to the Centers for Disease Control, and ensuring of medical competence.[28]

Most efforts at regulation of this field in the United States to date have been made by medical societies such as the American Society of Reproductive Medicine and its subgroup, the Society for Assisted Reproductive Technologies (the latter has developed a reporting process that lends legitimacy to participating programs), and by individual practices. Physicians and bioethicists have called for the regulation of technology, including more guidelines, laws, and technology assessment. Some especially favor impetus from professional associations, with participation from the public.[29]

In contrast to the U.S. approach, numerous European governments have attempted to regulate new reproductive technologies, and those efforts have emphasized social policy issues, such as how the family should be constituted.[30] The emphasis on family creation in numerous European nations illustrates how a nation's moral economy shapes its priorities. In those countries such policies reflect the precedence of social priorities over economic priorities. Both the American and European models, however, seek to control access to new reproductive technologies. In both models, heterosexual, married couples are privileged over single women and gay couples.

The lack of controls for infertility treatment illustrates how cultural tensions over value conflicts are expressed through society's institutions. In infertility treatment, physicians become the protagonists when they are viewed as making profits at consumers' expense. It is considered a moral responsibility *not* to use power, privilege, and knowledge against those who are less advantaged. For physicians, whose expert knowledge is considered to give them power, this ethos is reflected in the medical code of ethics. But physicians in private practice are also businesspeople. In conflicts of interest between business and medicine, medicine is supposed to come first. When consumers view practitioners as violating this principle, physicians become suspect, and a potential conflict arises in the doctor-patient relationship. Although consumer organizations acknowledge that consumers are a force in driving new reproductive technologies,[31] patients expect physicians to maintain a disinterested stance as they guide their patients through medical treatment. When patients infer that business has the upper hand in physicians' recommendations, the doctor-patient relationship is compromised, resulting in conflicts between individual physicians and patients.

Social and economic disparities are increasingly apparent as new reproductive technologies come to dictate practice trends. The consumers who are the targets of these technologies are predominantly white, college-educated Americans who are economically well off and own their own homes. These technologies are tailored to them. Although much has been said about the limits of collective forms of resistance in influencing powerful systems that have been institutionalized, these individuals can wield considerable power in asserting their own interests when they learn how to use the system effectively. Of great concern, however, are the women who are bypassed by lack of access to these technologies: low-income women who, because they have no access to these technologies and hence no place at the bargaining table, become invisible.[32]

We thus see a major dichotomy emerging in the treatment of infertility: at one end of the spectrum, people who have low incomes are unable to locate the most basic evaluative services.[33] At the other end, couples whose income exceeds $100,000 a year are spending $10,000 or more per cycle for in vitro fertilization. This trend reflects moral economy views about who is deserving and who is not, thus emphasizing the importance of improving the health of middle-class persons but not of those who are poor. Utilizing assisted reproductive technologies thus becomes a prerogative of the upper classes.

The use of new reproductive technologies in the United States reflects dominant cultural phenomena: the complex combination of institutional power, cultural ideologies, and actions that is uniquely American. While the stance on individual freedom has led to a lack of government regulation and contributes to the exacerbation of class, ethnic, and racial discrimination in access to services, this same stance enables women and men to utilize these technologies regardless of marital status, sexual orientation, or religion, leading to new ways of conceptualizing family. In

most other countries, access to these technologies may be restricted on
such grounds, illustrating how widely the need is perceived globally to
oversee and control the use of these technologies.[34]

The use of new reproductive technologies is subject to the particular
cultural configurations of individual societies. At the same time, global
interaction is occurring in the development of new technologies, dissem-
ination of technologies and their clinical applications, the trend for people to travel internationally to utilize these technologies, forms of resistance such as feminist coalitions, government decisions on a spectrum
of issues, such as the provision of access to these technologies, and international policy debates, such as the debate about the disclosure of
gamete donors' identity to offspring.[35] Policy decisions made in one
country inevitably inform policy debates in another country. Examining
new reproductive technologies globally is one route to understanding
the global landscape and the intertwining of cultures through technology.

THE LIMITS OF AGENCY

I have repeatedly drawn attention to ways in which the cultural ideology
of biological parenthood affects and impairs people's ability to move on
with their lives. But I have also tried to show that, in one way or another,
most people are eventually able to move beyond biology. Using new
reproductive technologies provokes women and men to resist the status
quo, rethink meanings of normalcy, and find other means to express and
enact gender.

Finding and developing new ways to define family is one significant
arena of action because of its potential to rework cultural ideologies,
break down old ideas, and develop more comprehensive views. The family is the context in which such ideologies are contested and reworked.[36]
But such debate threatens the moral order; hence the condemnation of
the use of donors by many organized religions and the efforts by biomedicine to regulate donor use. This is but one example of how deviating from the status quo challenges various cultural domains, and it
shows how overarching ideologies are expressed in different arenas.

Because they challenge cultural notions about what is natural, and,
indeed, experiment with technologies that explicitly defy such notions,
consumers of new reproductive technologies threaten the status quo—
the cultural ideologies and institutional forces that exert power over
people's lives and that resist change. At the same time, people's reactions

to and resistance against biological interpretations, of personhood for example, simultaneously reinforce those interpretations.[37] People in this book were resistant only up to a point—the point at which they created a workable solution for themselves. For many, however, the solution they found promised to involve them in a lifetime of resistance through advocacy, in order to remake the world to accommodate their child or to assert their moral authority. I have chosen to highlight resistance because it is deep and pervasive, and, even if partial, is contributing to social change.

In the midst of experimenting with new reproductive technologies, rethinking cultural ideologies, and breaking with cultural traditions about families as biologically based, people continue to strive for continuity and normalcy. No radically different family forms are being introduced by the people in this book. Most of them still subscribe to the American ideal of the two-parent family. They still want to fit into the world as they know it, and their actions reflect that desire. From that perspective, the changes they are trying to bring about are not earth-shaking; they are ordinary and expectable. In short, they reflect cultural imperatives about normalcy and how ideologies of normalcy are embodied in moral dialogues from which people are loath to—indeed, unable to—stray too far. Technology, as a template of culture, is one arena in which normalcy is both resisted and reaffirmed and through which the enactment and transformation of cultural practice occurs.

About the Research

This book is based on data from a large, primarily qualitative study funded by the National Institute on Aging, National Institutes of Health. In *Healing the Infertile Family,* I reported on an earlier pilot study funded by the Academic Senate, University of California, San Francisco. Although we collected various kinds of data in the larger study, the greatest volume of data was collected from couples going through infertility treatment, including new reproductive technologies. I describe those data first.

SAMPLING AND INTERVIEWING

The plan of this study was to capture the full range of experiences of infertility and its treatment. The potential sample was divided at the outset into four categories: people who had experienced infertility for less than a year; people who had been in infertility treatment for between one and three years; people who had been in medical treatment for three years or more, or who had utilized new reproductive technologies; and people who had ended medical treatment within the past three years. We tried to recruit approximately equal numbers of people in all four categories, but it was soon apparent that we had many fewer recruits in the first category. Based on this experience and that of the previous study, it appears that people do not recognize a problem at this early stage, or, if they do, they are not ready to talk about it. The study quickly turned into a study of people who had been in infertility treatment for over a year, and at the completion of recruitment the sample was divided almost equally among the other three categories.

Because of the nature of our sample, we did not focus exclusively on new reproductive technologies, although we anticipated that a sizable proportion of the sample would sooner or later decide to use them. We often interviewed people long before they even contemplated using such treatments. We followed them through treatment, and often beyond, with three in-depth interviews conducted over one or two years.

This approach was much preferable to the alternative, which was to begin talking with people only when they had made their treatment decision and begun using these technologies. It enabled us to elicit people's stories in the broad context of their lives and their experiences with unwanted childlessness and also to capture in detail the experience of infertility treatment, including sequences of medical treatments and the phases women and men went through as they undertook treatment and considered other possibilities. Over the four years of data collection, we conducted over five hundred interviews. The thrust of the interviews was on the meanings and interpretations people placed on infertility.

Although we first recruited from medical practices, we later expanded our recruitment to adoption counseling services, low-income clinics, and a self-help group (Resolve). Participants also volunteered after hearing about the study from others who had already volunteered. We eventually recruited 277 people, 143 women and 134 men.

Women were more willing to volunteer than men; and the fact that the study focused on couples rather than women only slowed down the recruitment process considerably. We had found the same pattern in the pilot study but felt that it was important to include men, first because we were studying gender, not simply women, and second because men significantly affect the process their partners go through. Leaving them out would have been a significant omission and altered the study in a variety of ways.

The interview format, following ethnographic interviewing methods, included both directive and nondirective strategies.[1] All interviews were recorded on tape and transcribed shortly afterward. Within the framework provided by the interview, the respondent's narration of the experience gives structure not only to the experience but also to the research encounter. While research questions may be used to guide the research overall, too much structure would inhibit the respondent from speaking of those matters that most concern her or him. A careful balance is therefore necessary. Respondents must be given freedom to discuss their experiences and ideas in their own terms, and an interviewer must listen with great care. In this study, the exact wording of interview questions and the sequence of the questions emerged during the interview. Interviewers made extensive use of probes to explain unclear responses and to supplement sparse comments.

Interviews were designed so that respondents could, by telling their story in their own words, develop their own structure.[2] Because people in this study experienced disruption to bodily functioning and bodily expectations, the interview questions encompassed many queries that led to responses about bodily perceptions.

Partners were first interviewed together in detailed interviews lasting two hours or more; followup individual interviews took place six to twelve months later, with final interviews with both partners taking place twelve to twenty-four months after that. Data were collected by six interviewers (four women and two men); I collected half the data myself. We conducted interviews in English, except with one couple who were interviewed in Spanish. Interviews addressed the events that led up to medical treatment, each person's experience of medical treatment, and related events, feelings, and experiences. The interview schedule was designed with two goals in mind: to explore the personal experience of infertility in order to gain new insights; and to collect data that could be coded and used in qualitative analysis. Probes were used during the interviews to elicit specific information about emotional reactions to infertility, attitudes about adoption, effect of infertility on the marital relationship, and related topics.

COLLECTION OF DATA
ON REPRODUCTIVE MEDICINE

When I began studying infertility in the early 1980s, I initiated what is now referred to as "multisited" ethnography as a matter of course. I wanted to understand infertility from various standpoints—those of physicians and others working in the field as well as those of patients. Reproductive medicine was then still a relatively new subspecialization, and I therefore undertook to understand its clinical practices and standpoints in relation to the general practice of obstetrics and gynecology. I spent over five years attending grand rounds on a weekly basis at two teaching hospitals in my area. For a year I sat in on teaching sessions for residents and medical students at one hospital where much of the teaching was done by infertility specialists. During the four years of the study I report here, I attended all grand rounds that addressed infertility in both hospitals. I formally interviewed five infertility specialists about their perspectives on the changing nature of reproductive medicine, and I talked informally with many others.

During that time I also attended almost every meeting sponsored by Resolve in which physicians presented their perspectives to prospective patients and answered questions. Because of its in-depth approach and its long-term nature, this fieldwork enabled me to observe how practice trends were changing and to track changes in reproductive medicine in relation to the broader field of obstetrics and gynecology. As new reproductive technologies took hold in my geographic area, I watched the growth of reproductive medicine as a subspecialty. I also observed practitioners without subspecialty training increasingly identify infertility as one of their areas of expertise. This work enabled me to understand the shifts that were taking place within the practice of medicine as a result of physicians' increased awareness of infertility.

DATA ANALYSIS

A qualitative data analysis was undertaken prior to the narrative analysis that I conducted specifically for this book. The first step was the development of core categories.[3] Coding categories are generated from meanings inherent in the data themselves.[4]

Paradigm cases were used to develop the analysis in terms of range and variation in the data.[5] A paradigm case is a case that is a strong instance of a particular observation or trend that appears to be prototypical in the early stages of data analysis, before it can be categorized.

We also coded the data by specific topics: for example, perceptions of risk. The material on risk awareness and experiences in chapter 5 resulted from an in-depth analysis on this topic midway through data collection and has been subject to further analysis since the completion of the study.

A case-by-case analysis was also carried out following an approach developed by Sharon Kaufman. The process begins with a close reading of each case for (1) repetition of specific words, phrases, and general thought patterns; (2) the structure of the overall case; and (3) topics that dominated respondents' reports as well as topics that were not raised at all.[6] In addition to these analyses, people were grouped by type of medical treatment and then compared across groups.

The process by which I analyzed narratives for this book extended the case-study approach and is described in detail in *Disrupted Lives*. I built on this approach in my subsequent analyses, scrutinizing clues to embodied distress, all statements about the body and bodily distress, all episodes of health problems and medical interventions, and all expressions of emotion. I also scrutinized narratives for links between bodily distress and social concerns, such as the distaste people expressed for some aspects of medical treatment and medical practices. I made an effort to work with all of the relevant data, which was a challenge because the body of data is so large. I believe that the stories in this book accurately represent the views of people who participated in this study.

DEMOGRAPHIC INFORMATION

Of the 277 respondents, demographic characteristics are available for 118 couples. The majority of respondents lived in a five-county urban and suburban area, but 44 lived in rural areas. The age range for women was 25 to 52 years (the mean was 36.13 years). For men the age range was 27 to 71 (mean 38.04). The sample was predominantly middle-class and college-educated. The cost of living in this area is among the highest in the United States, and salaries are correspondingly high. The majority had yearly family incomes of $60,000 or more and owned their own homes; but thirty-five couples had family incomes below $60,000, and four families had incomes below $20,000. Eighty percent of couples had some form of health insurance, but less than half of those had any coverage for the medical treatment of infertility. Respondents were primarily in professional, management, and white-collar employment. Ninety-seven women were employed outside the home, and 21 were not employed; 114 men were employed, and 4 were not employed. Forty respondents (15 percent of the sample) were nonwhite or Latino (4 Native Americans, 14 Asian Americans, 12 African Americans, 6 Latinos, 2 East Indians, and 2 Pacific Islanders). Forty-three were Catholic, 48 were Jewish, 55 were Protestant, 35 were members of other religions, 40 reported they had no religion, and 15 did not respond.

Glossary

Information about treatment modalities in the glossary follows standard biomedical explanations. It is not my intent in this book to question particulars of the science of reproductive medicine, except in instances where widespread treatment policies have been politicized, as evidenced by dissenting voices in the literature.

Artificial insemination. The placement of sperm within the genital tract of a woman by a method other than intercourse. The sperm is most commonly placed in the vagina or cervix but more recently has been injected directly into the uterine cavity (a procedure known as intra-uterine insemination, or IUI). Older terminology specified the source of the sperm: AIH referred to artificial insemination with the husband's sperm and AID to insemination with donor sperm.

Basic infertility workup. The traditional diagnostic procedures involve tests that examine the man's sperm and the woman's fallopian tubes, cervical mucus, and ovulation. These tests include a semen analysis, a postcoital test (PCT), a hysterosalpingogram (HSG), and three tests of ovulation: (1) basal body temperature (BBT), measured each morning for a month or more, which rises during ovulation; (2) serum progesterone level, which indicates whether the ovary has ovulated and is secreting sufficient hormone for optimal fertility; (3) an endometrial biopsy, an office procedure in which a small amount of tissue is removed from the lining of the uterus and analyzed by a pathologist to determine its "readiness" to accept a fertilized egg. See individual entries in glossary for more information.

Clomiphene. While not a hormone itself, clomiphene causes the pituitary gland to secrete an increased amount of follicle stimulating hormone (FSH), which acts on the ovary to enhance egg development and ovulation. (Because of this increased stimulation, there is a 10 percent chance of conceiving twins when taking clomiphene.) One to five pills are taken orally for five days to stimulate ovulation and make the menstrual cycle more predictable. The side effects of clomiphene, although not permanent or dangerous, may be bothersome; they include hot flashes, mild blurring of vision, ovulation pain, and mood swings and heightened feelings of emotion, sometimes with irritability or increased sensitivity. The major advantages of clomiphene are that few office visits per cycle are required, it is taken orally rather than injected, and it is relatively inexpensive. The alternative, therapy with human menopausal gonadotropins (hMG), is more powerful in that more follicles usually develop, it has a less pronounced effect on mood, and pregnancy rates are generally higher. However hMG is much more expensive, requires daily injections and more office visits for ultrasound monitoring, and is more likely to result in multiple gestation. Severe hyperstimulation, although relatively uncommon, represents a greater threat than any of clomiphene's side effects. *See also* hMG.

DES (diethylstilbestrol). A synthetic estrogen originally prescribed to women at risk for miscarriage (although its efficacy was never evaluated in a clinical trial). A small percentage of women whose mothers took DES during pregnancy developed a rare form of vaginal cancer in childhood. Others were found to have cervical and uterine abnormalities associated with elevated risks for infertility, miscarriage, and premature labor.

Donor egg technologies. Although originally developed to allow young women who were born without functioning ovaries to become pregnant, the use of another woman's eggs (donor eggs) has expanded to women whose ovaries are unable to produce fertile eggs for various other reasons, including chromosomal abnormalities; endometriosis, infection, or tumors; or autoimmmune diseases. Treatment has also been extended to women of any age whose eggs did not fertilize through IVF, and women in their late thirties and early forties for whom treatment has been unsuccessful because of ovarian aging. The egg donor may be a relative, a friend, or an anonymous donor from an agency. After the donor has been selected and screened for general health, infectious and inheritable diseases, and psychological suitability, the donor and recipient have their menstrual cycles synchronized. The donor receives injections of pituitary hormone to stimulate her ovaries, while the recipient receives injections of estrogen to prepare the lining of her uterus. When the donor's eggs are mature, they are removed with a small needle, using ultrasound imaging. The eggs are then combined with the recipient's partner's (or donor) sperm and allowed to fertilize in the laboratory. Two or three days later, the fertilized eggs are transferred into the recipient's uterus. A pregnancy test performed two weeks later indicates whether the procedure was successful. Each cycle has a 30 to 50 percent chance of success.

Donor insemination. The use of sperm from a man other than the recipient's partner for the purpose of achieving a pregnancy. In the past, the donor was frequently a college student recruited by the physician, but most donor sperm today is provided by commercial sperm banks. The donor's physical characteristics and various details of the medical history may be selected by the couple or single woman, but the identity of the donor is usually not revealed. The cost of frozen sperm from a sperm bank is generally $200–$400 per cycle. This does not include the cost of the insemination, which may be intravaginal, intracervical, or intrauterine, at an additional cost of $250–$1,000. Donor sperm may also be used for IVF.

Ectopic pregnancy. A condition in which a fertilized egg begins to develop within the fallopian tube instead of being transported to and implanting in the uterus. Ectopic pregnancy can be caused by scarring within the tube, as from pelvic inflammatory disease. The condition is painful, and if ignored or misdiagnosed it can result in rupture of the tube with catastrophic and sometimes fatal internal bleeding. Unless diagnosed in its earliest stage, when delicate surgery or medication can sometimes salvage the tube, an ectopic pregnancy is usually treated by surgically removing the affected fallopian tube.

Endometriosis. A condition in which the retrograde flow of menstrual blood allows cells from the lining of the uterus to implant and grow in the peritoneal lining of the pelvic and, less commonly, abdominal cavities. This tissue responds to the hormonal fluctuations of the menstrual cycle with pain, bleeding, inflammation, and scarring. Depending on the woman's age and the severity of the disease, endometriosis may be treated using hormones or with surgery. Endometriosis can be assessed with a numerical score that takes into account the presence, location, size, and severity of adhesions, tubal blockage, or endometriotic cysts of the ovary (endometriomas) and the probable effect on tubal or ovarian function. There is no convincing evidence that mild endometriosis causes infertility. In the past, almost all moderate and severe endometriosis was treated with a procedure known as "conservative" surgery. This surgery was meant to "conserve" as much normal tissue and function as possible while excising as much of the endometriosis and scar tissue as was surgically feasible. The adhesions that result from the inflammation of endometriosis can be extremely difficult to remove and the surgery challenging. In recent years, the trend has been to perform such surgery through the laparoscope.

GIFT (gamete intrafallopian transfer). A technique for removing, fertilizing, and implanting eggs in which the ovaries are visualized through a laparoscope. The retrieved eggs and washed sperm are placed into the fallopian tube or tubes as in natural reproduction. When IVF egg retrieval was performed by laparoscopy, GIFT offered some advantage to women with normal tubes. Since the advent of transvaginal ultrasonically guided egg retrieval, IVF no longer requires laparoscopy, which makes GIFT a more expensive and invasive procedure, albeit one with a somewhat higher pregnancy rate.

GnRH (gonadotropin-releasing hormone). The hypothalamic hormone that controls the release of FSH and LH (gonadotropins) from the pituitary gland during the menstrual cycle. In IVF treatment cycles, synthetic analogs of GnRH (marketed as Lupron and Synarel) are used to block the release of pituitary LH before the follicles have reached the optimal size for oocyte retrieval.

hCG (human chorionic gonadotropin). A hormone produced by the embryo immediately after implantation that is required for the continued production of ovarian progesterone during the first trimester. hCG levels usually double every forty-eight hours in the first two to three months of a normal pregnancy and are used in conjunction with ultrasound to detect early fetal problems, including nonviable and ectopic pregnancies.

hMG (human menopausal gonadotropins). Medications that mimic the pituitary hormones that stimulate egg development. They are sold under a variety of brand names and are given by injection. Using hMG helps ensure that multiple mature eggs are released during each cycle, thus increasing the chances for fertilization. Blood tests and ultrasound exams must be performed every few days to ensure that the ovaries are receiving neither too little nor too much stimulation. The two complications of hMG use are the greatly increased possibility of multiple gestation and the possibility of overstimulating the ovaries. If hyperstimulation occurs, the ovaries become enlarged and tender, with abdominal bloating and fluid retention. Mild cases last about a week and usually respond to bedrest at home. Severe hyperstimulation occurs in about 1 percent of cycles and has been associated with a few fatalities.

Hysterosalpingogram (HSG). An X-ray test, using a dye injected into the uterus and fallopian tubes, that detects a blockage in the fallopian tubes that would prevent the union of a sperm and egg or irregularity or scarring of the lining of the uterus. The risks of an HSG include an allergic reaction to iodine (rare) and pelvic infection.

Intracytoplasmic sperm injection (ICSI). A procedure performed in conjunction with an IVF cycle in cases where the man has very low numbers of normal sperm. Performed in the laboratory under a microscope with an extremely fine glass needle, ICSI involves the injection of a single sperm into the cytoplasm of an oocyte. Fertilization occurs in approximately two-thirds of injected eggs, and the technique achieves the same pregnancy rate as IVF when performed with normal sperm: approximately 20–40 percent per cycle. The procedure adds approximately $1,000–$2,000 to the cost of an IVF treatment cycle.

Intrauterine insemination (IUI). The technique of placing sperm directly into the uterine cavity. Less expensive than advanced procedures such as IVF and GIFT, IUI is used as a first step in cases of infertility where there is a "cervical" factor (inadequate or "hostile" mucus), anti-sperm antibodies, or unexplained infertility. Because the seminal plasma that makes up most of the ejaculate is irritating to the uterus, the sperm cells themselves must be separated from the seminal plasma by filtration or through multiple dilutions with physiologically sterile culture media (referred to as "sperm washing"), after which the sperm are placed through the cervix into the uterus using a thin plastic tube. The IUI procedure is usually painless, requiring only a few minutes. Although IUI can be performed within a natural menstrual cycle by using simple urine testing kits that detect the preovulatory luteinizing hormone release ("LH surge") to determine the best day for insemination, most studies have found that IUI is more effective if the ovaries are first stimulated with oral (clomiphene) or injectable (hMG) medications. IUI is usually attempted for three to six cycles. Depending on whether ovulation stimulants are used, the cost of an IUI cycle ranges from $350 to $2,500.

In vitro fertilization (IVF). Literally, in vitro fertilization means fertilization in glass—as in a test tube—but the technique actually involves a sequence of steps using injectable pituitary hormones (hMG) to stimulate the development of multiple eggs (usually ten to thirty depending on age and ovarian responsiveness), removing the mature eggs through the back wall of the vagina using an ultrasonically guided needle, combining the eggs and sperm in the laboratory under conditions designed to enhance fertilization, and transferring several of the two- or three-day-old embryos directly into the uterus through the vagina and cervix. IVF was initially developed to allow pregnancies in cases where the sperm was prevented from coming into contact with the egg because the woman's fallopian tubes were blocked, absent, or damaged beyond surgical repair. Gradually, however, its applications have expanded so that IVF is now offered as the final treatment option for almost all infertile couples.

Laparoscopy. A same-day surgical procedure that is commonly recommended if the tubal X ray is abnormal, if the patient has a history of IUD use, ectopic pregnancy, or pelvic infection, or when the basic infertility evaluation has not determined the cause for infertility. After a small incision is made in the lower fold of the navel, the lens and fiber-optic light source of the laparoscope are inserted through the abdominal wall, allowing a detailed evaluation of the pelvic organs, including the uterus, tubes, and ovaries. Corrective surgery may then be performed with electrocautery or lasers. The procedure takes twenty minutes if the pelvis is normal, but removal of extensive scarring may take several hours.

Lupron. See GnRH.

Male infertility. Infertility may be attributed to the male partner if one or more parameters of the semen analysis (i.e., volume, concentration, motility, morphology) are found to be repeatedly abnormal or if the sperm have failed to fertilize oocytes under laboratory conditions. Although identifiable causes of male infertility include genetic defects, semineferous tubular failure, obstruction of the seminal ducts, varicocele, chemotherapy, and infection, a specific diagnosis cannot be found for the majority of infertile men with abnormal semen analysis.

Pelvic inflammatory disease (PID). A term referring to a variety of infections that can contribute to female infertility. Pelvic infection usually spreads from the vagina through the cervix and uterus and into the fallopian tubes. Although in the past PID was believed to be synonymous with a gonococcal infection of the fallopian tubes, it is now believed that the presence of an intrauterine device can make it easier for infection to spread from the vagina into the uterus and fallopian tubes. As result, as many as 1 percent of all IUD wearers may have suffered tubal damage.

Polycystic ovary syndrome. A poorly understood, genetically inherited condition marked by irregular or absent menstrual cycles, excess facial and body hair, and infertility. Altered patterns of pituitary stimulation result in the failure of mature eggs to develop each month, along with the overproduction of male hormone by the ovaries. Treatment with hormones succeeds in bringing about pregnancy in approximately 50 percent of patients.

Postcoital test (PCT). Evaluates the interaction of sperm and cervical mucus. Each month the mucus increases in quantity and becomes more runny as ovulation approaches. The postcoital test is scheduled for a morning judged to be within a day or two prior to ovulation and is initiated by the couple's having intercourse at home. In the physician's office, a small amount of mucus is removed in a way similar to a Pap smear. The mucus is then immediately examined under a microscope to evaluate the mucus quality and to assess the number of motile sperm.

Premature ovarian failure. The cessation of ovarian function prior to age forty. The most common causes are an abnormality or absence of one of a woman's two X chromosomes and a poorly understood form of autoimmune disease affecting the ovary. No treatment can restore ovarian function; however, the ovarian hormones estrogen and progesterone can be replaced with oral medication, allowing a woman to carry a pregnancy using a donated egg.

Selective reduction. The reduction of one or more embryos in the event of multiple gestation. To maximize the chances for at least one embryo implanting, all advanced reproductive technologies attempt to produce multiple embryos in the laboratory. It has been common to transfer four embryos into the uterus at a time, but this figure may be higher or lower depending on the patient's age, the quality of the embryos, the experience of the laboratory, and the patient's willingness to assume the risk of multiple gestation. Although IVF is responsible for less than 1 percent of total births in the United States, it accounts for 22 percent of triplets. Patients carrying a triplet or

larger multiple pregnancy may be offered the option of selective reduction, a procedure in which a needle is inserted through the abdominal wall into the uterus under ultrasonic guidance and potas-
sium chloride is injected to stop the heart of one or more individual
fetuses.

Semen analysis. Measures the volume of the ejaculate, the sperm concentration measured in millions of sperm per cubic centimeter of semen, the percentage of sperm that are moving (motility), and the
percentage of sperm that are normally formed (morphology).

Varicocele. Formation of varicose veins around the testicle. The condition is found in 10 per cent of all men but in more than 33 percent
of infertile men. Because the optimal temperature for sperm production is lower than internal body temperature, it is believed that the
dilated veins of the varicocele keep the testicle too warm by surrounding it with body-temperature blood. The varicocele is usually repaired
by minor surgery through an incision in the groin. About two-thirds
of men show an improvement in sperm count or motility after surgical
varicocele repair.

Zygote intrafallopian transfer (ZIFT). Following controlled ovarian
hyperstimulation, oocyte retrieval, and in vitro fertilization, the early
embryo (zygote) is placed in the fallopian tube via laparoscopy. ZIFT
attempts to combine the advantages of IVF-ET and GIFT by utilizing
the fallopian tubes in their physiological role as the site of zygote
transport, at the cost of subjecting the patient to two separate anes-
thesias.

Notes

INTRODUCTION.
FROM PERSONAL EXPERIENCE TO RESEARCH

1. See Becker, *Healing the Infertile Family,* for discussion of how I moved from personal experience to conducting research on infertility.

2. I discuss my personal experience of disruption in Becker, *Disrupted Lives.*

CHAPTER 1. CONSUMING TECHNOLOGIES

1. All names and identifying characteristics have been changed to protect the anonymity of the interviewees.

2. See the glossary entry on "in vitro fertilization." For further discussion of IVF, see Turiel, *Beyond Second Opinions.*

3. Clarke, *Disciplining Reproduction,* traces the development of the reproductive sciences in the laboratory during the twentieth century.

4. Anthropologists continue to debate what constitutes culture. Implied in most definitions has been the idea that culture represents order (see, for example, Geertz, *Interpretation of Cultures,* 90; Hallowell, *Culture and Experience,* 94–95), but over the last twenty years there has been an increasing emphasis on examining culture as disorderly, for instance in the investigation of power, resistance, and agency (see, for example, Gupta and Ferguson, "Culture, Power, Place," 4–5). Gramsci's image of culture encompasses qualities that resonate with anthropological thinking and is distinct from concepts of hegemony and ideology. Following Gramsci, Comaroff and Comaroff define culture as "the space of signifying practice, the semantic ground on which human beings seek to construct and represent themselves and others—and, hence, society and history" (*Revelation and Revolution,* 21). They note that culture is empowered,

and the two dominant forms through which power enters are hegemony and ideology.

5. Technology embodies culture. That is, science, technology, and medicine are seen as culture by social scientists working in this field. See, for example, Casper and Koenig, "Reconfiguring Nature and Culture"; Franklin, "Science as Culture"; Haraway, *Modest_Witness;* Strathern, *Reproducing the Future* and "Displacing Knowledge." Haraway (*Modest_Witness,* 66) notes that science is both cultural practice and practical culture.

6. Many feminist scholars have examined the question of what is considered "natural," especially with respect to women. See especially Balsamo, *Technologies;* Franklin, *Embodied Progress;* Hartouni, *Cultural Conceptions;* Schiebinger, *Nature's Body;* Strathern, *After Nature;* and Yanagisako and Delaney, *Naturalizing Power.* Franklin observes, "Ideas of the natural comprise one of the most important 'cultural logics' that recent theorists have sought to analyze. . . . Developmental models with which to theorize both the levels of coherence, and of contradictory tensions, within the domain of the natural constitutes an ongoing and expanding area of social theory" (*Embodied Progress,* 57). Kinship is one arena in which cultural views about what is natural shape attitudes about new reproductive technologies. See Edwards et al., *Technologies of Procreation,* for discussions of how the challenge posed by new reproductive technologies to ideas of what is natural renders those technologies "dangerous."

7. Ong and Peletz address the body as a site of disruption in *Bewitching Women.* Throughout *Disrupted Lives* I discuss the experience of bodily distress arising out of disruption to life. Ginsburg and Tsing (*Uncertain Terms,* 2) observe that because of pervasive uncertainties over gender constructs, gender meanings are subject to constant negotiation at both the personal and the political levels. The contestation of meanings is most intensive, for example, at borders of communities, classes, cultures, and nationalities (de Lauretis, *Technologies of Gender;* Ginsburg and Tsing, *Uncertain Terms;* Ong and Peletz, *Bewitching Women*). In this study, that border lies between technology and the body, and technology can be seen as a catalyst for disruption.

8. Lock and Kaufert ("Introduction") also address the issue of women approaching technology as a pragmatic means to an end.

9. Franklin *(Embodied Progress)* has analyzed how new reproductive technologies are represented by organizations offering these services as "natural." She also found that women in England viewed these technologies as natural, but that finding was not echoed in this research. Instead, women in this study viewed these technologies as a necessary, but alien, means to an end.

10. Paul Rabinow refers to the process of transforming cultural phenomena by naturalizing them as "biosociality." He anticipates that a critical step in breaking down the nature/culture split will be the dissolution of the category of "the social." He suggests that in the future nature will be modeled on culture and that it will be understood as ordinary practices of daily life: "Nature will be known and remade through technique and will finally become artificial, just as culture becomes natural" (*Essays,* 99). Several feminists have explored the process by which technology is naturalized. Franklin (*Embodied Progress,* 68–69) observes the current effort by feminist anthropologists to denaturalize re-

production. See also Clarke, *Disciplining Reproduction;* Franklin and Ragone, "Introduction"; Haraway, *Modest_Witness;* Lock and Kaufert, "Introduction"; Yanagisako and Delaney, *Naturalizing Power.*

11. Giddens, *Consequences of Modernity,* 60.

12. The growing literature on cyborgs addresses the many ways in which culture is taken into the body through technology and the ways in which people embrace those developments. See Balsamo, *Technologies;* Gray, *Cyborg Handbook;* Davis-Floyd and Dumit, *Cyborg Babies;* Haraway, *Modest_Witness.*

13. Clarke *(Disciplining Reproduction)* views new reproductive technologies as transformative. They introduce the possibility that technology can assume the biological function of fertility (Franklin, *Embodied Progress,* 208–10), leading to a conflation of scientific knowledge with life itself.

14. Giddens, *Modernity and Self-Identity,* 33. See Becker, *Disrupted Lives,* for an exploration of this process.

15. This study explores the dominant model of heterosexual men and women, which is a starting place for examining cultural assumptions about gender and sexuality and the roots of those assumptions. By focusing exclusively on this model I am not suggesting that it is the only model or that it is better than others. See Lewin, *Lesbian Mothers;* Ludtke, *On Our Own;* Tober, "Romancing the Sperm"; and Weston, *Families We Choose,* for discussions of family creation by lesbian couples and single women. The nine women in the study who were interviewed without partners either were single or had partners who declined to be interviewed.

16. The response of couples in the second study to IVF programs has been as follows: Of 134 couples, 31 have attempted one or more cycles of IVF, and 5 have had successful pregnancies (excluding pregnancies created with a donor egg). Of those who did not have successful cycles, half planned to try again. People who had not attempted IVF often reported they would consider it or planned to try it if nothing else worked. Only a few couples said they would not consider these technologies. Those who ruled out IVF technologies cited the high cost, planned to spend their money on adoption, were concerned about the risks, were "burned out" on medical treatment, would explore other options such as surrogacy, or would remain childless.

17. This is Slater's suggestion *(Consumer Culture,* 210). Bijker and Law ("General Introduction," 3–4) observe that technologies mirror society—in that they reproduce and embody social, historical, economic, political, and psychological factors—and comment that the idea of a "pure" technology is nonsense.

18. Slater, *Consumer Culture,* 2.

19. Slater, *Consumer Culture.* Hirsch ("Negotiated Limits") concluded from his research on couples' views of new reproductive technologies in England that respondents were working out their attitudes toward commodities and consumption to find a balance between the market and the state that would prevent the equation of childbirth with shopping and would give people a reasonable amount of choice.

20. Appadurai, "Introduction"; Slater, *Consumer Culture,* 148.

21. See Brandt, "Behavior, Disease, and Health"; Katz, "Secular Morality"; Leichter, "Lifestyle Correctness"; Williams, "Health as Moral Performance."

22. Slater, *Consumer Culture*, 4–5.

23. The beginning of the modern era coincides with that of the Enlightenment. Harvey (*Condition of Post-Modernity*, 12) observes that Enlightenment thought embraced progress and actively sought the break with history and tradition that modernity espouses. Accumulated knowledge was to be used to pursue human freedom and enrich daily life, with an emphasis on rational modes of thought and social organization.

24. The establishment of the United States was taken in Europe to prove that many ideas of the Enlightenment were practical. The Constitution seemed to demonstrate the social contract because of its emphasis on rights and equality before the law, an emphasis Europeans themselves desired (Palmer and Colton, *History of the Modern World*, 331–32). Ultimately it gave rise to a form of radical individualism (Bellah et al., *Habits of the Heart*).

25. Harvey (*Condition of Post-Modernity*, 27–29) points to the importance of the Enlightenment axiom that there was only one possible answer to any question, which implied that the world could be controlled and rationally ordered if it were represented rightly. This idea did not begin to break down until after the revolutions of 1848.

26. Bellah et al. (*Habits of the Heart*, xxvi) note an overwhelming value consensus in spite of fundamental divisions within U.S. society. They observe that individualism is deeply embedded in U.S. social institutions and moral traditions (viii). Discussing how individualism is borne out in the current strength of neocapitalism, they state, "The neocapitalist vision is viable only to the degree to which it can be seen as an expression—even a moral expression—of our dominant ideological individualism, with its compulsive stress on independence, its contempt for weakness, and its adulation of success" (xxvi). Rapp ("Constructing Amniocentesis," 139) observes that the cultural and medical importance of individualism may make women particularly vulnerable to its effects. Bordo (*Unbearable Weight*) suggests that ostensibly liberatory practices are constantly in danger of being reabsorbed into the dominant cultural discourse of liberal individualism.

27. Williams defines ideology as "an articulated system of meanings, values, and beliefs of a kind that can be abstracted as [the] 'worldview' [of a social group]. . . . It is the fully articulate and systematic forms which are recognized as ideology" (*Marxism and Literature*, 109). In an extensive discussion of the relationships among ideology, hegemony, culture, and agency, Comaroff and Comaroff identify the basic difference between hegemony and ideology (*Revelation and Revolution*, 1:24–25). Following Gramsci and Williams, they suggest that hegemony consists of constructs and conventions that have been shared and naturalized throughout a political community, while ideology is the expression and the possession of a particular social group (although it may be disseminated beyond that group). Whereas hegemony is nonnegotiable, ideology may be perceived as a matter of opinion and therefore contested. They suggest that hegemony "exists in reciprocal interdependence with ideology: it is that part of a dominant worldview which has been naturalized and, having hidden itself in orthodoxy, no more appears as ideology at all."

28. Bellah et al. (*Habits of the Heart*, xxvi–xxviii) observe that neocapitalism

has been able to turn policy failures into ideological successes, and they show how people's ideas have been shaped by neocapitalism.

29. See, for example, Sandelowski, "Compelled to Try"; Tymstra, "Imperative Character."

30. See Appadurai, *Modernity at Large;* Giddens, *Consequences of Modernity;* Harvey, *Condition of Post-Modernity.*

31. See Lock and Kaufert, "Introduction," on the counterdiscourse on technology. Strathern ("Regulation, Substitution," 189) observes that when the commercial idiom substitutes for other ways of expressing preference or exercising reproductive choice, boundaries between the domains of kinship and commerce are crossed.

32. Koenig, "Technological Imperative."

33. Slater, *Consumer Culture,* 3.

34. Over 80 percent of the sample had some form of health insurance. The majority had little or no coverage for even the most basic infertility care, however, and only a few had insurance that covered any assisted reproductive technologies.

35. Kramon, "Fertility Center."

36. Slater (*Consumer Culture,* 162–63) discusses how commodities are defined by class. See also Bourdieu *(Distinction),* for whom taste and the class system are the mechanisms through which classes establish domination in society.

37. "$10,000 Eggs for Sale."

38. Blackwell et al., "Are We Exploiting the Infertile Couple?"

39. Ginsburg and Rapp ("Introduction," 5) suggest that analyses of reproductive health should focus on "nexes of power" shaping reproduction and not on the technologies themselves. Investigating the multiple loci of power that make up this industry is beyond the scope of this work.

40. The point at which consumers become a force in technological development and the strength of consumer influence are subject to debate. Cowan ("Consumption Junction," 278) suggests that consumers become a force in the diffusion stage of technological development by becoming the means through which it is diffused, whereas Bijker ("Social Construction of Fluorescent Lighting") suggests that innovation and diffusion may take place simultaneously. Bijker and Law ("General Introduction," 3) suggest that users themselves reshape technologies and influence future social, economic, and technical decisions. Miller ("Consumption as the Vanguard," 10–11), suggests that power is located in the consumer, and that it is central to the constitution of desire. Drawing on Foucault and de Tocqueville to suggest that power is simultaneously liberating and oppressive, diffuse and ambivalent, Miller concludes that power is located in ourselves, as a mass.

41. Giddens, *Modernity and Self-Identity,* 30.

42. For the majority of people in the second, larger study, infertility treatment was prolonged by the consideration and use of new reproductive technologies. The majority of participants in the second study did not go through pre-IVF medical treatment for infertility any faster than participants in the first study in the 1980s, when new reproductive technologies were unavailable in this geo-

graphic area. The few who did go through medical treatment quickly in the second study were women in their forties who, realizing the low likelihood that they would conceive on their own or with more basic treatments, turned quickly to these technologies.

43. The age of women undertaking IVF is the major determinant of success, with women over the age of forty having a greatly reduced chance of conceiving a viable pregnancy except with donor egg technology. Success rates overall are currently reported as 27.5 percent per cycle nationwide for a viable fetus that is carried to term for women less than thirty-five years old, compared to 10.6 percent for women over thirty-nine (American Society for Reproductive Medicine, "Assisted Reproductive Technology").

44. After fertilization in the laboratory, the zygote (early embryo) is observed until it completes two cell divisions and reaches the four-cell stage. Using a fine glass needle under a microscope, the DNA from one of the four cells is removed and the chromosomal complement is analyzed. If genetically normal, the remaining cells can be transferred to the recipient's uterus forty-eight hours later. This procedure is still in early clinical development and is currently limited to the evaluation of only a few of the human chromosomes linked to known genetic defects, such as X, Y, 11, 19, and 21.

45. Williams (*Marxism and Literature*, 112) observes that a lived hegemony is always a process, that it is not, except analytically, a system or a structure.

46. Collins, in a discussion of the social forces underlying this phenomenon ("Will the 'Real' Mother Please Stand Up?"), illustrates how ideology is borne out in policies that favor white women and discriminate against African American women. See also Davis, "Surrogates and Outcast Mothers." For an overview of the inaccessibility of infertility treatment to low-income women, see Nsiah-Jefferson and Hall, "Reproductive Technologies." Although this work was published in 1989, little has changed in the intervening years, except that the problem has become more pronounced.

47. For discussions of both compulsory and "voluntary" sterilization of women in the United States, in particular African American and Puerto Rican women, see Davis, *Women, Race, and Class* and "Surrogates and Outcast Mothers"; May, *Barren in the Promised Land*; and Lopez, "Agency and Constraint." On more subtle aspects of discriminatory policies against African American women, see Collins, "Will the 'Real' Mother Please Stand Up?"

48. Infertility, as a medical condition, exists at a higher rate among ethnic minorities than among whites; for example, married African American women have an infertility rate one and a half times that of married white women (Mosher and Pratt, "Fecundity, Infertility"). But ethnic minorities and those who are poor are seen as having too many children, not too few; the problem of infertility is thus unacknowledged. This situation reflects a particular ideology about reproduction among ethnic minorities and low-income people, one with a "logic of eugenics" at its base (Collins, "Will the 'Real' Mother Please Stand Up?" 267). See also Becker, "Advanced Reproductive Technologies"; Davis, "Surrogates and Outcast Mothers"; May, *Barren in the Promised Land*; and Nsiah-Jefferson and Hall, "Reproductive Technologies."

49. Minkler and Estes, *Critical Gerontology*, 2. The concept of moral econ-

omy, developed by E. P. Thompson (*Making of the English Working Class*) and building on the work of Mauss and Durkheim, has been used especially to demonstrate how premarket economies were grounded in social and moral terms. Scott's work (*Moral Economy of the Peasant*), for example, demonstrates through the group that he studied that the moral economy of the subsistence ethic in precapitalist peasant societies dictated that all members of a community had a right to a living. Recently, it has been argued that a dichotomy between moral and market economy is false (Kohli, "Retirement and the Moral Economy"), and the concept of moral economy has been applied to a range of contemporary issues in industrial societies (Hermann, "Women's Exchange"; Holstein, "Women and Productive Aging"; Minkler and Estes, *Critical Gerontology*). Booth ("On the Idea of the Moral Economy") suggests that all economies are moral economies because they are embedded in the ethical frameworks of their respective communities. Minkler and Cole ("Political and Moral Economy," 42–43) observe that the moral economy perspective enables social analysts to examine the preoccupation of United States social policies in distinguishing between "deserving" and "undeserving" populations.

50. This is suggested by Gupta and Ferguson, who view the world as a global space of relations ("Culture, Power, Place"). Appadurai (*Modernity at Large*) goes further suggesting that the world consists of "deterritorialized ethnoscapes."

51. This is the oldest woman known to have conceived and delivered using this technique. See Sauer, "Motherhood at Any Age?" Bijker and Law ("General Introduction," 8) observe that technologies are sometimes subverted by users and used in ways they were not originally intended.

52. For information on ICSI, see the glossary. Inhorn ("Money, Marriage, and Mortality" and "Missing Motherhood") reports a surge in use of new reproductive technologies in Egypt as a result of the development of ICSI. See Turiel, *Beyond Second Opinions,* for additional discussion of ICSI.

53. See Handwerker ("Hen That Can't Lay an Egg," "Consequences of Modernity for Childless Women," and "Social and Ethical Implications") for discussion of how policies governing reproductive technologies interact with other policies in China.

54. On a recent trip to Guatemala I encountered a number of couples from the United States and European countries who had come to adopt a child. That year, Guatemala had been identified as the "hot" place for international adoption. European couples from countries with socialized medicine were awaiting their turn for IVF but meanwhile had decided to adopt a child, whereas those from the United States were finished with medical treatment. I interviewed these couples on different occasions when we traveled together.

55. See Bellah et al., *Habits of the Heart,* on effects of individualism in the United States. Meirow and Schenker differentiate the U.S. position on reproductive technologies from the policies of all other nations, observing, "American law follows the American tradition of individual choice. . . . The American legal approach to ART [assisted reproductive technologies] is facilitative rather than regulatory" ("Reproductive Health Care Polices," 134). Annas ("Shadowlands") observes that the United States has been slow to regulate this industry

272 Notes to Pages 22–23

because of continuing controversies over abortion and embryo research, as well as a basic belief that decisions should be left to couples and their physicians. Whereas regulation, wherever it exists, has been left to states, he advocates federal regulation on a wide range of issues.

56. See Edwards et al., *Technologies of Procreation,* and especially Strathern, "Regulation, Substitution," for discussions of kinship and regulation. Strathern notes that at the heart of the Warnock Report is the notion that limits are not set by technologies but must come from other domains of social life ("Regulation, Substitution," 174). Meirow and Schenker ("Reproductive Health Care Policies"), drawing on their survey on policies about assisted reproductive technologies and gamete donation in sixty-two countries, detail specific regulations. The lack of regulation in the United States is apparently unique. This informative article is flawed by the authors' statements about their own beliefs, which they present in an apparent attempt to influence policy internationally.

57. For Great Britain, see Cannell, "Concepts of Parenthood"; Edwards et al., *Technologies of Procreation;* Franklin, *Embodied Progress;* Haimes, "Issues of Gender"; Shore, "Virgin Births"; Strathern, *After Nature* and *Reproducing the Future.*

58. Although there are no national regulations making access to the new reproductive technologies explicitly dependent on the sexual orientation of consumers, state laws on adoption may discriminate against gay and lesbian couples by requiring the nonbiological parent to go through second-parent adoption to become a legal parent. If the nonbiological parent is denied legal parenthood, he or she has no legal rights with respect to the child. Courts in only twenty states have allowed such adoptions. Recently a lesbian couple in California circumvented this difficulty by using new reproductive technologies: one partner supplied the egg, which was fertilized in a lab by sperm from an anonymous donor, and the other partner received the embryo and became the gestational mother. In a prebirth decree, a Superior Court judge ruled that both women have a biological claim to parenthood and both are legal parents. This ruling went beyond biology because it recognized the women's intent to create a child together. For further details of this case and the broader issues surrounding it, see Ness, "Lesbian Mothers' Legal Gains."

59. See Marcus, "Ethnography," for a discussion of multisited ethnography. Information on the various sites utilized in this research can be found in the appendix.

60. Resolve, Inc., a nonprofit membership organization, was founded in Boston in 1973 by Barbara Menning. After being diagnosed as infertile, Menning sought emotional support and quality medical care. Today, fifty-five affiliated chapters offer monthly programs, telephone counseling, formal support groups, and medical information to infertile couples. The national office, supported by Resolve membership fees and the sale of literature, produces written medical information used by chapters and members, a national listing of fertility specialists for referrals, and information on programs that perform advanced reproductive techniques. The national headquarters is located at 1310 Broadway,

Somerville, MA 98144–1731, phone (617) 623–0744. Resolve's website is resolve.org.

61. Recent efforts to problematize ethnography within anthropology have led to a worry about tendencies to "overvalorize resistance, 'experience,' and the 'authentic voices' of selected others" (Franklin and Ragone, "Introduction," 5). See also Marcus, "Ethnography." While the need to problematize ethnography is understandable, such analyses may, in searching for balance, instead overbalance and miss the main purpose of studies that begin with "experience," which, in my view, is to attend to the phenomenological foundations of cultural practices.

62. Most of the interviews with members of ethnic minorities were carried out by Seline Szkupinski Quiroga and form a central part of her dissertation work ("The Experience of Infertility: Identity, Subjectivity, and Meaning"). Analysis and publication of this material await her completion of this project.

63. See Becker, *Disrupted Lives,* for discussion of the relationship between bodily distress and the social order.

64. Such performances constitute action. People project images of themselves and the world to their audiences through performance (see, for example, Palmer and Jankowiak, "Performance and Imagination"). See also Becker, *Disrupted Lives;* Connerton, *How Societies Remember;* Laderman and Roseman, *Performance and Healing;* Stoller, "Embodying Colonial Memories." Butler (*Bodies That Matter* and "Performative Acts") suggests that the materiality of the body can be linked to the performativity of gender.

CHAPTER 2. CONFRONTING NOTIONS OF NORMALCY

1. Cussins, "Ontological Choreography," explores the issue of objectification of women's bodies in infertility clinics and demonstrates how objectification can also be seen as an element of women's agency that is tied to personhood.

2. For information on donor egg technology, see the glossary and Turiel, *Beyond Second Opinions.*

3. Medicalization, a term coined by Irving Zola ("Medicine as an Institution of Social Control"), refers to the process by which human experiences are redefined as medical problems. It is epitomized by the growth of medical treatment for infertility, a condition that was formerly viewed as a social problem but is now viewed as a medical condition (Becker and Nachtigall, "Eager for Medicalization"). The medicalization process may be initiated either from within biomedicine or by members of the public who seek legitimacy for a social condition (McLean, "Contradictions"). Moreover, consumers may embrace medicalization at the same time that they resist it. See also Lock and Kaufert, *Pragmatic Women,* and Wilkerson, *Diagnosis: Difference,* for discussions of medicalization and its management in the lives of women.

Reflecting the medicalization of the issue, the term *infertility* has replaced the commonly used term "involuntary childlessness" in the social sciences. Steinberg

(*Bodies in Glass,* 41–42) suggests that *infertility* has an inherent gender bias because it carries cultural resonances with earlier notions of "barrenness," a concept of failure firmly associated with women.

4. The basic infertility workup (see glossary) involves several tests that examine the fallopian tubes, sperm, cervical mucus, and ovulation. See Olive, "Clinical Fertility Trials," for a discussion of the tendency toward empirical treatment in the practice of reproductive medicine.

5. See, for example, Balsamo, *Technologies,* 10–11. Balsamo views technology as the stage for the enactment of gender. Judith Butler (*Gender Trouble,* 33) suggests the need to understand the process whereby "naturalized" gender identities are socially and culturally produced as part of new technological formations.

6. Butler, "Performative Acts," 411–12. As Butler further observes, the fact that "culture so readily punishes or marginalizes those who fail to perform the illusion of gender essentialism should be sign enough that on some level there is social knowledge that the truth or falsity of gender is only socially compelled and in no sense ontologically necessitated. . . . Performing it well provides the reassurance that there is an essentialism of gender identity after all."

7. Angela Davis suggests that, following the nineteenth-century cult of motherhood, we are now in a new era that mythologizes motherhood, leading to a "motherhood quest" that has become more compulsive and more openly ideological than in the nineteenth century ("Surrogates and Outcast Mothers," 211).

8. For more on gender identity with respect to infertility, see Becker, *Disrupted Lives* and *Healing the Infertile Family.*

9. Rethinking the gendered body has entailed a feminist critique of phenomenology (such as the work of Maurice Merleau-Ponty). Feminists argue that there is an implicit bias in phenomenology, that the body in question is the *male* body and that the phenomenology portrayed is one of maleness. These authors call for redefinitions of the body and for a reconsideration of phenomenology in relation to women's bodies. See Allen and Young, *Thinking Muse;* Bigwood, "Renaturalizing the Body"; Butler, *Bodies That Matter,* "Performative Acts," and "Sexual Ideology"; Grosz, *Volatile Bodies;* and Young, "Throwing Like a Girl." For an overview of feminist theories on embodiment, see Kathy Davis, "Embody-ing Theory."

10. Bodily experience reflects the culture in which it occurs. Every nuance of our lives is thus gendered through the reflexivity of being-in-the-world. Merleau-Ponty (*Phenomenology of Perception*) refers to automatic bodily functioning as the preobjective self, a culturally constituted way of being-in-the-world. In *The Visible and the Invisible* he attributes a transcendental function to the body-subject: the body is the basis of the constitution of the human world. In interpreting Merleau-Ponty's work, Martin Dillon observes, "The body contributes to the world we live in but the reverse is also true: the world contributes to the constitution of our body" ("Preface," xv–xvi). He notes that both the subject and its transcendent function, though preserved, are transfigured to be responsive to worldly conditions. According to Laurence Kirmayer ("The Body's Insistence on Meaning,") two orders are affected by people's experience: the order of the body and the order of the text (or narrative). An inescapable cir-

cularity exists between the two: expectations about the order of the body are expressed in the order of the text. See also Becker, *Disrupted Lives,* for a discussion of how the cultural ordering of meaning and narrative emerges out of this complicated process.

11. Connerton, *How Societies Remember.*

12. Merleau-Ponty, *The Visible and the Invisible.* Ricoeur (*Time and Narrative,* 67–68) observes that everyday praxis orders the present of the future and the present of the past, that is, how practice in the current moment in time orders one's view of past, present, and future. See also Carr, *Time, Narrative, and History;* Heidegger, *History of the Concept of Time.*

13. Dillon ("Preface," xvi) notes that in *The Visible and the Invisible,* Merleau-Ponty develops the thesis of reversibility of the flesh, a circular process in which the body comes to terms with its environment and then returns to the world by acquiring that environment in a sedimented form that structures the world with a habitus derived from the body. David Michael Levin observes that "intercorporeality and reversibility are categories derived from the flesh of our experience; and they bespeak a social order that calls into question all social systems where domination prevails over principles of mutual recognition and participatory justice" ("Visions of Narcissism," 74). Pierre Bourdieu's work (*Outline; Distinction; Logic of Practice*) represents a shift from a focus on the body as a source of symbolism to an awareness of the body as the locus of social practice. Recent work in anthropology examines embodiment and social practice. See, for example, Csordas, "Embodiment as a Paradigm," "Somatic Modes," and *Sacred Self.*

14. For further discussion of transformative action, see Becker, *Disrupted Lives;* Ginsburg and Rapp, "Introduction"; Haber, *Beyond Postmodern Politics;* Lock and Kaufert, "Introduction"; and Ortner, "Resistance."

15. Feminists view gender practices as sites of critical agency, reacting against the postmodern tendency to deny the role of agency. See, for example, Balsamo, *Technologies;* Butler, *Bodies That Matter* and *Gender Trouble;* Grosz, *Volatile Bodies;* Haber, *Beyond Postmodern Politics;* Moore, *Passion for Difference;* and Ortner, *Making Gender.* Although addressing the body is essential to my task, doing so poses a dilemma. The body as experienced has appeared infrequently in feminist writings because feminists have been intent on breaking free of the body and its long-term associations, such as the equation of women with nature (see, for example, Balsamo, *Technologies).* Recent feminist writings, however, have moved the body to the center of these debates (see especially Butler, *Bodies That Matter,* and Grosz, *Volatile Bodies).*

16. The metaphor of life as journey is a root metaphor. See Turner, *Dramas, Fields, and Metaphors,* 50–51, for a discussion of root metaphors. See Becker, *Disrupted Lives,* for further discussion of organizing metaphors in people's lives, including their use with reference to infertility.

17. Synthesis has practical implications for reorganizing life when a major disruption occurs, a view akin to Michael Jackson's view of metaphor as praxis. See Jackson, "Thinking through the Body" and *Paths toward a Clearing.* Metaphors help people to make sense of disruptions in life and mediate efforts to create continuity in the face of change. They also enable people to change their

view of cultural phenomena that impede resolution of disruption. Metaphor, observes James Fernandez ("Mission of Metaphor" and "Argument of Images"), has the ability to bind the past and future together and to give the impression of coherence.

18. In *Disrupted Lives* I address the transcendental experience of a long journey as an expression of Western cultural beliefs. Notions of transcendence and transformation are embodied in the Judeo-Christian tradition and in Western philosophy. The idea of continuity can be traced by examining how concepts such as development and transformation appear in Western cultural traditions and how people use them in their efforts to create continuity. See also Cohler, "Personal Narrative"; Luborsky, "Retirement Process."

19. In 1984, six years after the first successful IVF birth, Ricardo Asch described a variation of this technique which he called GIFT (gamete intrafallopian transfer—see glossary). For further discussion of GIFT, see Turiel, *Beyond Second Opinions*. IVF using donor eggs has become the treatment of last resort for many cases of refractory infertility, especially those felt to be the result of ovarian aging.

Research suggests that fertility in women begins to decline after age thirty and becomes clinically detectable after age thirty-seven. Other than signs of impending menopause, that is, an elevated blood level of pituitary follicle stimulating hormone or cessation of menstrual function, there is no absolute way for a woman to know when she can no longer conceive. Because the aging effect can be subtle in women still in their thirties, genetic analysis can be performed on embryos fertilized through an IVF procedure. The detection of chromosomal abnormalities in these embryos is believed to be an indication of ovarian aging and suggests that further attempts at pregnancies using the woman's own eggs are unlikely to be successful. Because older eggs become increasingly resistant to fertilization, implantation, and normal embryo development, very few women over the age of forty-three will successfully carry a pregnancy using their own eggs.

20. I use "American" and "U.S." interchangeably throughout this book. Marcel Mauss ("Category of the Human Mind") contrasts the concept of the self, which he defines as consciousness of the self—the awareness of body and spirit—with the social concept of the person as a compound of jural rights and moral responsibility. Grace Gladys Harris ("Concepts of Individual, Self, and Person") observes that in the United States, working conceptions of the person are shaped by a concern with the self. For further discussion of concerns about self and personhood with respect to infertility, see Becker, *Disrupted Lives* and *Healing the Infertile Family*.

21. Elsewhere I have used the term *cultural discourses* (Becker, *Disrupted Lives*). The term *discourse* derives from Foucault's notion of discursive formations, apparatuses, and technologies and "is meant to refuse the distinction between ideas and practices or text and world" (Abu-Lughod, "Writing against Culture," 147). Yanagisako and Delaney point out that "discourse" is not an adequate substitute for the concept of culture, however: "Culture is what makes the boundaries of domains seem natural, what gives ideologies power, and what makes hegemonies appear seamless. At the same time, it is what enables us to

make compelling claims for connections between supposedly distinct discourses" ("Naturalizing Power," 19).

22. Lewin ("On the Outside Looking In") captures the essence of cultural assumptions about women and normalcy in her discussion of "goodness" and motherhood.

23. See Becker, *Disrupted Lives,* for extensive discussions of normalcy.

24. Angela Davis, "Surrogates and Outcast Mothers," 220.

25. Cultural dialogues are moral discourses. That is, they embody how society views morality. Ideologies are embedded in moral discourses. See Becker, *Disrupted Lives,* for discussion of ideology in everyday life, and Howell, *Ethnography of Moralities,* for discussion of morality as culture.

26. This view is widespread among those conducting science studies. See, for example, Casper and Koenig, "Reconfiguring Nature and Culture"; Franklin, "Science as Culture"; and Lock and Kaufert, *Pragmatic Women.* The hegemonic aspects of technology are of particular concern. Comaroff and Comaroff define hegemony as "that order of signs and practices, relations and distinctions, images and epistemologies—drawn from a historically situated cultural field— that come to be taken for granted as the natural and received shape of the world and everything that inhabits it" (*Revelation and Revolution,* 1:23). They further note that hegemony is constantly being made and can be unmade; it is a process as much as a thing (25).

27. This is Foucault's suggestion *(Power/Knowledge).* Comaroff and Comaroff (*Revelation and Revolution,* 1:22) suggest that power is entailed in culture through ideology and hegemony, and that this is how the relationship between power and culture can be grasped.

28. This is Lock and Kaufert's suggestion ("Introduction," 23).

29. It has been repeatedly demonstrated that people are unable to develop new categories outside the known culture (Anderson, *Imagined Communities;* Quinn, "Cultural Basis"; Brackette Williams, "A Class Act"; Lewin, "On the Outside Looking In"; Weston, "Forever is a Long Time"). Agency, including resistance, is shaped by these limits.

30. Quinn, "Cultural Basis," argues that cultural models form the basis when people reorganize their thinking.

31. See Becker, *Disrupted Lives,* for discussion of this process.

32. For further discussion of men and gender identity with respect to infertility, see Becker, *Disrupted Lives* and *Healing the Infertile Family;* Nachtigall et al., "Effects of Gender-Specific Diagnosis."

33. Fry and Keith, "Life Course as a Cultural Unit"; Fry, "Life Course in Context"; Luborsky, "Romance with Personal Meaning"; Meyer, "Levels of Analysis"; Rubinstein, "Nature, Culture, Gender, Age."

34. See Becker, *Healing the Infertile Family,* for discussion of marital relationships and infertility.

35. See Cancian, *Love in America.*

36. David Schneider (*American Kinship*) points to two bases of the U.S. kinship system: relationships through blood and relationships through marriage.

37. There is no way to attribute statistics on divorce specifically to infertility. Clinicians and mental health practitioners working with this population, how-

ever, generally concur that there is a preponderance of long-term, committed relationships.

CHAPTER 3. THE EMBATTLED BODY

1. Yanagisako and Delaney, "Naturalizing Power," 2–9.

2. Franklin ("Postmodern Procreation," 68) notes that the project of feminists in the 1990s is "denaturalization and defamiliarization," challenging the equation of the known and familiar with the "natural" or "biological." Part of this challenge is to show the operations of biology as a cultural system or as a discourse. See also Balsamo, *Technologies*.

3. Bodily order reflects a state referred to by Merleau-Ponty as being-in-the-world. From a phenomenological perspective, social agents constitute social reality and are constituted by it. Although phenomenology appears to privilege the acting subject, this is a reflexive perspective that acknowledges that the person is also a recipient, or object, in a cultural world (Merleau-Ponty, *Phenomenology of Perception*). Judith Butler, in arguing that gender is not expressive of natural phenomena but is socially and culturally constructed, draws on Simone de Beauvoir's conception of gender as a historical situation. Butler argues that gender is not a stable identity, a locus of agency from which various acts proceed, but an identity tenuously constituted in time through a "stylized repetition of acts" ("Performative Acts," 403).

4. Butler, "Performative Acts," 412.

5. In contrast to previous feminist work, which conceptualized gender and sexuality separately, recent work has suggested that sexuality be theorized as part of gender. See, for example, Butler, *Gender Trouble* and *Bodies That Matter*; Grosz, *Volatile Bodies*. The work of Kulick *(Travesti)* on Brazilian transgendered prostitutes challenges traditional North American and European notions of gender. He finds that whereas the northern Euro-American gender system is based on anatomical sex, the gender system that structures *travestis'* perceptions and actions is based on sexuality (227), and suggests that these different notions about sex, sexuality, and gender may be widespread throughout much of Latin America and possibly the Mediterranean (237).

6. Rethinking the gendered body also entails thinking of gender in relation to sex. That is, instead of thinking of gender in opposition to sex, Butler *(Bodies That Matter)* suggests that gender absorbs and displaces sex. See also Grosz, *Volatile Bodies,* and Ortner, *Making Gender*.

7. Zolla, *Androgyne*.

8. See Becker, *Disrupted Lives* and *Healing the Infertile Family;* Luborsky, "Romance with Personal Meaning."

9. See also Becker, *Healing the Infertile Family,* 6–20.

10. Kaufman and Raphael, *Coming out of Shame,* call attention to various gender ideologies, or "cultural scripts," that evoke shame when people cannot live up to them.

11. Ibid.

12. Barnstone et al. (*Calvinist Roots,* xvii–xxii) note that particular Calvinist beliefs, such as the notion that humanity is innately depraved, were transformed in the late eighteenth and nineteenth centuries when liberal theologians rejected eternal damnation for the many and redemption for the few and deemphasized sin as the crucial, tormenting spiritual concern of Christians. Ultimately this shift led to a convergence of Calvinism and modernism in which modernism is a kind of Calvinism manqué: it maintains Calvinism's harshness and despair without its visionary idealism and its suffering without salvation. This transformation from theological doctrine to secular ideology has meant that the modern era has inherited the Calvinist paradox of insistence on both individualism and conformity.

13. See Nachtigall et al., "Effects of Gender-Specific Diagnosis." See also Snowden et al., *Artificial Reproduction,* and Greil et al., "Infertility."

14. Nachtigall et al., "Effects of Gender-Specific Diagnosis."

15. Ibid.

16. Regarding the medical gaze, see Armstrong, "Rise of Surveillance Medicine," and Foucault, *Birth of the Clinic.*

17. Katharine Young, *Presence in the Flesh,* 1. See also Toombs, *Meaning of Illness.* Allan Young ("Creation of Medical Knowledge") contrasts medical knowledge with lay knowledge and discusses the hierarchical ordering of different kinds of knowledge. Patients' and physicians' rights and responsibilities in medical treatment are delineated in part by the different knowledge they hold and the disparities in the types of information available to them. These differences have been found to influence the course of infertility treatment (Becker and Nachtigall, "Ambiguous Responsibility").

18. Although infertility is clinically defined as failure to conceive after one year of unprotected intercourse, a more meaningful definition of the problem is the point when one or both partners decide that conception is not occurring and seek help. Women in their mid- to late thirties or older should be especially mindful of decreasing fertility over the age of thirty. See also Becker, *Healing the Infertile Family.*

19. Seibel and Taymor, "Emotional Aspects of Infertility."

20. "Hostile" mucus is a term no longer in common use in infertility treatment. It was loosely applied to the finding in the postcoital test that sperm were not surviving in the cervical mucus, a problem often erroneously attributed to poorly identified antisperm antibodies. A variation involved the woman being told that she was "allergic" to her partner's sperm.

21. See also Becker, *Healing the Infertile Family.*

22. Control over the environment, and above all the environment of the body, is a key value in the United States. The need for control is rooted in the American ethic of individualism. See Becker, "Dilemma of Seeking Urgent Care" and *Disrupted Lives;* Kirmayer, "Mind and Body"; Lowenberg, *Caring and Responsibility;* and Reiser, "Responsibility for Personal Health." Kathy Davis ("Embody-ing Theory," 2) observes that with technologies such as IVF, the body has become the ultimate cultural metaphor for control. See also Crawford, "Cultural Account of 'Health,' " and Bordo, *Unbearable Weight.*

23. For discussions of gynecological practices in relation to experiencing the body and its manipulation, see, for example, Katharine Young, *Presence in the Flesh*, 46–79; Kapsalis, *Public Privates*.

24. See Armstrong, "Rise of Surveillance Medicine"; Foucault, *Birth of the Clinic*; Arney and Bergen, *Management*, 125.

25. Until recently, the medical treatment of infertility was the sole province of obstetrics and gynecology, and hence the medical gaze was fixed primarily on women. This phenomenon was part of a historical emphasis on the scrutiny of women's bodies by men, in male-dominated medical settings. See, for example, Arney, *Power*; Jordanova, *Sexual Visions*; Lacqueur, "Orgasm, Generation"; Martin, *Woman in the Body*; and Van den Wijngaard, *Reinventing the Sexes*. With recent further specialization, new attention is being paid to male infertility by urologists. Treatment of male infertility nevertheless continues to be carried out on women's bodies.

26. See also Nachtigall et al., "Effects of Gender-Specific Diagnosis"; Becker, *Healing the Infertile Family*.

27. Because approximately one-third of infertile men with reduced sperm concentration or motility are found to have a varicocele, that is, varicose veins that surround one or both testicles, a surgical procedure to "correct" this abnormality was considered a treatment option. Thousands of varicocelectomies were performed (and are still offered) despite the lack of controlled clinical trials demonstrating the procedure's effectiveness in increasing pregnancy rates.

CHAPTER 4. GENES AND GENERATIONS

1. In *Barren in the Promised Land* (140), Elaine Tyler May documents successive waves of pronatalism in the United States and their cultural roots. She calls the era in which most baby boomers were raised the "era of compulsory parenthood."

2. This is the view of Margaret Clark and Barbara Anderson: see Clark and Anderson, *Culture and Aging*.

3. For discussion of the relationship of values to memories, life experiences, and social ideologies, see Quinn, "Motivational Force"; Holland, "How Cultural Systems Become Desire"; and Claudia Strauss, "What Makes Tony Run?"

4. For a discussion of the relationship between values and culturally specific direction, see D'Andrade, "Cultural Meaning Systems." For a discussion of how values become the basis for commonsense constructions of the world, see Quinn and Holland, "Culture and Cognition," 11.

5. See Bellah et al., *Habits of the Heart*; Dumont, *Essays on Individualism*; Hewitt, *Dilemmas of the American Self*; Wilkinson, *Pursuit of American Character*.

6. See Becker, *Disrupted Lives*.

7. Efforts to ensure continuity, in cases of infertility, are made through use of reproductive technologies. See Becker, ibid.

8. In *Disrupted Lives* I outline the contemporary Western conception of the course of life as predictable, knowable, and continuous.

9. The postmodern turn challenges notions that the world is an ordered place. See, for example, Derrida, *Of Grammatology*. Nevertheless, people view their worlds as ordered. According to Hallowell (*Culture and Experience*, 94–95), order lies at the foundations of structures of meaning in human life, and it permeates social life. Geertz (*Interpretation of Cultures*, 90) observes that identities are secured when individual lives are anchored to some kind of larger, cosmic order. See also Lyon, "Order and Healing," 260, and Becker, *Disrupted Lives*.

10. Yanagisako and Delaney, "Naturalizing Power," 2.

11. See Wilkinson, *Pursuit of American Character*, 19, 50; Bellah et al., *Habits of the Heart*, 56, 206.

12. Self-determination is an important aspect of individualism in the United States. See Bellah et al., *Habits of the Heart*.

13. See Sandelowski, "Compelled to Try."

14. Collier and Yanagisako, "Introduction," 7. To understand women's and men's responses to infertility and their actions, we must tease apart the folk model of reproduction. Yanagisako and Collier ("Toward a Unified Analysis," 40–42), suggest that the first step is to examine cultural meanings that play into the symbolic construction of categories of people.

15. See Franklin, *Embodied Progress*; Edwards et al., *Technologies of Procreation*; Schneider, *American Kinship*; Strathern, *After Nature* and *Reproducing the Future*; Weiner, "Reproductive Model" and "Trobriand Kinship."

16. See Lewin, *Lesbian Mothers*; Ludtke, *On Our Own*; Thorne and Yalom, *Rethinking the Family*; Tyler May, *Barren in the Promised Land*; Weston, *Families We Choose*.

17. See Collier and Yanagisako, "Introduction," for discussion of culturally imposed differences. Biological sex becomes socially significant through the constitution of gender in social institutions and through social organization (Butler, *Bodies That Matter*; Grosz, *Volatile Bodies*). Identities, cultural meanings, and social relationships all emanate from the structural aspects of gender (Brenner and Laslett, "Social Reproduction"). See Edwards et al., *Technologies of Procreation*, and Strathern, *After Nature* and *Reproducing the Future*, for discussions of how kinship is viewed as natural.

It is not simply the general public that is entrenched in thinking of gender and kinship as "natural," however. Social scientists, and specifically anthropologists, have a long history of confusion about the role of biology in kinship. See Franklin, *Embodied Progress*, for a cogent discussion of how anthropologists have conceptualized kinship historically by dichotomizing culture and biology and thus viewing kinship in all societies through the lens of Western notions about reproduction.

18. See Franklin, *Embodied Progress*, 58; Weiner, "Reproductive Model," "Trobriand Kinship," and "Reassessing Reproduction." See also Franklin, *Embodied Progress*, 57–65, for a synopsis of Weiner's work.

19. Strathern ("Regulation, Substitution," 172–73) observes that Euro-American ideas about kinship rest on multiple orderings of knowledge and that people move between orders of knowledge. Examples abound of the cultural importance of biology in American life, the most striking of which have been

the eugenics movements. See Duster, *Backdoor to Eugenics;* Nelkin and Lindee, *DNA Mystique;* and May, *Barren in the Promised Land.*

20. Martin, "Egg and the Sperm."

21. Nelkin and Lindee, *DNA Mystique.* See also Duster, *Backdoor to Eugenics.*

22. See Davis, "Surrogates and Outcast Mothers" and *Women, Race, and Class;* May, *Barren in the Promised Land.*

23. Nelkin and Lindee, *DNA Mystique, 2.* Haraway *(Modest_Witness)* refers to the current preoccupation with genetics as "gene fetishism."

24. Nelkin and Lindee, *DNA Mystique, 58.*

25. Victor Turner, who developed notions of liminality and being "in between" in his work on ritual, observed in *Ritual Process* that liminal people are suspended in social space. See Becker, *Disrupted Lives,* 119–35, for discussion of living in limbo. Angela Davis ("Surrogates and Outcast Mothers") addresses how adulthood and womanhood are equated with motherhood.

26. Victor Turner *(Ritual Process)* refers to the conclusion of the ritual process as "communitas" to signify the communal nature of ritual.

27. Using a donor egg alleviates age-related worries about Down's syndrome because egg donors are invariably young (in their early twenties to early thirties).

CHAPTER 5. EXPERIENCING RISKS

1. For detailed discussion of the notion of risk, see Becker and Nachtigall, "Born to Be a Mother." See also Beck, *Risk Society;* Douglas, *Risk and Blame;* Douglas and Wildavsky, *Risk and Culture;* Short, "Social Fabric at Risk."

2. Douglas and Wildavsky *(Risk and Culture)* and Douglas *(Risk and Blame)* note that risk relations have been defined with respect to specific health outcomes without attending to the social, cultural, political, and economic constraints that affect such outcomes. See also Hayes, "Epistemology of Risk." Nelkin ("Communicating Technological Risk") observes that defining risk can be a way of explaining the failure of existing political and social relationships, voicing mistrust and delegating blame. Lash and Wynne ("Introduction") suggest that although discourses of risk have taken on an aura of liberal pluralism, such discourses portray an idealized model of risk that is instrumental and reductionistic, while Douglas *(Risk and Blame)* notes that risk analyses are presented as if they are "innocent" and value-free and concludes that risk analysis cannot exclude moral ideas and politics. Beck *(Risk Society)* goes further, to suggest that risks are uncontrollable scientific, technical, or social developments that in effect create a "risk society" by shifting industrial societies' focus from questions about the allocation of wealth to questions about the allocation of risks. Questions have been raised from within medicine about how social biases pervade risk analyses, for example, in cultural values and beliefs held by practitioners that affect medical decision making (see Forrow et al., "Science, Ethics," and Gullick, "Talking with Patients").

3. Bell, "The Meaning of Risk"; Ince, "Fertility Rites"; Short, "Social Fabric at Risk"; and Shrader-Frechette, "Producer Risk." For general discussion of

risks in infertility treatment, see Turiel, *Beyond Second Opinions*. Since the data for this study were collected, epidemiological studies have raised a question about the relationship between fertility drugs and ovarian cancer (Whittemore et al., "I: Methods"; Whittemore et al., "II: Invasive Epithelial Cancers"; Harris et al., "III: Epithelial Tumors"; Whittemore et al., "Pathogenesis"). While these studies are cautious in their interpretation of findings and have been criticized for their limitations, they have also been acknowledged as worthy of attention, and the American Society for Reproductive Medicine has consequently made suggestions to physicians for advising patients about potential risks (Spirtas et al., "Fertility Drugs"). Although the National Cancer Institute has not advocated any changes regarding the use of fertility-enhancing drugs, the FDA has requested that drug firms add the potential risk of ovarian cancer to the drug label. The FDA stated that "this labeling change is being made in one section of the label without a conclusion about causality; no change is being made in prescribing directions."

Ordinarily, 1.5 percent of women develop ovarian cancer, most commonly after age fifty. Known risk factors for ovarian cancer include family history, a high-fat diet, and infertility. Family history is by far the strongest risk; the increased risk from infertility was noted before the use of fertility drugs became widespread. It is uncertain whether ovulation makes the ovary more susceptible to cancer. Women who have many pregnancies or take oral contraceptives ovulate less frequently and have a lower incidence of ovarian cancer, whereas fertility drugs work to induce ovulation.

4. Physicians view risk within a biomedical ideology, as an intrinsic part of the practice of medicine. Two types of risk assessment are routine in medical treatment: (1) the epidemiological construct of relative risk used to help make diagnoses and guide the choice of diagnostic tests; and (2) weighing risks and benefits when a test or procedure may have its own adverse outcome. Some risks may be acknowledged but denigrated. Risk taking is sanctioned by biomedicine in the form of medical aggressiveness and rewarded in a variety of ways, for example, when a physician publishes papers on successful outcomes in cases that involve considerable medical risks. Inaction, conversely, may be construed as overly conservative, or even negligent, medical behavior. Risk is balanced against two medical responsibilities: first, the value of patients' well-being requires physicians to protect them from potentially harmful consequences of choices; and second, the value of respecting patients' rights to make decisions about their own lives when they are able requires physicians to give patients some control over decision making. See Forrow et al., "Science, Ethics," and Brock and Wartman, "When Competent Patients Make Irrational Choices."

5. Connors ("Risk Perception") defines lived risk as situated in the circumstances and constraints that impinge on daily life at any given time. Parsons and Atkinson ("Lay Constructions") note that perceptions of being at risk are related to critical junctures in the life course, especially during the reproductive years.

6. See glossary for information on hMG (human menopausal gonadotropins) and laparoscopy.

7. Handwerker, "Medical Risk"; Whiteford and Poland, *New Approaches*.

8. Olive, "Clinical Fertility Trials."

9. The physician is referring to choriocarcinoma, a rare cancer of the tissue that normally forms the placenta.

10. In an analysis midway through the research, only eight of fifty-three couples who were childless at that point reported they stopped treatment because of perceived risks, although ten women and eight men described refusing treatments they saw as too risky. IVF was most commonly seen as too risky because of its emotional and financial consequences.

11. Over one-third of successful IVF deliveries result in multiple births, so that IVF, while accounting for less than 1 percent of all births in the United States, accounts for 2.4 percent of all twins and 22 percent of all triplets (Wilcox et al., "Assisted Reproductive Technologies"). This translates into a fourfold increase in family costs for twins and an elevenfold increase in family costs for triplets compared to a single delivery (Callahan et al., "Economic Impact").

12. Becker and Nachtigall, "Ambiguous Responsibility."

CHAPTER 6. TAKING ACTION

1. In *Disrupted Lives* and *Healing the Infertile Family* I discuss the use of these other modalities and their role in resolving infertility and bodily distress, including efforts at self-healing that can help to bring life disruptions to a close.

2. Transformation through action is a specific focus of both *Disrupted Lives* and *Healing the Infertile Family*. See also Mullings, "Households Headed by Women," and Ginsburg and Rapp, "Introduction."

3. Comaroff and Comaroff (*Revelation and Revolution*, 1:10), define agency as "practice invested with subjectivity, meaning, and to a greater or lesser extent, power. It is, in short, motivated." While I acknowledge that hegemony constrains action, I reject the postmodern tendency to deny the significance of agency. Anthropological feminist writings address the issue of women's agency in abundance. See, for example, Behar and Gordon, *Women Writing Culture;* Ginsburg and Rapp, *Conceiving the New World Order;* Lock and Kaufert, *Pragmatic Women;* and Ong and Peletz, *Bewitching Women.* See Inhorn, *Quest for Conception,* for a discussion of how poor Egyptian women demonstrate activism and resistance in addressing their infertility. Lewin ("On the Outside Looking In," 117) shows how lesbians becoming mothers in the United States forged a path between resistance and accommodation, weaving them together into a rewarding definition of self. Cussins ("Ontological Choreography") addresses women's agency in her research on IVF clinics.

4. Along with a renewed attention to agency, recent work has scrutinized and deromanticized the concept of resistance. Ortner ("Resistance"), in reviewing resistance studies, examines these issues in depth. Lewin ("Wives, Mothers, and Lesbians") cautions that apparent acts of resistance may not be what they seem. Despite such admonitions, understanding resistance in a given social group is critical to an in-depth consideration of agency. See Becker, *Disrupted Lives,* on resistance and the introduction of new cultural themes. With respect to gender, see, for example, Lock and Kaufert, *Pragmatic Women,* and Ong and Peletz, *Bewitching Women.*

5. Although identity politics is not new (see Toch, *Social Psychology*, for example), it has received a surge of recent attention as an expression of modernity and a way of better understanding the intersection of agency and ideology: see, for example, Calhoun, "Social Theory," 21–22; Giddens, *Modernity and Self-Identity;* and Somers and Gibson, "Reclaiming the Epistemological 'Other.' " Calhoun observes that an emphasis on identity politics is giving way to an emphasis on the politics of difference. See Becker, *Disrupted Lives,* for further discussion of difference and its manifestations in everyday life, and Haber, *Beyond Postmodern Politics,* on the politics of difference from a feminist perspective.

6. See Johnston and Klandermans, "Cultural Analysis." Swidler ("Cultural Power," 25) suggests that traditional Weberian approaches to social movements, which emphasize powerful, internalized beliefs and values held by individual actors, may ultimately provide less explanatory leverage than newer approaches (such as those of Bourdieu and Foucault), which see culture as operating in the contexts that surround individuals, influencing action from the "outside in."

7. See especially Butler, *Bodies That Matter,* x.

8. Butler ("Performative Acts," 409), proposes a less individually oriented view of acts than the phenomenological notion of constitutive acts. She states that "the theatrical sense of 'act' forces a revision of individualist assumptions underlying the more restricted view of constituting acts within phenomenological discourse. . . . Just as within feminist theory the very category of the personal is expanded to include political structures."

9. See Bellah et al., *Habits of the Heart,* for a discussion of the tension between individualism and community in the United States, and Becker, *Disrupted Lives,* for further discussion of the collective as an antidote to the U.S. cultural emphasis on autonomy.

10. Becker and Nachtigall, "Eager for Medicalization." See also Lock and Kaufert, "Introduction," for a discussion of women's agency with respect to medicalization.

11. Epstein (*Impure Science,* 20) observes the significance of social class and the role of the middle class in fostering and sustaining social movements. Epstein also suggests that, in contrast to traditional working-class politics, new social movements do not emphasize class ("Construction of Lay Expertise," 412–13). Instead they emphasize personal and intimate aspects of life (see Johnston, Larana, and Gusfield, "New Social Movements," 6–9).

12. These meetings are referred to as awareness meetings.

13. See Epstein, "Construction of Lay Expertise" and *Impure Science,* for a discussion of how this process has evolved in AIDS activism.

14. Emphasis may sometimes be on adoption rather than on medical treatment, for example.

15. Ortner, "Resistance," 191.

CHAPTER 7. SELLING HOPE

1. See Becker, *Disrupted Lives,* for discussion of the disruptive effect of infertility.

2. See Good et al., "American Oncology," on the role of hope in the practice of oncology, and Becker, *Disrupted Lives,* on the recurrence of the hope metaphor in issues of health and illness.

3. See Figge, "Tyranny of Technology."

4. Sandelowski, "Compelled to Try"; Tymstra, "Imperative Character."

5. Brock and Wartman, "Competent Patients"; Tymstra, "Imperative Character"; Tversky and Kahneman, "Framing of Decisions."

6. Current IVF practice involves the use of GnRH agonists that block the woman's natural pituitary function and prevent ovulation until the physician is ready to retrieve the eggs. After retrieval, eggs are isolated under a microscope and prepared for fertilization. Both the eggs and the fertilized eggs (embryos) can be qualitatively analyzed on their appearance and the speed with which they divide. In general, the more cells that make up the embryo (representing the number of times it has divided), the better the chance for implantation and a successful pregnancy.

7. Franklin *(Embodied Progress)* has also observed how success is redefined.

8. Franklin, ibid., also addresses the central role of hope in decisions to continue medical treatment.

9. Sandelowski, *With Child in Mind;* Modell, "Last Chance Babies."

10. Under pressure from congressional regulators, for the past several years the Society of Assisted Reproductive Technologies has published the pooled statistics of its 281 voluntarily participating IVF clinics in the United States, and these data are filed with the Centers for Disease Control. Data is broken down by patient's age, presence of male infertility factor, type of embryo transfer (fresh or frozen), donor or patient egg source, and type of assisted procedure (e.g., IVF or GIFT). The statistics are two years old by the time they are compiled, analyzed, and published.

11. Because the success rate is calculated as the pregnancy rate per egg retrieval, an IVF clinic could impose very strict requirements for patients who proceed to the retrieval stage in order to maximize its published success rate. Although discouraging challenging patients may be considered a cost-effective measure, the practice does not take account of the disappointment and financial loss of patients who are either not accepted or later dropped from treatment.

12. Nationwide statistics from 1995 indicate that of 41,087 cycles of IVF (excluding frozen embryo and donor egg cycles), 22.5 percent of retrievals led to delivery (American Society for Reproductive Medicine, "Assisted Reproductive Technology"). See also Turiel, *Beyond Second Opinions.*

13. The incidence of pregnancy loss from amniocentesis complications is generally less than 1 percent.

14. Figge suggests that such "tyranny in medical technology may be the decisive factor in whether medical practice, as it is currently construed, will survive" ("Tyranny of Technology," 1368). See also McDonough, "Need for Technology Assessment."

15. McDonough, "Need for Technology Assessment," 1082.

16. Figge, "Tyranny of Technology."

17. Appadurai, "Introduction." Clarke ("Modernity, Postmodernity," 142) also discusses the commodification of children in new reproductive technologies.

18. Mauss, *The Gift*. Douglas ("Foreword") highlights Mauss's central thesis, observing that there are no free gifts, that gifts are part of a system of reciprocity, and that the theory of the gift is a theory of human solidarity. Three important aspects of Mauss's theory are the view of the individual as social being, the assertion that social relations change with changes in the mode of production, and the moral role of political participation. These ideas were central in the later development of the concept of moral economy. Layne ("Introduction") points to the idea of the gift with respect to reproduction and demonstrates that the ideology of the gift is deeply rooted in traditions of western Christianity, permeating people's interpretations of children as gifts. This theme is explored by contributors to Layne's *Transformative Motherhood* with respect to a range of situations such as adoption, children with disabilities, surrogate motherhood, foster parenthood, and pregnancy loss.

19. See Bellah et al., *Habits of the Heart*.

20. Slater, *Consumer Culture*, 28.

21. Bellah et al., *Habits of the Heart*.

CHAPTER 8. DECISIONS ABOUT DONORS

1. Martin, "The Egg and the Sperm," ridicules the cultural meanings associated with masculinity and femininity that are attached to egg and sperm and the ways they are conveyed in science writing.

2. Different approaches to donor insemination and egg donation are readily apparent in the literature on the use of donors. See, for example, Haimes, "Issues of Gender"; Lamport, "Genetics of Secrecy"; Lessor, "All in the Family"; Nachtigall, "Secrecy"; Nachtigall et al., "Disclosure Decision" and "Stigma, Disclosure"; and Schover, "Psychological Aspects."

3. See Snowden et al., *Artificial Reproduction;* Nachtigall et al., "Effects of Gender-Specific Diagnosis."

4. Even though donor insemination has been widely practiced in this country for over fifty years, only twenty-eight states have adopted laws stipulating that the DI offspring is the legal child of the couple (Nachtigall, "Secrecy"). For further discussion, see Becker, "Deciding Whether to Tell."

5. Haimes, "Issues of Gender."

6. For an overview of some of the major issues in donor insemination, see Daniels and Haimes, *Donor Insemination*.

7. Although the husband's sperm quality is the suspected or contributing cause of infertility in 40 to 50 percent of infertile couples, little effective treatment or medication to increase sperm counts was available until the development of ICSI in 1992. Prior to that time most infertile couples were offered the choice of varicocelectomy (for the one-third of infertile men in whom a varicocele can be detected), donor insemination, or adoption. New technologies that attempt to treat male infertility, such as ICSI, must be used in conjunction with assisted reproductive technologies such as IVF and cost between $10,000 and $15,000 per cycle; the average cost of a donor insemination cycle is $700. An estimated thirty thousand or more children are conceived each year in the United States through donor insemination (Nachtigall, "Secrecy"), yet the public has

almost no knowledge of this practice because it is a private interaction involving only the couple and the health practitioner. Donor insemination is practiced by heterosexual couples as well as by single women and lesbian couples. The issues are quite different for each group.

8. In a study of donor insemination and family functioning, Becker and Nachtigall ("The Disclosure Decision," and Becker, "Deciding Whether to Tell") found that a wife's deferral to the husband's feelings (and thus his wishes) was a dominant pattern.

9. The stigma of male infertility has been a major factor affecting men's willingness to use donor insemination. See Nachtigall et al., "Effects of Gender-Specific Diagnosis" and "Stigma, Disclosure"; Snowden et al., *Artificial Reproduction.*

10. Robert Nachtigall reports this pattern from his large group practice, noting that since the introduction of ICSI, men who have oligospermia (low sperm count) turn to donor insemination only when ICSI fails.

11. See Nachtigall, "Donor Insemination."

12. Ibid.

13. Ibid. Meirow and Schenker ("Reproductive Health Care Policies") have erroneously interpreted these guidelines as mandatory in the United States. They state that the use of frozen sperm is mandatory in all sixty-two of the countries they surveyed that allow sperm donation. It may be, however, that the United States is the only country where the use of frozen sperm is *not* mandatory.

14. Nachtigall, "Donor Insemination."

15. A recent review of policies for new reproductive technologies and gamete donation worldwide reflects this ambivalence when it states that "Donor sperm should not be used in ART [assisted reproductive technologies] before fertilization attempts with the husband's sperm have failed following application of micromanipulation [ICSI] methods" (Meirow and Schenker, "Reproductive Health Care Policies," 133).

16. Haimes, "Issues of Gender."

17. Pregnancy rates for donor insemination are generally thought to be between 5 and 20 percent per cycle, with a cumulative rate of 40 to 70 percent. Factors that influence these rates include the use of fresh or frozen sperm and intrauterine insemination (Robert Nachtigall, personal communication). In our general study of infertility, of twenty-one couples who used donor insemination, fourteen became parents through this method.

18. This was the dominant experience reported by men. The few men who did not express this dramatic alteration to their perspective were men who felt coerced or were never willing to use this method. Their feelings of resentment intruded on the fathering experience, but even that reaction diminished over time as they became emotionally involved in fathering the child and came to see themselves as the father.

19. In most countries these policies tend to affirm confidentiality (see Meirow and Schenker, "Reproductive Health Care Policies," 136–37). One exception is Australia, where confidentiality is a matter of intense debate and the policy may soon be altered to one of mandatory openness (Walker and Broderick, "Psychology of Assisted Reproduction").

20. Both patterns were found in the analysis of data in this research. See also Tober, "Romancing the Sperm."

21. See Kolata, "Old Mother Hubbard," and Angell, "Pregnant at Sixty-Three?"

22. The concept of normalizing in the social sciences was first developed by Anselm Strauss in relation to the experience of chronic illness (*Chronic Illness*), and normalization has subsequently become a key term with respect to surveillance techniques (Foucault, *Birth of the Clinic*). See Arney and Bergen, *Management;* Arney, *Profession.* Most recently, Cussins ("Producing Reproduction") has applied this concept to her study of IVF clinics.

23. Many people in this study who have considered adoption and decided either to postpone it or not to pursue it would agree with this statement. In California, where the study took place, and where private adoption is a primary route to adoption, finding a child is an expensive, challenging, and potentially long-term undertaking.

24. Statistics nationwide for 1997 indicate that 4,498 donor oocyte cycles were initiated, with an overall success rate of 40 deliveries per 100 transfers (American Society of Reproductive Medicine, "Assisted Reproductive Technology"; see also Turiel, *Beyond Second Opinions*). Eleven women in this study attempted one or more cycles of IVF using a donated egg; eight conceived and gave birth.

25. Mead ("Eggs for Sale") addresses this burgeoning market and the rising price of donor eggs; the Kaiser Daily Reproductive Health Report summarizes the recent mixed response to the appearance of the availability of "model" eggs on the Internet.

26. Numerous theorists (for example, Bourdieu and Marx) have observed that class is significant in shaping consumption patterns and that one class benefits at the expense of another. See Slater, *Consumer Culture*, for an overview of the embeddedness of class in theories of consumption. Recent work on organ donation implicates poverty as a key factor in the selling of body parts worldwide. See, for example, Cohen, "Where It Hurts," and Scheper-Hughes, "Theft of Life." Hogle addresses how the conceptualization of bodies and body parts as human waste, or refuse, facilitated Nazi ideologies during the Third Reich (*Recovering the Nation's Body*). This notion of body parts as refuse has a modern-day parallel in the view that human eggs might as well be sold, or "donated," because they would otherwise be "wasted" by the body. See Mead, "Eggs for Sale," 60.

27. For an in-depth discussion of the eugenics question in donor insemination, see Hanson, "Donor Insemination."

CHAPTER 9. EMBODIED TECHNOLOGY

1. Clarke, *Disciplining Reproduction.*

2. Haraway (*Modest_Witness*) calls attention to the role of touch and vision in transforming the fetus. She observes that there is a continual interplay of sacred and secular through narratives and metaphor. All of these factors con-

tribute to the transformative process that occurs. See also Becker, *Disrupted Lives*, for discussion of narrative and metaphor in relation to infertility, embodied experience, and transformation, with respect to the image of a baby as a transformer and the transformative process women and men undergo.

3. Petchesky, "Fetal Images," 144–45. The tendency to collect, save, and memorialize these images was widespread among women and men in this study. Rapp ("Constructing Amniocentesis") addresses the different responses to visual technologies she found with respect to class and ethnicity.

4. Ginsburg and Rapp, "Introduction," 6–7. They further note: "Through such erasure, the separation of infertility treatments from women's bodies is made to appear natural, and scientific procedures become almost miraculous" (7). Novaes and Salem ("Embedding the Embryo") examine the complex circumstances in new reproductive technologies and the underlying legal, moral, and social issues that facilitate the privileging of the embryo.

5. Turner, *Dramas, Fields, and Metaphors* and *Ritual Process*.

6. Sandelowski *(With Child in Mind)* also notes the use of the roller coaster metaphor. This metaphor has become part of a common framework used by members of Resolve to describe the experience of infertility.

7. Rapp ("Constructing Amniocentesis") has called attention to the widespread deployment of sonographic images and their political uses, both specifically in the discourse on abortion and more generally in shaping women's responses to the fetus and societal views about technology.

8. The fetal heart can often be seen on transvaginal ultrasound within four weeks of conception.

9. See Becker, *Disrupted Lives*, 66–67.

10. See also Lock and Kaufert, "Introduction," 19–20, for a discussion of technologies of naturalization.

11. Franklin ("Postmodern Procreation," 335) summarizes the feminist perspective on new reproductive technologies when she says, "A male dominated and quintessentially patriarchal system of power and knowledge was deployed to name, define, and control a territory located inside women's bodies." The cultural elaboration of this territory with medical-scientific discourse is a major source of concern. See Inhorn *(Infertility and Patriarchy)* for analysis of the relationship between infertility and patriarchy in Egypt and of how women's actions mediate this relationship.

CHAPTER 10. SHIFTING GEARS

1. See Becker, *Disrupted Lives*, 136–41, for discussion of this process.

2. The term *childfree* is used by people associated with Resolve because it is viewed as less negative than the term *childless* and is intended to connote a sense of choice.

3. Progress is a core aspect of American individualism. See Bellah et al., *Habits of the Heart;* Wilkinson, *Pursuit of American Character;* and Becker, *Disrupted Lives,* 178. See also Franklin, *Embodied Progress;* Layne, "How's

the Baby Doing?" and Lock and Kaufert, "Introduction," for discussion of "narratives of progress."

4. For further discussion, see Becker, *Disrupted Lives*, 149–51. Issues of hope in infertility treatment are also taken up by Franklin *(Embodied Progress)* and Sandelowski *(With Child in Mind).*

5. Because the freezing process itself is so harmful to sperm, the freezing of multiple sperm samples in the hope of combining and concentrating them is usually not successful.

6. See Becker, *Disrupted Lives*, and Bellah et al., *Habits of the Heart*. Franklin, in her study of English women undergoing IVF *(Embodied Progress)*, addresses at length the cultural meaning of overcoming obstacles.

7. See Becker, *Disrupted Lives*, for discussion of continuity as a cultural ideology.

8. See Bellah et al., *Habits of the Heart*, and Dumont, *Essays on Individualism.*

CHAPTER 11. REDEFINING NORMALCY

1. Carr *(Time, Narrative, and History*, 29) observes that temporal experience has a crucial component, a forward reference in which past and present are experienced as a function of what will be. See Becker, *Disrupted Lives* and *Healing the Infertile Family*, for discussions of the temporal dimension in relation to the experience of infertility.

2. Modell, in *A Sealed and Secret Kinship*, analyzes cultural assumptions underlying American adoption practices and suggests that a completely new way of thinking about adoption is needed. In "Freely Given," Modell considers how the idea of the gift transforms adoption in the United States.

3. See Becker, *Disrupted Lives;* Sandelowski, "Compelled to Try."

4. See Becker, *Healing the Infertile Family*, 139–40, 277–78, for a discussion of rituals that help with bringing this era of life to a close.

5. See Becker, ibid., for discussions of friendship and infertility.

6. Anthropological perspectives on adoption may help people to view adoption without the cultural blinders that Americans often have about the subject, as adoption is accepted—even routine—in many cultures around the world. See Terrell and Modell, "Anthropology and Adoption." For an in-depth look at the adoption process, see Modell, *Kinship with Strangers.*

7. Becker, *Healing the Infertile Family*, 227–35.

CHAPTER 12. WOMEN
RETHINKING PARENTHOOD

1. See Becker, *Disrupted Lives*, for discussion of the cultural ideology of continuity.

2. Ireland, *Reconceiving Women*. Ireland discusses women's identity and life

without children in depth. See Carter and Carter, *Sweet Grapes,* for discussion of rethinking the question of having children.

CHAPTER 13. REWRITING THE FAMILY

1. Some couples continued to pursue medical treatment after adopting. Without exception, this group stated that medical treatment was much less stressful and they were much less invested in it than they had previously been because they already had a child.

2. Few others in this study had any further contact with the birth mother once they took the child home. A few people sent pictures of the child to the birth mother, usually on an annual basis. One other person reported the birth mother visited her and her husband on invitation. Most women and men reported that birth mothers did not wish to have ongoing contact any more than they did; the birth mothers expressed a wish to get on with their lives. Couples who had not yet adopted and were contemplating it, however, often joked anxiously about the worst-case scenario—having the birth mother come to dinner. These anxieties reflect the preadoption worry about having control over the process. Adoption, in the words of a two-time adoptive mother, is "an out-of-control situation when you already feel out of control [because of infertility treatment]."

3. Adding gifts to a substantial amount of money is one of the most recent innovations that potential users of donated eggs have adopted to entice donors. These gifts include vacations and college tuition. See Mead, "Eggs for Sale," 62.

4. See Rapp, "Heredity," 7. See also Schneider, *American Kinship.*

5. Yanagisako and Delaney, "Naturalizing Power," 9–12.

6. Ibid.

7. Becker, *Disrupted Lives.*

8. Yanagisako and Delaney suggest that reading across domains is a critical way to denaturalize gender and reproduction because of the insights it produces. Reading across domains not only demonstrates their interrelatedness but also dislodges their apparent "naturalness" and reveals how dominant notions about reproduction and gender, for example, are perpetuated: "Culture is what makes the boundary of domains seem natural, what gives ideologies power, and what makes hegemonies appear seamless. At the same time, it is what enables us to make compelling claims for connections between supposedly distinct discourses" *(Naturalizing Power,* 19). See also Strathern, *Reproducing the Future* and "Regulation, Substitution," for discussion of crossing domain boundaries with respect to reproductive technology.

9. See Duster, *Backdoor to Eugenics;* Nelkin and Lindee, *DNA Mystique.*

10. Giddens, *Social Theory,* 216.

CHAPTER 14. PERFORMING GENDER

1. Casper and Koenig, "Reconfiguring Nature and Culture," 529; Strathern, *Reproducing the Future* and "Displacing Knowledge."

2. Balsamo (*Technologies,* 9) addresses at length the effects of these technological developments on cultural enactments of gender.

3. Clarke ("Cyborg," 141) notes that the distinction between human and nonhuman is of decreasing relevance to reproductive and genetic scientists.

4. Clarke, "Cyborg," 149. This represents a shift from Fordist to flexible post-Fordist modes of production (Lury, *Consumer Culture,* 94).

5. Davis, "Surrogates and Outcast Mothers," 220.

6. Judith Butler ("Performative Acts," 409–10) draws on Victor Turner's perspective in articulating the concept of gendered performance as social action that requires repeated performance. Turner *(Dramas, Fields, and Metaphors)* states, "This repetition is at once a reenactment and reexperiencing of a set of meanings already socially established—it is the mundane and ritualized form of their legitimation." Butler concludes, "Gender is an act which has been rehearsed, much as a script survives the particular actors who make use of it, but which requires individual actors in order to be actualized and reproduced as reality once again."

7. Butler states, "Certain kinds of acts are usually interpreted as expressive of a gender core or identity, and . . . these acts either conform to an expected gender identity or contest that expectation in some way" ("Performative Acts,"411).

8. I also demonstrate such efforts with respect to infertility in *Disrupted Lives.* People work within the confines of culture as they know it in undertaking this process.

9. See Haber, *Beyond Postmodern Politics,* and Slater, *Consumer Culture,* for discussion of choice as a political activity. Numerous feminists have discussed the constraints on choice. Riessman ("Stigma and Everyday Resistance Practices") discusses choice and resistance among childless women in India. Lopez ("Agency and Constraint," 160) observes that the ideology of choice is based on the assumption that people have options, and implicit in this view is the belief that the higher their social and class status, the more numerous their options. She points out that choices are primed by larger institutional structures and ideological messages: the choices Puerto Rican women make about sterilization reflect the constraints in their lives. Rapp ("Constructing Amniocentesis," 138) notes that all Americans prize choice as a political and cultural value and that it is middle-class women who have been able to maintain the illusion of control over their lives, but nevertheless medical technology transforms their "choices" on an individual level.

10. The collective force of such actions has been called counter-hegemony or alternative hegemony. Williams, following Gramsci (*Keywords,* 145), defines alternative hegemonies as "a new predominant practice and consciousness . . . distinct, for example, from the idea that new institutions and relationships will of themselves create new experience and consciousness." Williams further suggests (*Marxism and Literature,* 112) that hegemonic forces are not only continually renewed, recreated, defended, and modified, but they are also continually resisted, limited, altered, and challenged.

11. A new hegemonic order may be established through counter-hegemonic forces (see, for example, Comaroff and Comaroff, *Revelation and Revolution,*

1:26). But even efforts to destabilize existing institutions may function to uphold and maintain those institutions. In this study, for example, although women challenged the biomedical status quo, they wanted better services, not a different system.

12. Slater (*Consumer Culture,* 132) notes that we produce and reproduce cultures, social relations, and society through culturally specific forms of consumption, and by doing so we demonstrate membership in a particular social order.

13. Slater (*Consumer Culture,* 30) suggests that status and identity are negotiated through consumer culture. Regulation of these issues by tradition is replaced by negotiation and construction and promotes a new flexibility in the relations among consumption, communication, and meaning. The structure of status and the structure of meaning become unstable, flexible, and highly negotiable. Somers and Gibson ("Reclaiming the Epistemological 'Other' ") argue that ontological and "public narratives" are a vehicle for identity politics.

14. See Franklin, *Embodied Progress;* Layne, "How's the Baby Doing?" and Lock and Kaufert, "Introduction," for discussions of "narratives of progress."

15. See Duster, *Backdoor to Eugenics,* and Nelkin and Lindee, *DNA Mystique.* Davis ("Surrogates and Outcast Mothers," 219) observes that ideological representations of motherhood are manipulated differently depending on attributions of race and class.

16. Balsamo, *Technologies,* 9.

17. Douglas, *Purity and Danger.*

18. Here I am referring to the phenomenological sense of natural order, keeping in mind Butler's observation that embodied selves do not preexist the cultural conventions that signify bodies: the gendered body acts its part in a culturally restricted corporeal space and enacts interpretations within the confines of already existing directives ("Performative Acts," 410). See also Becker, *Disrupted Lives.*

19. Strathern ("Disembodied Choice," 76–77) notes the persuasiveness of consumer attitudes that choice must always be enhancing of the self and that to choose to do something about infertility is a more enterprising choice than to choose not to.

20. Tymstra, "Imperative Character."

21. Katz, *Silent World.*

22. See Armstrong, "Rise of Surveillance Medicine"; Arney, *Power;* Foucault, *Birth of the Clinic.* Rabinow (*Essays,* 100) observes a shift from the older face-to-face surveillance of individuals and groups viewed as dangerous or ill toward projecting risk factors that deconstruct and reconstruct the individual or group subject.

23. Ortner, "Resistance," 179.

24. Bellah et al., *Habits of the Heart;* Holstein, "Women and Productive Aging."

25. Comaroff and Comaroff (*Revelation and Revolution,* 1:30) observe that the hegemonic is inscribed largely in enduring forms, such as the commodity form. While they last, such forms lay down the implicit ground within which the meaningful world may be subjectively constructed, negotiated, and actively

empowered. Arguing that hegemony is to ideology as form is to content, they observe that innovation depends on the play of culture with form and content.

26. Minkler and Cole ("Political and Moral Economy," 42–43), discuss an underlying element of the moral economy: some persons are viewed as deserving while others are not, based on ideas about who is productive in society.

27. Hendricks and Leedham ("Dependency or Empowerment?") propose two types of moral economy: moral economies grounded in use value are characterized as meeting human needs and creating social arrangements that maximize life chances for all, whereas moral economies grounded in exchange value take a utilitarian approach to the public good and ignore both problematic issues of distributive justice and the existence of goods not easily measured in economic terms.

28. U.S. House Committee on Small Business, Subcommittee on Regulation, Business Opportunities, and Energy, *Hearing on Consumer Protection Issues.*

29. Figge, "Tyranny of Technology"; McDonough, "Need for Technology Assessment"; Elias and Annas, "Social Policy Considerations."

30. Herz, "Infertility and Bioethical Issues"; Annas, "Shadowlands."

31. U.S. House Committee on Small Business, Subcommittee on Regulation, Business Opportunities, and Energy, *Hearing on Consumer Protection Issues.*

32. See Collins, "Will the 'Real' Mother Please Stand Up?" and Davis, "Surrogates and Outcast Mothers," on the privileging of white, middle-class women, the disenfranchisement of other women, and the risk of perpetuating a racist, classist society.

33. Health care providers can offer limited infertility services to low-income populations through funds that the federal government distributes to the states for use in community health clinics. One clinic was doing so in this area during this study. When that clinic closed, another family planning clinic serving low-income women began offering these services. However, such clinics are few and far between, and their offerings are completely inadequate. They usually operate on a weekly basis, but most infertility treatments need to be available on a daily basis. A further problem in this instance was the difference in target populations. The first clinic was located in a predominantly Spanish-speaking neighborhood, while the second was in a predominantly Cantonese-speaking area. There were no funds in either case to do outreach or develop ways to accommodate cultural and language differences. Therefore, Latinas used the first clinic but did not go to the second clinic, located a great distance from the first, when the first clinic shut down.

34. See Meirow and Schenker, "Reproductive Health Care Policies," for an overview of the positions of sixty-two countries on issues relating to new reproductive technologies.

35. In some countries the anonymity of donors is mandated, whereas in others parents are urged to disclose to their children; in some countries donor offspring have the right to access their donor's genetic information. See Becker, "Deciding Whether to Tell."

36. Collier et al. ("Is There a Family?") view the family as an ideological unit, a moral statement about the place of family in society.

37. Comaroff and Comaroff observe that "unlike explicit ideologies that can

be traced to people with particular social position and interests, hegemonic understandings are more difficult to trace to human agents" (*Revelation and Revolution,* 1:24).

APPENDIX. ABOUT THE RESEARCH

1. Hammersley and Atkinson, *Ethnographic Principles in Practice.*
2. Ibid.
3. Wiener, *Politics of Alcoholism.*
4. Mishler, *Research Interviewing.*
5. Benner, *From Novice to Expert.*
6. Kaufman, *Ageless Self.*

References

Abu-Lughod, Lila. 1991. "Writing against Culture." In *Recapturing Anthropology: Working in the Present,* ed. Richard G. Fox, 137–62. Santa Fe: School of American Research.

Allen, Jeffner, and Iris Marion Young, eds. 1989. *The Thinking Muse: Feminism and Modern French Philosophy.* Bloomington: Indiana University Press.

American Society for Reproductive Medicine/Society for Assisted Reproductive Technology Registry. 1998. "Assisted Reproductive Technology in the United States and Canada: 1995 Results Generated from the American Society for Reproductive Medicine/Society for Assisted Reproductive Technology Registry." *Fertility and Sterility* 69:389–98.

Anderson, Benedict. 1991. *Imagined Communities: Reflections on the Origin and Spread of Nationalism.* London: Verso.

Angell, Marcia. 1997. "Pregnant at Sixty-Three? Why Not?" *New York Times,* op-ed column, April 25.

Annas, George J. 1998. "The Shadowlands: Secrets, Lies, and Assisted Reproduction." *New England Journal of Medicine* 339:935–39.

Appadurai, Arjun. 1986. "Introduction: Commodities and the Politics of Value." In *The Social Life of Things: Commodities in Cultural Perspective,* ed. Arjun Appadurai, 3–63. Cambridge: Cambridge University Press.

———. 1996. *Modernity at Large: Cultural Dimensions of Globalization.* Minneapolis: University of Minnesota Press.

Armstrong, David, 1995. "The Rise of Surveillance Medicine." *Sociology of Health and Illness* 17:393–404.

Arney, William Ray. 1982. *Power and the Profession of Obstetrics.* Chicago: University of Chicago Press.

Arney, William Ray, and Bernard J. Bergen. 1984. *Medicine and the Management of Living: Taming the Last Great Beast.* Chicago: University of Chicago Press.

Balsamo, Anne. 1996. *Technologies of the Gendered Body: Reading Cyborg Women.* Chapel Hill: Duke University Press.

Barnstone, Aliki, Michael Tomasek Manson, and Carol J. Singley, eds. 1997. "Introduction." In *The Calvinist Roots of the Modern Era,* ed. Aliki Barnstone, Michael Tomasek, and Carol J. Singley, xiii–xxii. Hanover: University Press of New England.

Beck, Ulrich. 1992. *Risk Society: Towards a New Modernity.* Beverly Hills: Sage.

Becker, Gay. 1997 (1990). *Healing the Infertile Family: Strengthening Your Relationship in the Search for Parenthood.* Berkeley: University of California Press.

———. 1997. *Disrupted Lives: How People Create Meaning in a Chaotic World.* Berkeley: University of California Press.

———. 1998. "Advanced Reproductive Technologies and the New Eugenics: The Impact of Structural Inequities on Upper- and Lower-Income Infertility Populations in the U.S." Paper given at the annual meeting of the American Anthropological Association, Philadelphia.

———. Forthcoming. "Deciding Whether to Tell Children about Donor Insemination: An Unresolved Question in the United States." In *Infertility around the Globe: New Thinking on Childlessness, Gender, and Reproductive Technologies,* ed. Marcia C. Inhorn and Frank van Balen. Berkeley: University of California Press.

Becker, Gay, Susan Janson-Bjerklie, Patricia Benner, Kathleen Slobin, and Sandra Ferketich. 1993. "The Dilemma of Seeking Urgent Care: Asthma Episodes and Emergency Service Use." *Social Science and Medicine* 37:305–13.

Becker, Gay, and Robert D. Nachtigall. 1991. "Ambiguous Responsibility in the Doctor-Patient Relationship: The Case of Infertility." *Social Science and Medicine* 32:875–85.

———. 1992. "Eager for Medicalization: The Social Production of Infertility as a Disease." *Sociology of Health and Illness* 14:456–71.

———. 1994. " 'Born to Be a Mother': The Cultural Construction of Risk in Infertility Treatment." *Social Science and Medicine* 39:507–18.

Behar, Ruth, and Deborah A. Gordon, eds. 1995. *Women Writing Culture.* Berkeley: University of California Press.

Belkin, Lisa. 1997. "Pregnant with Complications." *New York Times Magazine,* October 26.

Bell, Susan E. 1989. "The Meaning of Risk, Choice, and Responsibility for a DES Daughter." In *Healing Technology: Feminist Perspectives,* ed. Kathryn Strother Ratcliff, 245–61. Ann Arbor: University of Michigan Press.

Bellah, Robert N., Richard Madsen, William M. Sullivan, Ann Swidler, and Steven M. Tipton. 1996 (1985). *Habits of the Heart: Individualism and Commitment in American Life.* Berkeley: University of California Press.

Benner, Patricia. 1984. *From Novice to Expert: Excellence and Power in Clinical Nursing Practice.* Reading, Mass.: Addison-Wesley.

Bigwood, Carol. 1991. "Renaturalizing the Body (with the Help of Merleau-Ponty)." *Hypatia* 6 (3). Special Issue: Feminism and the Body.

Bijker, Wiebe E. 1992. "The Social Construction of Fluorescent Lighting, or How an Artifact Was Invented in Its Diffusion Stage." In *Shaping Technol-*

ogy/Building Society: Studies in Sociotechnical Change, ed. Wiebe E. Bijker and John Law, 75–102. Cambridge: MIT Press.

Bijker, Wiebe E., and John Law. 1992. "General Introduction." *In Shaping Technology/Building Society: Studies in Sociotechnical Change,* ed. Wiebe E. Bijker and John Law, 1–14. Cambridge: MIT Press.

Blackwell, Richard E., Bruce R. Carr, R. Jeffrey Chang, Alan H. DeCherney, Arthur F. Haney, William R. Keye, Jr., Robert W. Rebar, John A. Rock, Zev Rosenwaks, Machelle M. Seibel, and Michael R. Soules. 1987. "Are We Exploiting the Infertile Couple?" *Fertility and Sterility* 48:735–39.

Booth, William James. 1994. "On the Idea of the Moral Economy." *American Political Science Review* 88:653–68.

Bordo, Susan. 1993. *Unbearable Weight: Feminism, Western Culture, and the Body.* Berkeley: University of California Press.

Bourdieu, Pierre. 1977. *Outline of a Theory of Practice.* Translated by Richard Nice. Cambridge: Cambridge University Press.

———. 1984. *Distinction: A Social Critique of the Judgment of Taste.* Translated by Richard Nice. Cambridge: Harvard University Press.

———. 1990. *The Logic of Practice.* Translated by Richard Nice. Stanford: Stanford University Press.

Brandt, Allan M. 1997. "Behavior, Disease, and Health in the Twentieth-Century United States: The Moral Valence of Individual Risk." In *Morality and Health,* ed. Allan M. Brandt and Paul Rozin, 53–78. New York: Routledge.

Brock, Dan W., and Steven A. Wartman. 1990. "When Competent Patients Make Irrational Choices." *New England Journal of Medicine* 322:1595–99.

Butler, Judith. 1989. "Sexual Ideology and Phenomenological Description: A Feminist Critique of Merleau-Ponty's Phenomenology of Perception." In *The Thinking Muse: Feminism and Modern French Philosophy,* ed. Jeffner Allen and Iris Marion Young, 85–100. Bloomington: Indiana University Press.

———. 1990. *Gender Trouble: Feminism and the Subversion of Identity.* New York: Routledge.

———. 1993. *Bodies That Matter: On the Discursive Limits of "Sex."* New York: Routledge.

———. 1997. "Performative Acts and Gender Constitution: An Essay in Phenomenology and Feminist Theory." In *Writing on the Body: Female Embodiment and Feminist Theory,* ed. Katie Conboy, Nadia Medina, and Sarah Stanbury, 401–17. New York: Columbia University Press.

Calhoun, Craig. 1994. "Social Theory and the Politics of Identity." In *Social Theory and the Politics of Identity,* ed. Craig Calhoun, 8–36. Oxford: Blackwell.

Callahan, T. L., J. E. Hall, S. L. Etner, C. L. Christiansen, M. F. Greene, and W. F. Crowley. 1994. "The Economic Impact of Multiple-Gestation Pregnancies and the Contribution of Assisted-Reproduction Techniques to Their Incidence." *New England Journal of Medicine* 331:244–49.

Cancian, Francesca M. 1987. *Love in America: Gender and Self-Development.* New York: Cambridge University Press.

Cannell, Fenella. 1990. "Concepts of Parenthood: The Warnock Report, the Gillick Debate, and Modern Myths." *American Ethnologist* 17:667–86.

Carr, David. 1986. *Time, Narrative, and History*. Bloomington: Indiana University Press.

Carter, Jean W., and Michael Carter. 1989. *Sweet Grapes: How to Stop Being Infertile and Start Living Again*. Indianapolis: Perspectives Press.

Casper, Monica J., and Barbara A. Koenig. 1996. "Reconfiguring Nature and Culture: Intersections of Medical Anthropology and Technoscience Studies." *Medical Anthropology Quarterly* 10: 523–36.

Clark, M. Margaret, and Barbara Anderson. 1967. *Culture and Aging*. Springfield, Ill.: Charles C. Thomas.

Clarke, Adele. 1995. "Modernity, Postmodernity and Reproductive Processes ca. 1890–1990, or, 'Mommy, Where Do Cyborgs Come from Anyway?' " In *The Cyborg Handbook*, ed. Chris Hables Gray, with Heidi J. Figuerroa-Sarriera and Steven Mentor, 139–55. Routledge: New York and London.

———. 1998. *Disciplining Reproduction: Modernity, American Life Sciences, and the Problem of Sex*. Berkeley: University of California Press.

Cohen, Lawrence. 1999. "Where It Hurts: Indian Material for an Ethics of Organ Transplantation." *Daedalus* 128:135–65. Special Issue: Bioethics and Beyond.

Cohler, Bertram. 1982. "Personal Narrative and Life Course." In *Life Span Development and Behavior*, ed. Paul Baltes, 4:205–41. New York: Academic Press.

Collier, Jane, Michelle Z. Rosaldo, and Sylvia Yanagisako. 1997. "Is There a Family? New Anthropological Views." In *The Gender/Sexuality Reader*, ed. Roger N. Lancaster and Micaela di Leonardo, 71–81. New York: Routledge.

Collier, Jane Fishburne, and Sylvia Junko Yanagisako. 1987. "Introduction." In *Gender and Kinship: Essays Toward a Unified Analysis*, ed. Jane Fishburne Collier and Sylvia Junko Yanagisako, 1–13. Stanford: Stanford University Press.

Collins, Patricia Hill. 1999. "Will the 'Real' Mother Please Stand Up? The Logic of Eugenics and American National Family Planning." In *Revisioning Women, Health, and Healing: Feminist, Cultural, and Technoscience Perspectives*, ed. Adele E. Clarke and Virginia Olesen, 266–82. New York: Routledge.

Comaroff, Jean, and John Comaroff. 1991. *Of Revelation and Revolution: Christianity, Colonialism, and Consciousness in South Africa*, volume 1. Chicago: University of Chicago Press.

Connerton, Paul. 1989. *How Societies Remember*. New York: Cambridge University Press.

Connors, Margaret M. 1992. "Risk Perception, Risk Taking, and Risk Management among Intravenous Drug Users: Implications for AIDS Prevention." *Social Science and Medicine* 34:591–601.

Cowan, Ruth Schwartz. 1987. "The Consumption Junction: A Proposal for Research Strategies in the Sociology of Technology." In *The Social Construction of Technological Systems: New Directions in the Sociology and History of Technology,* ed. Wiebe E. Bijker, Thomas P. Hughes, and Trevor Pinch, 261–80. Cambridge: MIT Press.

Crawford, Robert. 1984. "A Cultural Account of 'Health': Control, Release and the Social Body." In *Issues in the Political Economy of Health Care,* ed. J. McKinlay, 60–103. New York: Tavistock.

Csordas, Thomas. 1990. "Embodiment as a Paradigm for Anthropology." *Ethos* 18:5–47.

———. 1993. "Somatic Modes of Attention." *Cultural Anthropology* 8:135–56.

———. 1994. *The Sacred Self: A Cultural Phenomenology of Charismatic Healing.* Berkeley: University of California Press.

Cussins, Charis. 1996. "Ontological Choreography: Agency through Objectification in Infertility Clinics." *Social Studies of Science* 26:575–610.

———. 1998. "Producing Reproduction: Techniques of Normalization and Naturalization in Infertility Clinics." In *Reproducing Reproduction: Kinship, Power, and Technological Innovation,* ed. Sarah Franklin and Helena Ragone, 118–31. Philadelphia: University of Pennsylvania Press.

D'Andrade, Roy. 1984. "Cultural Meaning Systems." In *Culture Theory: Mind, Self, and Emotion,* ed. Richard A. Shweder and Robert A. LeVine, 88–112. Cambridge: Cambridge University Press.

Daniels, Ken, and Erica Haimes, eds. 1998. *Donor Insemination: International Social Science Perspectives.* Cambridge: Cambridge University Press.

Davis, Angela. 1981. *Women, Race, and Class.* New York: Random House.

———. 1998. "Surrogates and Outcast Mothers: Racism and Reproductive Politics in the Nineties." In *The Angela Y. Davis Reader,* ed. Joy James, 210–21. Malden, Mass.: Blackwell.

Davis, Kathy. 1997. "Embody-ing Theory: Beyond Modernist and Postmodernist Readings of the Body." In *Embodied Practices: Feminist Perspectives on the Body,* ed. Kathy Davis, 1–26. London: Sage.

Davis-Floyd, Robbie, and Joseph Dumit, eds. 1998. *Cyborg Babies: From Techno-Sex to Techno-Tots.* New York: Routledge.

de Lauretis, Teresa. 1987. *Technologies of Gender: Essays on Theory, Film, and Fiction.* Bloomington: Indiana University Press.

Derrida, Jacques. 1976. *Of Grammatology.* Translated by Gayatri Chakravorty Spivak. Baltimore: Johns Hopkins University Press.

Dillon, Martin C. 1991. "Preface: Merleau-Ponty and Postmodernity." In *Merleau-Ponty Vivant,* ed. Martin C. Dillon, ix–xxxv. Albany: State University of New York Press.

———. 1997. *Merleau-Ponty's Ontology.* 2d ed. Evanston: Northwestern University Press.

Douglas, Mary. 1966. *Purity and Danger: An Analysis of the Concepts of Pollution and Taboo.* London: Routledge.

———. 1990 (1950). "Foreword: No Free Gifts." In Marcel Mauss, *The Gift: The Form and Reason for Exchange in Archaic Societies,* vii–xviii. New York: Norton.

———. 1992. *Risk and Blame: Essays in Cultural Theory.* London: Routledge.

Douglas, Mary, and Aaron Wildavsky. 1982. *Risk and Culture: An Essay on the Selection of Technological and Environmental Dangers.* Berkeley: University of California Press.

Dumont, Louis. 1986. *Essays on Individualism: Modern Ideology in Anthropological Perspective.* Chicago: University of Chicago Press.

Duster, Troy. 1990. *Backdoor to Eugenics.* New York: Routledge.

Edwards, Jeanette, Sarah Franklin, Eric Hirsch, Frances Price, and Marilyn Strathern. 1999. *Technologies of Procreation: Kinship in the Age of Assisted Conception.* 2d ed. London: Routledge.

Elias, Sherman, and George J. Annas. 1986. "Social Policy Considerations in Noncoital Reproduction." *Journal of the American Medical Association* 255:62–68.

Epstein, Steven. 1995. "The Construction of Lay Expertise: AIDS Activism and the Forging of Credibility in the Reform of Clinical Trials." *Science, Technology and Human Values* 20:408–37.

———. 1996. *Impure Science: AIDS, Activism, and the Politics of Knowledge.* Berkeley: University of California Press.

Fernandez, James. 1974. "The Mission of Metaphor in Expressive Culture." *Current Anthropology* 15:119–45.

———. 1986. "The Argument of Images and the Experience of Returning to the Whole." In *The Anthropology of Experience,* ed. Victor W. Turner and Edward M. Bruner, 159–87. Urbana: University of Illinois Press.

Figge, David C. 1988. "The Tyranny of Technology." *American Journal of Obstetrics and Gynecology* 162:1365–69.

Forrow, Lachlan, Steven A. Wartman, and Dan W. Brock. 1988. "Science, Ethics, and the Making of Clinical Decisions." *Journal of the American Medical Association* 259:3161–67.

Foucault, Michel. 1973. *The Birth of the Clinic: An Archeology of Medical Perception.* Translated by A. M. Sheridan Smith. New York: Vintage.

———. 1976. *The History of Sexuality, Volume 1: An Introduction.* Translated by Robert Hurley. New York: Random House.

———. 1979. *Discipline and Punish: The Birth of the Prison.* Translated by A. M. Sheridan Smith. New York: Vintage.

———. 1980. *Power/Knowledge.* New York: Pantheon Books.

———. 1986. *The History of Sexuality, Volume 3: The Care of the Self.* Translated by Robert Hurley. New York: Random House.

Franklin, Sarah. 1995. "Postmodern Procreation: A Cultural Account of Assisted Reproduction." In *Conceiving the New World Order: The Global Politics of Reproduction,* ed. Faye D. Ginsburg and Rayna Rapp, 323–45. Berkeley: University of California Press.

———. 1995. "Science as Culture, Cultures of Science." *Annual Review of Anthropology* 24: 163–84.

———. 1997. *Embodied Progress: A Cultural Account of Assisted Conception.* London: Routledge.

Franklin, Sarah, and Helena Ragone. 1998. "Introduction." In *Reproducing Reproduction: Kinship, Power, and Technological Innovation,* ed. Sarah Franklin and Helen Ragone, 1–14. Philadelphia: University of Pennsylvania Press.

Fry, Christine L. 1990. "The Life Course in Context: Implications of Comparative Research." In *Anthropology and Aging,* ed. Robert Rubinstein, 129–49. Dordrecht, The Netherlands: Kluwer.

Fry, Christine L., and Jennie Keith. 1982. "The Life Course as a Cultural Unit." In *Aging from Birth to Death: Volume 2, Sociotemporal Perspectives,* ed. Matilda White Riley, Ronald Abeles, and M. S. Teitelbaum. Boulder: Westview Press.

Geertz, Clifford. 1973. *The Interpretation of Cultures.* New York: Basic Books.

Giddens, Anthony. 1987. *Social Theory and Modern Sociology.* Stanford: Stanford University Press.

———. 1990. *The Consequences of Modernity.* Stanford: Stanford University Press.

———. 1991. *Modernity and Self-Identity: Self and Society in the Late Modern Age.* Stanford: Stanford University Press.

Ginsburg, Faye D., and Rayna Rapp. 1995. "Introduction: Conceiving the New World Order." In *Conceiving the New World Order: The Global Politics of Reproduction,* ed. Faye D. Ginsburg and Rayna Rapp, 1–18. Berkeley: University of California Press.

Ginsburg, Faye D., and Rayna Rapp, eds. 1995. *Conceiving the New World Order: The Global Politics of Reproduction.* Berkeley: University of California Press.

Ginsburg, Faye D., and Anna Lowenhaupt Tsing, eds. 1990. *Uncertain Terms: Negotiating Gender in American Culture.* Boston: Beacon Press.

Good, Mary-Jo DelVecchio, Byron J. Good, Cynthia Schaffer, and Stuart E. Lind. 1990. "American Oncology and the Discourse on Hope." *Culture, Medicine, and Psychiatry* 14:59–79.

Gray, Chris Hables, ed. 1995. *The Cyborg Handbook.* New York: Routledge.

Greil, Arthur L., T. A. Leitko, and K. L. Porter. 1988. "Infertility: His and Hers." *Gender and Society* 2:172–99.

Grosz, Elizabeth. 1994. *Volatile Bodies: Toward a Corporeal Feminism.* Bloomington: University of Indiana Press.

Gullick, Muriel R. 1988. "Talking with Patients About Risk." *Journal of General Internal Medicine* 3:166–70.

Gupta, Akhil, and James Ferguson. 1997. "Culture, Power, Place: Ethnography at the End of an Era." In *Culture, Power, Place: Explorations in Critical Anthropology,* ed. Akhil Gupta and James Ferguson, 1–29. Durham: Duke University Press.

Haber, Honi Fern. 1994. *Beyond Postmodern Politics: Lyotard, Rorty, Foucault.* New York: Routledge.

Haimes, Erica. 1993. "Issues of Gender in Gamete Donation." *Social Science and Medicine* 36:85–93.

Hallowell, A. Irving. 1955. *Culture and Experience.* New York: Schocken.

Hammersley, Martin, and Paul Atkinson. 1986. *Ethnographic Principles in Practice.* London: Tavistock.

Handwerker, Lisa. 1994. "Medical Risk: Implicating Poor Pregnant Women." *Social Science and Medicine* 38:665–75.

———. 1995. "The Hen That Can't Lay an Egg (Bu Xia Dan de Mu Ji): Conceptions of Female Infertility in Modern China." In *Deviant Bodies,* ed. Jennifer Terry and Jacqueline Urla, 358–86. Bloomington: Indiana University Press.

———. 1995. "Social and Ethical Implications of In Vitro Fertilization in Contemporary China." *Cambridge Quarterly of Healthcare Ethics* 4:355–63.

———. 1998. "The Consequences of Modernity for Childless Women in China: Medicalization and Resistance." In *Pragmatic Women and Body Politics,* ed. Margaret Lock and Patricia Kaufert, 178–205. Cambridge: Cambridge University Press.

Hanson, F. Allan. Forthcoming. "Donor Insemination: Eugenic and Feminist Implications." *Medical Anthropology Quarterly.*

Haraway, Donna J. 1997. *Modest_Witness @ Second_Millennium. FemaleMan©_Meets_Oncomouse™: Feminism and Technoscience.* New York: Routledge.

Harris, Gladys Grace. 1989. "Concepts of Individual, Self, and Person in Description and Analysis." *American Anthropologist* 91:599–612.

Harris, R., A. S. Whittemore, J. Intyre, and the Collaborative Ovarian Cancer Group. 1992. "Characteristics Relating to Ovarian Cancer Risk: Collaborative Analysis of Twelve U.S. Case-Control Studies. III: Epithelial Tumors of Low Malignant Potential in White Women." *American Journal of Epidemiology* 136:1204–11.

Hartouni, Valerie. 1997. Cultural Conceptions: *On Reproductive Technologies and the Remaking of Life.* Minneapolis: University of Minnesota Press.

Harvey, David. 1990. *The Condition of Postmodernity: An Enquiry into the Origins of Cultural Change.* Cambridge, Mass.: Blackwell.

Hayes, M. V. 1992. "On the Epistemology of Risk: Language, Logic, and Social Science." *Social Science and Medicine* 35:401–7.

Heidegger, Martin. 1985. *History of the Concept of Time: Prolegomena.* Translated by Theodore Kisiel. Bloomington: University of Indiana Press.

Hendricks, Jon, and Cynthia A. Leedham. 1991. "Dependency or Empowerment? Toward a Moral and Political Economy of Aging." In *Critical Perspectives on Aging: The Political and Moral Economy of Growing Old,* ed. Meredith Minkler and Carroll L. Estes, 51–64. Amityville, N.Y.: Baywood Publishing Company.

Herrmann, Gretchen M. 1996. "Women's Exchange in the U.S. Garage Sale." *Gender and Society* 10:703–28.

Herz, Elisabeth K. 1989. "Infertility and Bioethical Issues of the New Reproductive Technologies." *Psychiatric Clinics of North America* 12:117–31.

Hewitt, John P. 1989. *Dilemmas of the American Self.* Philadelphia: Temple University Press.

Hirsch, Eric. 1999 (1993). "Negotiated Limits: Interviews in South-East England." In *Technologies of Procreation: Kinship in the Age of Assisted Conception,* ed. Jeanette Edwards, Sarah Franklin, Eric Hirsch, Frances Price, and Marilyn Strathern, 91–121. London: Routledge.

Hogle, Linda F. 1999. *Recovering the Nation's Body: Cultural Memory, Medicine, and the Politics of Redemption.* New Brunswick, N.J.: Rutgers University Press.

Holland, Dorothy. 1992. "How Cultural Systems Become Desire." In *Human Motives and Cultural Models,* ed. Roy D'Andrade and Claudia Strauss, 61–89. Cambridge: Cambridge University Press.

Holstein, Martha. 1999. "Women and Productive Aging: Troubling Implications." In *Critical Gerontology: Perspectives from Political and Moral Economy,* ed. Meredith Minkler and Carroll L. Estes, 359–73. Amityville, New York: Baywood Publishing Company.

Howell, Signe, ed. 1997. *The Ethnography of Moralities.* London: Routledge.

Ince, Susan. 1988. "Fertility Rites and Wrongs." *Savvy,* 86–88, June.

Inhorn, Marcia C. 1994. *Quest for Conception: Gender, Infertility, and Egyptian Medical Traditions.* Philadelphia: University of Pennsylvania Press.

———. 1996. *Infertility and Patriarchy: The Cultural Politics of Gender and Family Life in Egypt.* Philadelphia: University of Pennsylvania Press.

———. 2000. "Missing Motherhood: Infertility, Poverty, and Technology in Egyptian Women's Lives." In *Ideologies and Technologies of Motherhood,* ed. Frances Winddance Twine and Helena Ragone. New York: Routledge.

———. Forthcoming. "Money, Marriage, and Morality: Constraints of IVF Treatment Seeking among Infertile Egyptian Couples." In *Cross-Cultural Perspectives on Reproductive Health,* ed. Carla Makhlouf Obermeyer. Oxford: Oxford University Press.

Ireland, Mardi S. 1993. *Reconceiving Women: Separating Motherhood from Female Identity.* New York: Guilford Press.

Jackson, Michael. 1983. "Thinking through the Body: An Essay on Understanding Metaphor." *Social Analysis* 14:127–49.

———. 1989. *Paths toward a Clearing: Radical Empiricism and Ethnographic Inquiry.* Bloomington: Indiana University Press.

Johnston, Hank, Enrique Larana, and Joseph R. Gusfield. 1994. "Identities, Grievances, and New Social Movements." In *New Social Movements: From Ideology to Identity,* ed. Enrique Larana, Hank Johnston, and Joseph R. Gusfield, 3–35. Philadelphia: Temple University Press.

Johnston, Hank, and Bert Klandermans. 1995. "The Cultural Analysis of Social Movements." In *Social Movements and Culture,* ed. Hank Johnston and Bert Klandermans, 3–24. Minneapolis: University of Minnesota Press.

Jordanova, Ludmilla. 1989. *Sexual Visions: Images of Gender in Science and Medicine between the Eighteenth and Twentieth Centuries.* Madison: University of Wisconsin Press.

Kapsalis, Terri. 1997. *Public Privates: Performing Gynecology from Both Ends of the Speculum.* Chapel Hill: Duke University Press.

Katz, Jay. 1984. *The Silent World of Doctor and Patient.* New York: Free Press.

Katz, Solomon. 1997. "Secular Morality." In *Morality and Health,* ed. Allan M. Brandt and Paul Rozin, 197–230. New York: Routledge.

Kaufman, Gershen, and Lev Raphael. 1996. *Coming Out of Shame: Transforming Gay and Lesbian Lives.* New York: Doubleday.

Kaufman, Sharon R. 1986. *The Ageless Self: Sources of Meaning in Late Life.* Madison: University of Wisconsin Press.

Kirmayer, Laurence. 1988. "Mind and Body as Metaphors: Hidden Values in

Biomedicine." In *Biomedicine Examined,* ed. Margaret Lock and Deborah Gordon, 57–93. Dordrecht, The Netherlands: Kluwer.

———. 1992. "The Body's Insistence on Meaning: Metaphor as Presentation and Representation in Illness Experience." *Medical Anthropology Quarterly* 6:323–46.

Koenig, Barbara. 1988. "The Technological Imperative in Medical Practice: The Social Creation of a 'Routine' Treatment." In *Biomedicine Examined,* ed. Margaret Lock and Deborah Gordon, 465–96. Dordrecht, The Netherlands: Kluwer.

Kohli, Martin. 1991. "Retirement and the Moral Economy: An Historical Interpretation of the German Case." In *Critical Perspectives on Aging: The Political and Moral Economy of Growing Old,* ed. Meredith Minkler and Carroll L. Estes, 273–92. Amityville, N.Y.: Baywood Publishing Company.

Kolata, Gina. 1997. "Old Mother Hubbard Was Never a Sex Pot." *New York Times,* April 27.

Kramon, Glenn. 1992. "Fertility Center Plans to Reproduce Itself." *San Francisco Chronicle,* June 20.

Kulick, Don. 1998. *Travesti: Sex, Gender, and Culture among Brazilian Transgendered Prostitutes.* Chicago: University of Chicago Press.

Laderman, Carol, and Marina Roseman, eds. 1996. *The Performance of Healing.* New York: Routledge.

Lamport, Ann. 1988. "The Genetics of Secrecy in Adoption, Artificial Insemination, and In Vitro Fertilization." *American Journal of Law and Medicine* 14:109–24.

Laqueur, Thomas. 1987. "Orgasm, Generation, and the Politics of Reproductive Biology." In *The Making of the Modern Body: Sexuality and Society in the Nineteenth Century,* ed. Catherine Gallagher and Thomas Laqueur, 1–41. Berkeley: University of California Press.

Lash, Scott, and Brian Wynne. 1992. "Introduction." In Ulrich Beck, *Risk Society: Towards a New Modernity,* 1–8. Beverly Hills: Sage.

Laslett, Barbara, and Johanna Brenner. 1989. "Gender and Social Reproduction: Historical Perspectives." *Annual Review of Sociology* 15:381–404.

Layne, Linda. 1996. "How's the Baby Doing? Struggling with Narratives of Progress in a Neonatal Intensive Care Unit." *Medical Anthropology Quarterly* 10:624–56.

———. 1999. "Introduction: The Child as Gift." In *Transformative Motherhood: On Giving and Getting in a Consumer Culture,* ed. Linda L. Layne, 1–28. New York: New York University Press .

———, ed. 1999. *Transformative Motherhood: On Giving and Getting in a Consumer Culture.* New York: New York University Press.

Leichter, Howard M. 1997. "Lifestyle Correctness and the New Secular Morality." In *Morality and Health,* ed. Allan M. Brandt and Paul Rozin, 359–78. New York: Routledge.

Lessor, Roberta. 1993. "All in the Family: Social Processes in Ovarian Egg Donation between Sisters." *Sociology of Health and Illness* 15:393–413.

Levin, David Michael. 1991. "Visions of Narcissism: Intersubjectivity and the

Reversals of Reflection." In *Merleau-Ponty Vivant,* ed. Martin C. Dillon, 47–90. Albany: State University of New York Press.

Lewin, Ellen. 1993. *Lesbian Mothers: Accounts of Gender in American Culture.* Ithaca: Cornell University Press.

———. 1995. "On the Outside Looking In: The Politics of Lesbian Motherhood." In *Conceiving the New World Order: The Global Politics of Reproduction,* ed. Faye D. Ginsburg and Rayna Rapp, 103–21. Berkeley: University of California Press.

———. 1998. "Wives, Mothers, and Lesbians: Rethinking Resistance in the U.S." In *Pragmatic Women and Body Politics,* ed. Margaret Lock and Patricia A. Kaufert, 164–77. Cambridge: Cambridge University Press.

Lock, Margaret, and Patricia A. Kaufert. 1998. "Introduction." In *Pragmatic Women and Body Politics,* ed. Margaret Lock and Patricia A. Kaufert, 1–27. Cambridge: Cambridge University Press.

Lock, Margaret, and Patricia A. Kaufert, eds. 1998. *Pragmatic Women and Body Politics.* Cambridge: Cambridge University Press.

Lopez, Iris. 1998. "An Ethnography of the Medicalization of Puerto Rican Women's Reproduction." In *Pragmatic Women and Body Politics,* ed. Margaret Lock and Patricia A. Kaufert, 240–59. Cambridge: Cambridge University Press.

Lowenberg, June S. 1989. *Caring and Responsibility: The Crossroads between Holistic Practice and Traditional Medicine.* Philadelphia: University of Pennsylvania Press.

Luborsky, Mark. 1993. "The Romance with Personal Meaning in Gerontology: Cultural Aspects of Life Themes." *Gerontologist* 33:445–52.

———. 1994. "The Retirement Process: Making the Person and Cultural Meanings Malleable." *Medical Anthropology Quarterly* 8:411–29.

Ludtke, Melissa. 1997. *On Our Own: Unmarried Motherhood in America.* Berkeley: University of California Press.

Lury, Celia. 1996. *Consumer Culture.* New Brunswick, N.J.: Rutgers University Press.

Lyon, Margot L. 1990. "Order and Healing: The Concept of Order and Its Importance in the Conceptualization of Healing." *Medical Anthropology* 12:249–68.

Marcus, George E. 1995. "Ethnography in/or the World System: The Emergence of Multi-Sited Ethnography." *Annual Reviews of Anthropology* 24:95–117.

Martin, Emily. 1987. *The Woman in the Body: A Cultural Analysis of Reproduction.* Boston: Beacon Press.

———. 1991. "The Egg and the Sperm: How Science Has Constructed a Romance Based on Stereotypical Male-Female Roles." *Signs* 16:485–501.

Mauss, Marcel. 1985. "A Category of the Human Mind: The Notion of Person, the Notion of Self." In *The Category of the Person: Anthropology, Philosophy, History,* ed. Michael Carrithers, Steven Collins, and Steven Lukes, 1–25. Cambridge: Cambridge University Press.

———. 1990 (1950). *The Gift: The Form and Reason for Exchange in Archaic Societies.* New York and London: Norton.

May, Elaine Tyler. 1995. *Barren in the Promised Land: Childless Americans and the Pursuit of Happiness.* Cambridge: Harvard University Press.

McDonough, Paul. 1992. "The Need for Technology Assessment in the Reproductive Sciences." *American Journal of Obstetrics and Gynecology* 166: 1082–90.

McLean, Athena. 1990. "Contradictions in the Social Production of Clinical Knowledge: The Case of Schizophrenia." *Social Science and Medicine* 9:969–85.

Mead, Rebecca. 1999. "Eggs for Sale." *New Yorker,* August 9, 56–65.

Meirow, D., and J. G. Schenker. 1997. "Reproductive Health Care Policies around the World. The Current Status of Sperm Donation in Assisted Reproduction Technology: Ethical and Legal Considerations." *Journal of Assisted Reproduction and Genetics* 14:133–38.

Merleau-Ponty, Maurice. 1962. *Phenomenology of Perception.* Translated by Colin Smith. New York: Routledge.

———. 1968. *The Visible and the Invisible.* Edited by Claude Lefort; translated by Alphonso Lingis. Evanston, Ill.: Northwestern University Press.

Meyer, John W. 1988. "Levels of Analysis: The Life Course as a Cultural Construction." In *Social Structures and Human Lives,* ed. Matilda White Riley, 49–62. Beverly Hills: Sage.

Miller, Daniel. 1995. "Consumption as the Vanguard of History: A Polemic by Way of an Introduction." In *Acknowledging Consumption: A Review of New Studies,* ed. Daniel Miller, 1–57. London and New York: Routledge.

Minkler, Meredith, and Thomas R. Cole. 1999. "Political and Moral Economy: Getting to Know One Another." In *Critical Gerontology: Perspectives from Political and Moral Economy,* ed. Meredith Minkler and Carroll L. Estes, 37-49. Amityville, N.Y.: Baywood Publishing Company.

Minkler, Meredith, and Carroll L. Estes, eds. 1999. *Critical Gerontology: Perspectives from Political and Moral Economy.* Amityville, N.Y.: Baywood Publishing Company.

Mishler, Elliott. 1986. *Research Interviewing.* Cambridge: Harvard University Press.

Modell, Judith S. 1989. "Last Chance Babies: Interpretations of Parenthood in an In Vitro Fertilization Program." *Medical Anthropology Quarterly* 3:124–38.

———. 1994. *Kinship with Strangers: Adoption and Interpretations of Kinship in American Culture.* Berkeley: University of California Press.

———. 1999. "Freely Given: Open Adoption and the Rhetoric of the Gift." In *Transformative Motherhood: On Giving and Getting in a Consumer Culture,* ed. Linda L. Layne, 29–64. New York: New York University Press.

———. 2000. *A Sealed and Secret Kinship: Policies and Practices in American Adoption.* Providence: Berghahn Press.

Moore, Henrietta. 1994. *A Passion for Difference: Essays in Anthropology and Gender.* Bloomington: Indiana University Press.

Mosher, William, and W. Pratt. 1987. "Fecundity, Infertility, and Reproductive Health in the United States, 1982." DHHS Pub. No. (PHS) 87–1990, Vital and Health Statistics, Series 23, No. 14. Hyattsville, Md.: National Center for Health Statistics.

Mullings, Leith. 1995. "Households Headed by Women: The Politics of Race, Class, and Gender." In *Conceiving the New World Order: The Global Politics of Reproduction,* ed. Faye D. Ginsburg and Rayna Rapp, 122–39. Berkeley: University of Calfornia Press.

Nachtigall, Robert D. 1993. "Secrecy: An Unresolved Issue in the Practice of Donor Insemination." *American Journal of Obstetrics and Gynecology* 168: 1846–53.

———. 1994. "Donor Insemination and Human Immunodeficiency Virus: A Risk/Benefit Analysis." *American Journal of Obstetrics and Gynecology* 170: 1692–96.

Nachtigall, Robert D., Gay Becker, and Mark Wozny. 1992. "The Effects of Gender-Specific Diagnosis on Men's and Women's Response to Infertility." *Fertility and Sterility* 54:113–21.

Nachtigall, Robert D., Gay Becker, Seline Szkupinski Quiroga, and Jeanne M. Tschann. 1998. "The Disclosure Decision: Concerns and Issues of Parents of Children Conceived through Donor Insemination." *American Journal of Obstetrics and Gynecology* 178:1165–70.

Nachtigall, Robert D., Jeanne M. Tschann, Seline Szkupinski Quiroga, Linda Pitcher, and Gay Becker. 1997. "Stigma, Disclosure, and Family Functioning among Parents of Children Conceived through Donor Insemination." *Fertility and Sterility* 68:83–89.

Nelkin, Dorothy. 1989. "Communicating Technological Risk: The Social Construction of Risk Perception." *Annual Review of Public Health* 10:95–113.

Nelkin, Dorothy, and M. Susan Lindee. 1995. *The DNA Mystique: The Gene as a Cultural Icon.* New York: W. H. Freeman.

Ness, Carol. 1999. "Lesbian Mothers' Legal Gains." *San Francisco Examiner,* May 2.

Novaes, Simone Bateman, and Tania Salem. 1998. "Embedding the Embryo." In *The Future of Human Reproduction: Ethics, Choice, and Regulation,* ed. John Harris and Soren Holm, 100–26. Oxford: Clarendon Press.

Nsiah-Jefferson, Laurie, and Elaine J. Hall. 1989. "Reproductive Technology: Perspectives and Implications for Low-Income Women and Women of Color." In *Healing Technology: Feminist Perspectives,* ed. Kathryn Strother Ratcliff, 93–118. Ann Arbor: University of Michigan Press.

Olive, David. 1986. "Analysis of Clinical Fertility Trials: A Methodological Review." *Fertility and Sterility* 45:157–70.

Ong, Aihwa, and Michael G. Peletz. 1995. "Introduction." In *Bewitching Women, Pious Men: Gender and Body Politics in Southeast Asia,* ed. Aihwa Ong and Michael G. Peletz, 1–18. Berkeley: University of California Press.

Ortner, Sherry B. 1995. "Resistance and the Problem of Ethnographic Refusal." *Comparative Studies in Society and History* 37:173–93.

———. 1996. *Making Gender: The Politics and Erotics of Culture.* Boston: Beacon Press.

Palmer, Gary B., and William R. Kankowiak. 1996. "Performance and Imagination: Toward an Anthropology of the Spectacular and the Mundane." *Cultural Anthropology* 11:225–58.

Palmer, R. R., and Joel Colton. 1965. *A History of the Modern World.* 3d. ed. New York: Alfred A. Knopf.

Parsons, Evelyn, and Paul Atkinson. 1992. "Lay Constructions of Genetic Risk." *Sociology of Health and Illness* 14:437–55.

Petchesky, Rosalind Pollack. 1997. "Fetal Images: The Power of Visual Culture in the Politics of Reproduction." In *The Gender/Sexuality Reader,* ed. Roger N. Lancaster and Micaela di Leonardo, 134–150. New York: Routledge.

Quinn, Naomi. 1991. "The Cultural Basis of Metaphor." In *Beyond Metaphor: The Theory of Tropes in Anthropology,* ed. James Fernandez, 56–93. Stanford: Stanford University Press.

———. 1992. "The Motivational Force of Self-Understanding: Evidence from Wives' Inner Conflicts." In *Human Motives and Cultural Models,* ed. Roy D'Andrade and Claudia Strauss, 90–126. Cambridge: Cambridge University Press.

Quinn, Naomi, and Dorothy Holland. 1987. "Culture and Cognition." In *Cultural Models in Language and Thought,* ed. Dorothy Holland and Naomi Quinn, 3–40. Cambridge: Cambridge University Press.

Rabinow, Paul. 1996. *Essays on the Anthropology of Reason.* Princeton: Princeton University Press.

Rapp, Rayna. 1990. "Constructing Amniocentesis: Maternal and Medical Discourses." In *Uncertain Terms: Negotiating Gender in American Culture,* ed. Faye Ginsburg and Anna Lowenhaupt Tsing, 28–42. Boston: Beacon.

———. 1995. "Heredity, or Revising the Facts of Life." In *Naturalizing Power: Essays in Feminist Cultural Analysis,* ed. Sylvia Yanagisako and Carol Delaney, 69–86. New York: Routledge.

Reiser, Stanley J. 1985. "Responsibility for Personal Health: A Historical Perspective." *Medical Philosophy* 10:7–17.

Ricoeur, Paul. 1984. *Time and Narrative.* Vol. 1. Chicago: University of Chicago Press.

Riessman, Catherine Kohler. 2000. "Stigma and Everyday Resistance Practices: Childless Women in South India." *Gender and Society* 14:111–35.

Rubinstein, Robert L. 1990. "Nature, Culture, Gender, Age." In *Anthropology and Aging,* ed. Robert L. Rubinstein, 109–15. Dordrecht, The Netherlands: Kluwer.

Ruzek, Sheryl Burt. 1988. "Gender and Medicine." In Health and Human Values Supplement, Pennsylvania Humanities Council, *Pittsburgh Post Gazette.* November 22.

Sandelowski, Margarete. 1991. "Compelled to Try: The Never-Enough Quality of Conceptive Technology." *Medical Anthropology Quarterly* 5:29–47.

———. 1993. *With Child in Mind: Studies of the Personal Encounter with Infertility.* Philadelphia: University of Pennsylvania Press.

Sauer, Mark V. 1998. "Motherhood at Any Age? Egg Donation Was Not Intended for Everyone." *Fertility and Sterility* 69:187–88.

Scheper-Hughes, Nancy. 1996. "Theft of Life: The Globalization of Organ Stealing Rumours." *Anthropology Today* 12:3–11.

Schiebinger, Londa. 1993. *Nature's Body: Gender in the Making of Modern Science*. Boston: Beacon.

Schneider, David. 1984 (1968). *American Kinship: A Cultural Account*. Englewood Cliffs, N.J.: Prentice-Hall.

Schover, L. R., R. L. Collins, and S. Richards. 1992. "Psychological Aspects of Donor Insemination: Evaluation and Follow-up for Recipient Couples." *Fertility and Sterility* 57:583–90.

Scott, James C. 1976. *The Moral Economy of the Peasant: Rebellion and Subsistence in Southeast Asia*. New Haven: Yale University Press.

Seibel, Machelle M., and Marvin L. Taymor. 1982. "Emotional Aspects of Infertility." *Fertility and Sterility* 37:137–45.

Shore, Cris. 1992. "Virgin Births and Sterile Debates: Anthropology and the New Reproductive Technologies." *Current Anthropology* 33:295–314.

Short, J. F. 1984. "The Social Fabric at Risk: Toward the Social Transformation of Risk Analysis." *American Sociological Review* 49:711–25.

Shrader-Frechette, Kristin. 1988. "Producer Risk, Consumer Risk, and Assessing Technological Impacts." *Impact Assessment Bulletin* 6:155–64.

Slater, Don. *Consumer Culture and Modernity*. Cambridge: Blackwell.

Somers, Margaret R., and Gloria D. Gibson. 1994. "Reclaiming the Epistemological 'Other': Narrative and the Social Constitution of Identity." In *Social Theory and the Politics of Identity,* ed. Craig Calhoun, 37–99. Oxford: Blackwell.

Snowdon, R., G. D. Mitchell, and E. M. Snowdon. 1983. *Artificial Reproduction: A Social Investigation*. London: George Allen and Unwin.

Spirtas, R., S. C. Kaufman and N. J. Alexander. 1993. "Fertility Drugs and Ovarian Cancer: Red Alert or Red Herring?" *Fertility and Sterility* 59:291–93.

Steinberg, Deborah. 1997. *Bodies in Glass: Genetics, Eugenics, Embryo Ethics*. Manchester: Manchester University Press.

Stoller, Paul. 1994. "Embodying Colonial Memories." *American Anthropologist* 96:634–48.

Strathern, Marilyn. 1992. *After Nature: English Kinship in the Late Twentieth Century*. Cambridge: Cambridge University Press.

———. 1992. *Reproducing the Future: Anthropology, Kinship, and the New Reproductive Technologies*. New York: Routledge.

———. 1999 (1993). "Regulation, Substitution, and Possibility." In *Technologies of Procreation: Kinship in the Age of Assisted Conception,* ed. Jeanette Edwards, Sarah Franklin, Eric Hirsch, Frances Price, and Marilyn Strathern, 171–202. London: Routledge.

———. 1995. "Displacing Knowledge: Technology and the Consequences for Kinship. In *Conceiving the New World Order: The Global Politics of Reproduction,* ed. Faye D. Ginsburg and Rayna Rapp, 346–63. Berkeley: University of California Press.

———. 1995. "Disembodied Choice." In *Other Intentions: Cultural Contexts and the Attribution of Inner States,* ed. Lawrence Rosen, 69–90. Santa Fe: School of American Research Press.

Strauss, Anselm, Juliet Corbin, Shizuko Fagerhaugh, Barney G. Glaser, David

Maines, Barbara Suczek, and Carolyn L. Wiener. 1984. *Chronic Illness and the Quality of Life.* 2d. ed. St. Louis: C. V. Mosby.

Strauss, Claudia. 1992. "What Makes Tony Run? Schemas as Motives Reconsidered." In *Human Motives and Cultural Models,* ed. Roy D'Andrade and Claudia Strauss, 191–224. Cambridge: Cambridge University Press.

Swidler, Ann. 1995. "Cultural Power and Social Movements." In *Social Movements and Culture,* ed. Hank Johnston and Bert Klandermans, 25–40. Minneapolis: University of Minnesota Press.

"$10,000 Eggs for Sale to Childless Women: Doctors Debate Ethics of a Growing Business." 1991. *San Francisco Chronicle,* November 11.

Terrell, John, and Judith Modell. 1994. "Anthropology and Adoption." *American Anthropologist* 96:155–61.

Thompson, E. P. 1966. *The Making of the English Working Class.* New York: Vintage Books.

Thorne, Barrie, and Marilyn Yalom, eds. 1992. *Rethinking the Family: Some Feminist Questions.* Boston: Northeastern University Press.

Tober, Diane. 1999. "Romancing the Sperm: Sexuality, Technology, and Alternative American Families." Ph.D. diss., University of California, Berkeley/San Francisco Joint Medical Anthropology Program.

Toch, Hans. 1965. *The Social Psychology of Social Movements.* Indianapolis: Bobbs Merrill.

Toombs, S. Kay. 1993. *The Meaning of Illness: A Phenomenological Account of the Different Perspectives of Physician and Patient.* Dordrecht, The Netherlands: Kluwer.

Turiel, Judith Steinberg. 1998. *Beyond Second Opinions: Making Choices about Fertility Treatment.* Berkeley: University of California Press.

Turner, Victor. 1969. *The Ritual Process: Structure and Anti-Structure.* Ithaca: Cornell University Press.

———. 1974. *Dramas, Fields, and Metaphors: Symbolic Action in Human Society.* Ithaca: Cornell University Press.

Tversky, Amos, and Daniel Kahneman. 1981. "The Framing of Decisions and the Psychology of Choice." *Science* 211:453–58.

Tymstra, Tjeerd. 1989. "The Imperative Character of Medical Technology and the Meaning of 'Anticipated Decision Regret.'" *International Journal of Technology Assessment in Health Care* 5:207–13.

U.S. House. 1989. Committee on Small Business, Subcommittee on Regulation, Business Opportunities, and Energy. *Hearing on Consumer Protection Issues Involving In Vitro Fertilization Clinics.* 101st Congress, March 9. Washington, D.C.: U.S. Government Printing Office, Serial No. 101–5.

Van den Wijngaard, Marianne. 1997. *Reinventing the Sexes: The Biomedical Construction of Femininity and Masculinity.* Bloomington: Indiana University Press.

Walker, Iain, and Pia Broderick. 1999. "The Psychology of Assisted Reproduction, or Psychology Assisting Its Reproduction?" *Australian Psychologist* 34:38–44.

Weiner, Annette B. 1978. "The Reproductive Model in Trobriand Society." *Mankind.* Special Issue: Trade and Exchange in Oceania and Australia.

————. 1979. "Trobriand Kinship from Another View: The Reproductive Power of Women and Men." *Man* 14:328–48.

————. 1995. "Reassessing Reproduction in Social Theory." In *Conceiving the New World Order: The Global Politics of Reproduction*, ed. Faye D. Ginsburg and Rayna Rapp, 407–24. Berkeley: University of California Press.

Weston, Kath. 1991. *Families We Choose: Lesbians, Gays, Kinship*. New York: Columbia University Press.

———— 1995. "Forever Is a Long Time: Romancing the Real in Gay Kinship Ideologies." In *Naturalizing Power: Essays in Feminist Cultural Analysis*, ed. Sylvia Yanagisako and Carol Delaney, 87–110. New York: Routledge.

Whiteford, Linda, and Marilyn Poland, eds. 1989. *New Approaches to Human Reproduction: Social and Ethical Dimensions*. Boulder: Westview Press.

Whittemore, A. S., R. Harris, J. Intyre, and the Collaborative Ovarian Cancer Group. 1992. "Characteristics Relating to Ovarian Cancer Risk: Collaborative Analysis of Twelve U.S. Case-Control Studies. I: Methods." *American Journal of Epidemiology* 136:1175–83.

Whittemore, A. S., R. Harris., J. Intyre,and the Collaborative Ovarian Cancer Group. 1992. "Characteristics Relating to Ovarian Cancer Risk: Collaborative Analysis of Twelve U.S. Case-Control Studies. II: Invasive Epithelial Ovarian Cancers in White Women." *American Journal of Epidemiology* 136: 1184–1203.

Whittemore, A. S., R. Harris, J. Intyre, and the Collaborative Ovarian Cancer Group. 1992. "Characteristics Relating to Ovarian Cancer Risk: The Pathogenesis of Epithelial Ovarian Cancer." *American Journal of Epidemiology* 136:1212–20.

Wiener, Carolyn. 1981. *The Politics of Alcoholism*. New Brunswick, N.J.: Transaction.

Wilcox, L. S., J. L. Kiely, C. L. Melvin, and M. C. Martin. 1996. "Assisted Reproductive Technologies: Estimates of their Contribution to Multiple Births and Newborn Hospital Days in the United States." *Fertility and Sterility* 65: 361–66.

Wilkerson, Abby L. *Diagnosis: Difference. The Moral Authority of Medicine.* Ithaca: Cornell University Press, 1998.

Wilkinson, Rupert. 1988. *The Pursuit of American Character*. New York: Harper and Row.

Williams, Brackette. 1989. "A Class Act: Anthropology and the Race to Nation across Ethnic Terrain." *Annual Review of Anthropology* 18:401–44.

Williams, Raymond. 1976. *Keywords: A Vocabulary of Culture and Society*. London: Oxford University Press.

————. 1977. *Marxism and Literature*. Oxford: Oxford University Press.

Williams, Simon J. 1998. "Health as Moral Performance: Ritual, Transgression, and Taboo." *Health* 2:435–57.

Yanagisako, Sylvia Junko, and Jane Fishburne Collier. 1987. "Toward a Unified Analysis of Gender and Kinship." In *Gender and Kinship: Essays Toward a Unified Analysis*, ed. Jane Fishburne Collier and Sylvia Junko Yanagisako, 14–50. Stanford: Stanford University Press.

Yanagisako, Sylvia, and Carol Delaney. 1995. "Naturalizing Power." In *Nat-

uralizing Power: Essays in Feminist Cultural Analysis, ed. Sylvia Yanagisako and Carol Delaney, 1–22. New York: Routledge.

Young, Allan. 1981. "The Creation of Medical Knowledge: Some Problems in Interpretation." *Social Science and Medicine* 15B:379–86.

Young, Iris. 1989. "Throwing Like a Girl: A Phenomenology of Feminine Body Comportment, Motility, and Spatiality." In *The Thinking Muse: Feminism and Modern French Philosophy,* ed. Jeffner Allen and Iris Marion Young, 51–70. Bloomington: Indiana University Press.

Young, Katharine. 1997. *Presence in the Flesh: The Body in Medicine.* Cambridge: Harvard University Press.

Zola, Irving K. 1972. "Medicine as an Institution of Social Control." *American Sociological Review* 20:487–504.

Zolla, Elemire. 1981. *The Androgyne: Fusion of the Sexes.* London: Thames and Hudson.

Index

Text: 10/13 Sabon
Display: Sabon
Composition: Binghamton Valley Composition
Printing and binding: Haddon Craftsmen

DATE DUE

JAN 1 4 2004		
OCT 1 3 2006		
MAR 1 1 2008		

Demco, Inc. 38-293